Managing for Success in Health Care

MANAGING FOR SUCCESS IN HEALTH CARE

Tim Porter-O'Grady, EdD, ScD(h), APRN, FAAN
Senior Partner
Tim Porter-O'Grady Associates, LLC
Otto, North Carolina;
Associate Professor, Leadership Scholar
Program in Health Innovation
School of Nursing
Arizona State University
Phoenix, Arizona

Kathy Malloch, PhD, MBA, RN, FAAN
President
Malloch & Associates, Inc.
Glendale, Arizona;
Program Director
Master's in Healthcare Innovation
ASU College of Nursing
Phoenix, Arizona

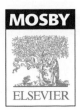

MOSBY
ELSEVIER

11830 Westline Industrial Drive
St. Louis, Missouri 63146

Managing for Success in Healthcare   ISBN-13: 978-0-323-03427-2
                                                          ISBN-10: 0-323-03427-6

Notice

Neither the Publisher nor the Authors assume any responsibility for any loss or injury and/or damage to persons or property arising out of or related to any use of the material contained in this book. It is the responsibility of the treating practitioner, relying on independent expertise and knowledge of the patient, to determine the best treatment and method of application for the patient.

                                                   The Publisher

---

Library of Congress Cataloging-in-Publication Data
Managing for success in health care / Tim Porter-O'Grady, Kathy Malloch.
   p. cm.
Includes bibliographical references and index.
ISBN-13: 978-0-323-03427-2
ISBN-10: 0-323-03427-6
 1. Health services administration. 2. Leadership. 3. Organizational change. I. Porter-O'Grady, Timothy. II. Malloch, Kathy.
RA971.M34635 2007
362.1068–dc22

                                     2006045781

Senior Editor: Yvonne Alexopoulos
Developmental Editor: Kristin Hebberd
Editorial Assistant: Sarah Vales
Publishing Services Manager: Jeff Patterson
Project Manager: Amy Rickles
Design Manager: Mark A. Oberkrom
Text Photographs: Copyright 2006, JupiterImages Corporation

Printed in China

Last digit is the print number: 9 8 7 6 5 4 3 2 1

REVIEWERS

Karen Brasfield, RN, MSN, CMSRN
Instructor
Department of Nursing
Everett Community College
Everett, Washington

Jacqueline Rosenjack Burchum, DNSC, APRN, BC
Assistant Professor
College of Nursing
University of Tennessee Health Science Center
Memphis, Tennessee

Lynda H. Crawford, PhD, RN, CAE
Associate Dean, Center for Nonprofit Management
Spertus Institute
Chicago, Illinois

Renee M. Jocson, RN, BSN
Nurse
Twin Cities Behavioral Health
Normal, Illinois

Marcia Sterk, RN, BSN
Director
OSF St. Joseph Medical Center
Bloomington, Illinois

James S. Vales, BA, BSN, MD, FAAFP, AAUCM
Physician
Urgent Care, St. Joseph Hospital
Bloomington, Illinois

Janice Womak, RN
Associate Nurse Executive
Northwest Georgia Regional Hosptial
Rome, Georgia

This book is dedicated to all of our leadership colleagues who every day demonstrate the meaning and value of good leadership and who confront the challenges of transformation with the spirit of hope and commitment that inspires and encourages all who care for others.

TPOG

KM

PREFACE

Books on management and leadership abound across every culture and relate to every work process. And there's a reason for this: Leadership is as dynamic as the processes and events of life and is best represented in the challenges and vagaries of the life experience. However, as leadership becomes more complex, reflecting the shifting character of work and relationships, the nuances, insights, and vagaries that relate to expressing it become equally more intricate. In the process, those of us who are involved in the various roles directed toward exercising leadership can often become so caught up in its multifaceted expression and subtle applications that we forget the very foundations upon which leadership practices are built.

Every so often, it is wise to remind ourselves how those basic principles of leadership influence leader thought and action. They form the substance and foundation upon which increasing levels and facets of expression are based. *Leadership should be founded on a clear understanding of basic human relationships and needs.* It is true that work realities are constantly shifting. Now, in the midst of the digital age, whole new conditions and circumstances are affecting the very design of work—how it is configured, distributed, assigned, linked and integrated across the global stage. Issues of virtual communication, mobility, outsourcing, technology applications, and a host of other considerations have transformed the very fabric of work. This is no less true in managing clinical services in a wide variety of organizational settings. As genetic, nano, chemo, pharma, and digital technologies become the cornerstones of the application of therapeutic modalities, shorter lengths of stay, increasing varieties of clinical options, high turnover related to patient activities, and an increasing level of synthesis are required to effectively manage the healthcare experience; all are challenging the provider with new ways of thinking and doing.

It is easy in these circumstances to get lost in the dynamics of change, the chaos of emerging configurations, the mosaic of intersecting and interacting clinical relationships, and the glamour of technology and in meeting the requirements of an increasingly evidence-based clinical environment. Yet, through it all, the leader must be encouraged and reinforced through her or his continual reengagement of the ever-constant fundamentals of human behavior, relationship, and action. Although the environment and the context for leadership thinking is challenged by constant movement and change, it is also strengthened and renewed by the consistency and validity of the core elements of human behavior that are best represented in engagement, openness, care, and good relationships. These factors may take many new forms in their expression, but their presence is a constant reminder to the leader of how important the fundamentals are to the success of any venture or enterprise and how seriously it can be compromised when these basic concepts are forgotten.

In an effort to reengage and touch on those fundamental issues in leadership, this book offers a unique design. It is not intended to be read from cover to cover. Managers and leaders have precious little time in today's fast-paced and Internet-moderated work environment to read leadership books page by page, cover to cover. This work is predominantly designed as a reference and guidebook for leaders, calling them back to foundational questions and issues but doing so by creating a more contemporary and applied context for their consideration. The latest thinking and research with regard to the application of leadership principles have been included, but the authors have done so in a way in which the information can be obtained quickly and used in real time. Each chapter is developed and designed so that readers can locate critical issues of leadership within a short space of time and immediately apply them to almost any leadership situation. In addition, the new circumstances and characteristics of the contemporary workplace related to the management of emotional issues, evidence-based practice, outcomes-driven accountability, and other critical elements that now play a central part of a leader's role have been addressed. The authors hope that this book will be used as a tool rather than simply a reference and that it can be an extension of the leader's day-to-day resources, specifically applicable to any contemporary leadership or management situation.

Of course, no work on leadership can fully address all of the subtleties and issues related to either the concepts of leadership or their applications. Leadership books should be seen as a mosaic of information and data that, once linked together, can create a substantial picture of the characteristics, expressions, roles, and relationships essential to good leadership. Each work on leadership is simply a small piece of this mosaic and can only seek to contribute to leadership knowledge within that defined set of parameters. However, the authors hope that this more practical and applied presentation of leadership principles and practices will not only add to that mosaic of leadership knowledge but will also provide an ongoing tool useful to any reader who uses it to inform and guide personal leadership practice. If the contemporary leader finds it relevant and useful, it will have fulfilled the authors' purpose. The reader is challenged to remember that, like any work of its kind, this book is a work in progress. It serves as one in a number of resources the leader should access. The authors hope that this book will provide one key in the array of resources that help leaders unlock potential in themselves and in those they lead. In a time of great change, the steady, consistent and faithful application of good leadership foundations offers perhaps the only source of consistency and stability in the workplace and creates the frame for hope and encouragement in a constantly transforming world.

Tim Porter-O'Grady

Kathy Malloch

ACKNOWLEDGMENTS

The authors would like to thank all those who contributed their own leadership insights and advice and who provided the inspiration and ideas for this book.

Special thanks go to

Mark Ponder, who represents the best in good leadership and who keeps our world organized and exciting and fills it will love and encouragement.

Bryan Malloch, who provides counsel, love and companionship in a way that makes this work always seem worthwhile even when it feels tedious and challenging.

CONTENTS

Managing for Success in Health Care

UNIT 1: TEAM DEVELOPMENT AND LEADERSHIP

1. EFFECTIVE TEAMS

2. MANAGING CONFLICT

3. TEAM PERFORMANCE: EVALUATING RESULTS

4. TRANSFORMATION AND TRANSITIONS

5. TRANSFORMING TEAMS FOR DECISIONS

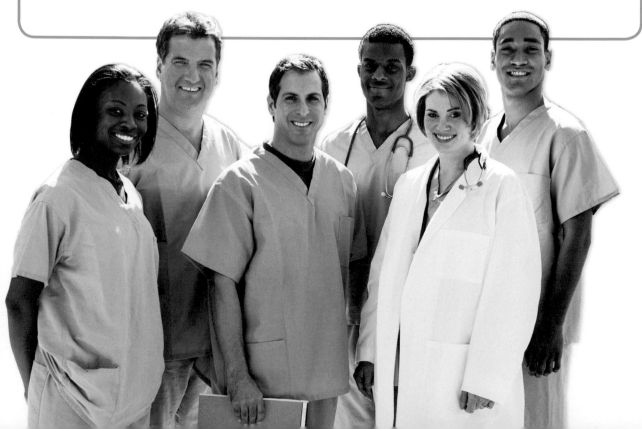

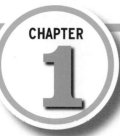

CHAPTER 1

EFFECTIVE TEAMS

Working together is the central point of all organizations.
Working in teams is the frame for all collective contribution at work.

TEAMS ARE EVERYTHING

In all work environments, in every unit of service, teams are central to the success of the organization. Teams are the basic unit of work, yet they conflict with almost every kind of traditional infrastructure in the workplace and across all work systems. Leaders give much lip service to the value of teams such that much value in the organization suggests individual performance almost at the expense of collective values. Teams represent the understanding of horizontal relationships in all human dynamics (Hackman, 2002). The value and implication of these horizontal relationships are critical to the success of any human system. Leaders must be familiar with the theory, processes, and dynamics that affect the collective action of work groups.

Organizational measures of performance and systems of rewards have always focused on the individual. As a result, individual activities and values have been articulated in reward systems, performance evaluation, and achievement of outcomes. However much of that which is sustainable is accomplished by collections of people committed together, contributing individual skills collectively, and aggregating the talents and abilities of many to achieve the necessary outcomes of organizations of which they are part. This is the contribution of teams and the central value of teams to all work effort.

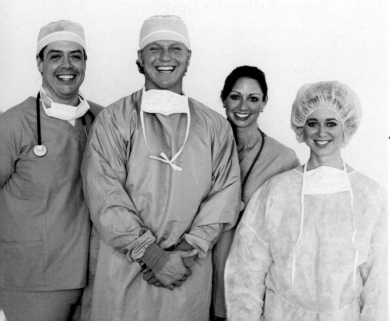

Teams, not individuals, are the basic units of work

All workplaces are successful because of the collective contribution of teams

Team Value

It is important teams reflect a specified level of performance and set of expectations.
All teams must reflect:

- Competence
- Performance capacity
- Good relationships
- Orientation to outcome
- Consonant set of values

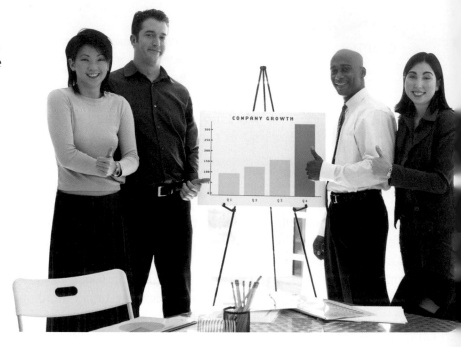

CONSTRUCTING TEAMS

Making teams work depends precisely on how well the teams are constructed in the first place. Managers often find themselves dealing with the vagaries of poor team construction later on when teams are in the midst of attempting to do their work. But these leaders often find out that failing to construct the team well and doing the preliminary work necessary to success ends up costing time and energy in attempting to manage these teams.

Good leaders know that careful thought to the formation, integration, and structuring of teams is important to the ultimate effectiveness of working teams. These leaders are concerned about ensuring appropriate rules of engagement and setting up the frames for behavior far in advance of expecting teams to perform. Establishing the framework for the team becomes a critical first step and should engage the full attentions of the potential team leader.

ESTABLISHING THE RULES OF ENGAGEMENT

Rules of engagement are simply the agreed-upon parameters around which the team process builds. Elements of the rules of engagement include those things that will help the team integrate well and work effectively together.

Some Rules to Consider

- Team member behavior patterns
- Processes of conflict resolution
- Agreement to role assignments
- Work rules
- Process methodology
- Outcome expectations
- Role and performance evaluation

Note:

Increasingly, decisions will be made at the point of service. This will require the full range of effectiveness embedded in team members' operating without close supervision.

The Basic Constructs for Good Work Teams

- Not individuals but members
- Must build on relationships
- Need to create strong work bonds
- Individuals valued as team
- Team evaluates effectiveness
- Teams control work expectations
- Teams problem solve
- Teams manage conflicts/crisis

"DECONSTRUCTING" THE CULTURE OF INDIVIDUALISM

Team-based approaches conflict with almost every kind of infrastructure currently operating in most organizations. In America, individual performance is emulated above all kinds of expectations. Many components of the traditional organizational infrastructure will have to be removed or "deconstructed," simply because they impede the creation and sustenance of point of service-driven decision making and team effectiveness.

Leaders will need to recognize that this long tradition of valuing individualism above the contribution of the team is also embedded deeply within the leadership role and relationship. In establishing the team, the basic unit of service calls for major shifts in sight and perspective with regard to performance, expectations, achievements, and outcomes. Furthermore, leaders must introduce structures and processes that are put in place and value team-based efforts, incorporating team processes into performance expectations, implementation, and evaluation.

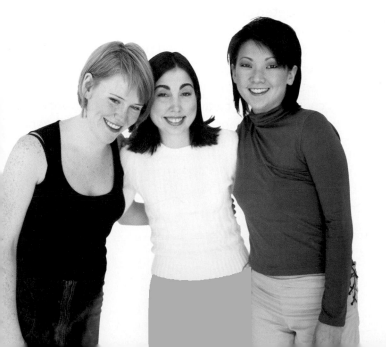

Team Members Must Always:

- Know their work
- Know their partners
- Know there are processes
- Know their expectations
- Know their values
- Know their outcomes

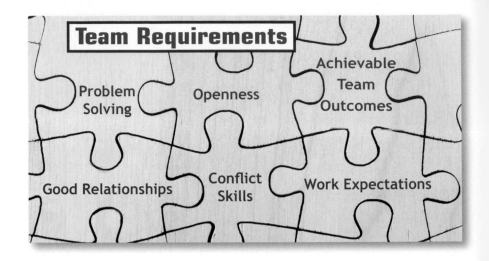

TEAMS THAT MAKE A DIFFERENCE

Structuring teams to be sustainable and to make a difference is a challenging experience. It is important the teams recognize the expectations for working together: performance expectations in the values and outcomes that are exemplified as products of their work. Teams must be able to reflect in their membership an understanding that the commitment of the team is to achieve the purposes, values, and outcomes of the organization.

Teams are not configured simply for the good of organization (Lencioni, 2002). They are designed as a way to more effectively undertake work and achieve outcomes. The team-based approach maximizes the skills and talents of individuals and integrates them, and through their cohesive energy and activities, achieves better results. Designing teams to do this work in a sustainable way calls for a careful construction of the team format, good linkage in relationship between team members, strong interface of diverse skills, and commitment on the part of team members to achieve the goals and outcomes of the team.

Rewards of systems, too, must also be incorporated into the valuing and structuring of teams. Traditionally, remuneration and rewards were allocated based on individual performance and work outcomes. In team-based approaches the valuation of work and the delineation of rewards aggregates to the team as a whole and demonstrates the effectiveness and productivity of the collective enterprise rather than individual performance. Any differentiation and distribution of rewards in a team-based approach is negotiated and determined between and among team members based on contribution, value, and previously determined team-based arrangements (Parker, 2003). The rules related to remuneration and rewards of teams must be well conceived and clearly established in advance of team performance, so the rules of engagement are clear to all the stakeholders.

MANAGEMENT SUPPORT FOR TEAMS

The traditional management structure does not allow for the development of the kinds of relationships essential for good management leadership of teams. Teams require more intensive cores onto relationship between leaders and members. The old superior-subordinate and hierarchical relationships between managers and individuals is no longer a successful format for good team leadership or team functioning.

Team leaders must be an integral part of the team process. These team leaders facilitate, coordinate, and integrate all of the components necessary for team effectiveness. Beginning with team relationships, interactions, and process, moving through the elements of creation, innovation, and outcomes, the team leader must be an integral part of the team's activities. This calls for a much "tighter" relationship between leader and team members reflecting a more intense and horizontal relationship between team members and the leader. Gone are the hierarchical expectations of role, the differentiation of leadership from membership, and the organizational aloofness that are often exhibited in the separation of leadership and management roles from those of the staff.

This intensity of relationship calls for a different mechanism and process for interaction, communication, and problem solving; the leader digs in, becomes a part of the team process, and guides the team toward creative and more unique methods of solution seeking, advancing performance, and achieving outcomes (Pedersen & Easton, 2005). These leaders balance the relational and directional skills necessary to guide a team in the achievement of its determined objectives and to link and integrate the human effort in a mosaic of activities that ultimately achieve the expectations and performance outcome of the team.

Usually leadership needs to be retrained to assume a much more active and facilitating relationship rather than a superior and directing relationship traditionally found in the manager role. This leadership program helps the individual leader tap into interpersonal relations skills, mentoring and monitoring behaviors, relational and directional problems, and mechanisms for advancing innovative practices within the team.

Note:
Teams require participation, not direction, with an expectation that their leaders are members and experience the same demands and obligations of all members of the team in a movement toward common goals.

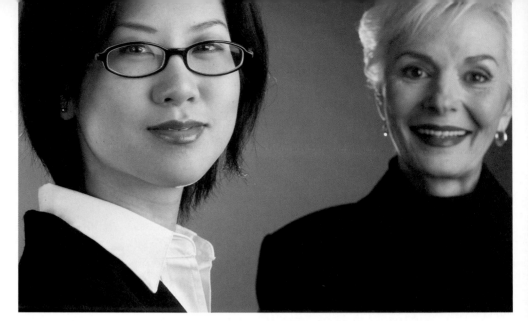

DETERMINING TEAMS' SKILL SETS

> Consider existing skills.

> Identify personal patterns of behavior.

> Base staffing numbers on team needs.

> Fit personalities together well.

> Don't forget the leader's personality characteristics.

> Make sure there's a good fit regarding number of team members.

> Make sure team members are developed well.

> Make sure all team members understand work expectations.

> Ensure that individual expectations and obligations are clear.

> Ensure that mechanisms for problem solving are well outlined.

> Determine that ultimately the team works well together.

PRINCIPLES FOR TEAMWORK AND A NEW AGE

Moving into a new paradigm suggests the ability to discern the essential principles of the new age that underpin and provide purpose for that new age of work. The principles that once characterized the 20th century workplace are diminishing, and organizations must shift to a new set of foundations upon which the social constructs and parameters of work unfold (Porter-O'Grady & Krueger Wilson, 1998).

First Principle: Partnership

Everywhere one looks today the evidence of partnership is apparent. As we move toward a more global community, the understanding that partnership is a driving force to building relationships will become even more critical. As work becomes more integrated with the digital technology of communication, we will find that the global community represents a more boundary-less framework within which to understand and to apply work.

Partnership simply represents the essential characteristic of relationship embedded in all levels of intensity and unfolding work. From international partnerships to regional communities to the linkage of work team goals and processes, partnership is embedded in every level of understanding regarding work relationships and productivity. As digitalization transforms the human community, every aspect of human relationships is altered to reflect the characteristics and effect of global considerations. Furthermore, as complexity theory and an understanding of the quantum nature of the universe becomes a more coherent concept, it will have an effect on every aspect of human life. The notion of the inherent relatedness of all things calls the human community to better understand the nature of relationships, the effect of decisions, and the synthesis of all action across a broad stage.

All of the issues affecting building relationships use partner-based principles as the framework for forming and structuring these relationships. From building international communities, to multinational corporations, to global work projects, to the Internet, and to every relationship between workers and with customers, partnership becomes the driving centerpiece.

> ### Note:
> Building partnerships is no longer an optional exercise. Instead, it is the central characteristic of all work roles and relationships in any work setting any place in the world. Indeed, building partnerships is the work of our time.

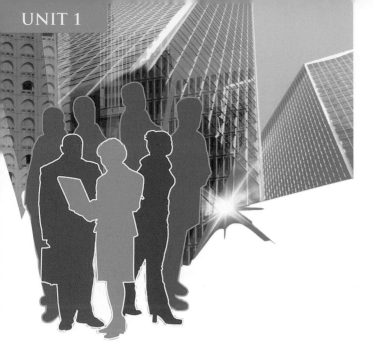

PARTNERING WITH A PURPOSE

Partnerships shouldn't be formed just because they are timely and a good thing to do. Partnerships must be driven by purpose and reflect some essential value that provides meaning for them. Individuals form partnerships in order to extend the values, skills, or outcomes that cannot be as effectively obtained without them. Partnerships are the aggregation of specific skills, resources, and work that when combined advance the value of each of the members of the partnership. It is here where the greatest challenges with regard to partnership unfold. The relationship must be negotiated with the rules and parameters affecting it clarified in advance so that all parties to the partnership are clear of expectations, roles, and contribution. Clarifying each party's activities and role with regard to the relationship upon which the other partners will depend is a critical foundation for building sustainable partnerships (Thompson et al, 2002).

Elements of Good Partnership

- A clear understanding of the reason for creating the partnership
- A clearly articulated foundation upon which to build a partnership
- Clearly enumerated rules of engagement for the partners
- Well-designed and clearly defined role expectations for each partner
- A delineation of the contributions of each partner to the whole
- A method of periodic evaluation of the progress of the partners
- A well-defined method of conflict resolution and problem solving
- Adaptability, discipline, and a willingness to change quickly
- An ability to terminate partnership when no longer relevant

Note:

Partnerships must always reflect the common values that bring people together. It is here where partnerships enumerate their meaning and refine their purpose.

CONFRONTING THE PAST: BUILDING NEW PARTNERSHIPS

Making partnerships work is the past practice of most organizations. In a highly competitive environment, it is often difficult to conceive of building partnerships with people who may have otherwise or previously been competitors. Recognizing the value of partnership may require leaders to overcome past attitudes and behaviors that created barriers and limitations to establishing different kinds of relationship.

The competitive environment remains competitive. However, the necessity to thrive in a much larger marketplace now depends on forming alliances and configurations that best position individuals and partners in a larger playing field. This means leaders must confront their own limitations and past practices. They must be willing to look at internal designs and infrastructure, identifying elements within that act as barriers to the formation of the kinds of partnerships that will be necessary for success.

Partnerships must be judiciously and carefully entered. Clearly, the agreements necessary to define the partnerships must protect the individuals in a way that does not allow them to be jeopardized or sacrificed under the rubric of partnership. However, at the same time, partners must recognize that they will be changed and transformed by the partnership and the results that emerge from new relationships and ways of doing business. Confronting past practices and behaviors and carefully constructing the foundations for future interactions in the context of a larger partnership will require patience, skill, and determination. Helping leadership and staff through the processes of forming new frameworks for work, changing relationships, and a shift in performance and role expectations will be the critical centerpiece of good leadership in the 21st century.

Eliminating Past Practices

- Check people's attitudes.
- Clearly enumerate expectations.
- Identify specific problems.
- Focus on new culture.
- Have staff in on the change.
- Delineate why this is better.
- Name new roles/behaviors.
- Give people time to adjust.
- Evaluate problems and progress.

EQUITY: VALUING EVERY PERSON

If every person in the enterprise attempting to contribute to the relationship is not valued to the extent of the contribution, partnership cannot be lasting. Equity is simply the measure of value attached to the contribution of each member in a relationship. Equity recognizes the essential need for every element and role in an organization to be clearly enumerated so that its value and contribution to the work and the outcomes of the organization are apparent to all.

In many organizations equity and value are often poorly understood. Creating a goodness-of-fit between individual roles and the purpose and productivity of an organization is critical to its long-term viability and success. Every member of an organization should know the value of all members in the organization. Productivity should simply be the measure of this value.

EQUITY: MAKING VALUE REAL

There is nothing more denigrating to the integrity of any group than diminishing the value of any one member. Yet for value to be real, it must be clear and understood by each team member. Value is something that can be articulated broadly with a measure that everyone understands and uses consistently. Equity suggests that value is clearly delineated in advance and understood by each participant in light of their individual obligations in their collective contribution.

Value eliminates the necessity for a hierarchical framework for organization and relationship. Delineating value in role and person as well as between and among the members of the team becomes a critical requisite of good leadership and the fundamental element of strong organizations. When one is clear about expectations, performance, and outcomes, the contribution that must be made to achieving those ends becomes a clear frame for the work and should be understood by all participants.

Note:

All people have value. This value must be translated into the larger value of the organization if both the people and the organization are to thrive.

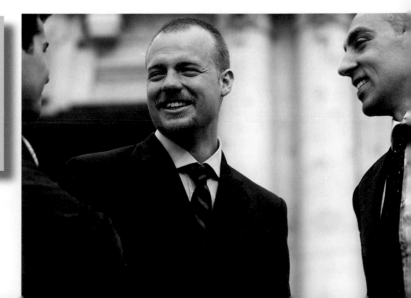

ESSENTIAL ELEMENTS OF EQUITY

> Everyone clearly understands his or her role.

> All workers understand their contribution.

> Expectations for performance are known ahead of time.

> Everyone's role is understood by everyone else.

> There are no secrets in the team.

> Conflict resolution and problem solving is the rule.

> If you don't have a value you shouldn't be there.

> Members give evidence of their contribution to the team.

> Equity dimishes hierarchy.

> Roles are always fluid, flexible, and changing.

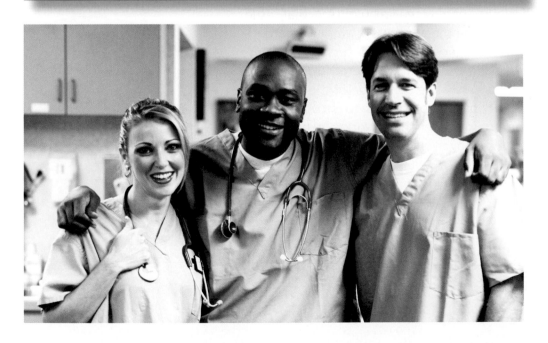

ACCOUNTABILITY:
THE CORNERSTONE OF EFFECTIVENESS

Accountability is the centerpiece around which all work performance is based regardless of the activity. It is important to differentiate accountability from responsibility in order to better understand how it is different and how it needs to be applied.

Responsibility as it's currently understood in the workplace is very much an industrial age concept. It usually reflects the relationship between the worker and his or her employer. Employees have historically been held responsible for performing certain tasks and activities consistent with delineated expectations, job descriptions, or position requirements. The content of their work and their jobs clearly defined their expectations for performance within which all workers were essentially required to perform. In a responsibility-based format, the relationship between all interactions requires that the employee fulfill the mandates of the organization as defined by its management in a subsequent and subordinating role. Decision making, authority, and appropriate action have historically always been determined by the leadership. Most communication has been essentially top-down (Porter-O'Grady & Krueger Wilson, 1998).

Employer-defined work responsibilities do not require the engagement of the worker in defining those responsibilities. It is the expectation of the worker that those responsibilities defined by the employer be carried out within the context and the expectations of those definitions. Missing from responsibility is any sense of ownership or investment in the individual elements of work for which the worker is responsible.

Responsibility Attributes

Responsibility is always employer driven. It is expected, in responsibility-based environments, that the employer will define the elements of work, the expectations for performance, the parameters for performing the work, and the results expected from accomplishing the work. It is the obligation of the employer in responsibility-based approaches to provide definitive parameters for the worker. Worker expectation, engagement, or involvement in the definition of responsibilities is not a requisite of the responsibility-driven environment. Finally, control in the hands of the employer is a fundamental characteristic and subset of responsibility-driven processes.

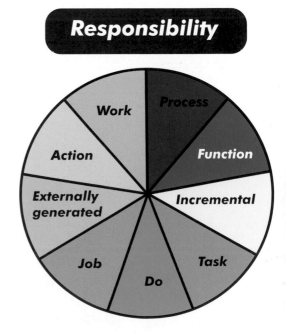

ACCOUNTABILITY BASICS

Accountability focuses more on results than it does on process. The primary element of accountability is its orientation to outcome, to the products of work rather than the process of working. Accountability assumes that the outcomes of work have been defined and that people are committed to the achievement of those outcomes. This orientation to outcomes changes the relationship of the worker to work and of workers to the workplace. As a result, there is a stronger orientation to ownership and investment and inclusion in defining the elements and processes of work relating to agreed-upon outcomes. The value of the work is aligned with the achievement of outcomes.

Accountability Elements

Accountability incorporates characteristics that reflect significant alterations in the organization's expectations for work performance:

- Work expectations are not a laundry list of performance functions.
- Performance evaluations reflect the achievement of work outcomes.
- Defining expectations is shared between workers and management.
- The relationship between workers and managers is around mutual expectations and outcomes.
- Defining relationships is as important as defining the work and performance expectations.
- Roles are defined by virtue of their contribution, not simply as indicators of their job classification.
- What individuals are accountable for is clearly defined before performance expectations are identified.
- Accountability is always generated from within the person and the role and expectations for performance reflect that level of ownership.
- Accountability is owned, not delegated.
- It is the obligation of every individual to clearly understand and articulate accountabilities with group expectations.

Accountability
(21st Century)

Product
Result
Outcome
Accomplish
Difference
Fit
Role
Sustainable
Internally generated

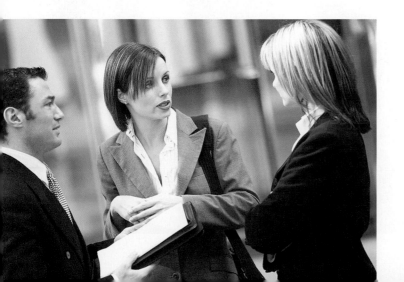

ACCOUNTABILITY IN ACTION

Accountability is a dynamic, not stable or inert, concept. It assumes that all in the organization are focused on the achievement of commonly defined and clearly enumerated outcomes and related work processes. It is important in understanding accountability that it is seen as an expression of the commitment to work values from within. One is "accountable for" rather than "responsible to." This results from the fact that there is an embedded relationship, indeed partnership, between the worker and the work. The worker shares with the workplace a defined set of expectations and outcomes negotiated around clearly understood values, purposes, and results.

Leaders come to understand they play a different role in an accountability-based organization. There's a different configuration of leadership role and relationships in a partnership-driven organization, where there is shared and mutual obligation for defining performance expectations, work processes, and mutual outcomes. Unlike responsibility, accountability is never delegated. Each accountable role is linked and connected with other roles that are equally accountable. Because accountability defines the role, each individual that performs within it plays a major part in determining the content of the accountability and achieving its performance outcomes. These products of the work are themselves the basic delineator of work value, productivity, and success. In this frame of reference, accountability is always shared; each person plays his or her part in clearly defining the foundations of a common set of expectations, roles, performance, and mutual outcomes (Stickler, 1995).

Ownership and accountability are essentially aligned. They reflect the seamless integration of roles and membership working together throughout the organization for common purposes and goals. All members of the organization commit their effort toward achieving common outcomes and ultimately having a mutually beneficial effect on the organization's success and achievement. In such a framework there is no secrecy or arbitrary behavior. Control, paternalism, and arbitrary or capricious behavior is eliminated as a foundation for work performance and relationships.

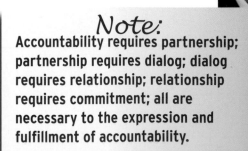

Note:
Accountability requires partnership; partnership requires dialog; dialog requires relationship; relationship requires commitment; all are necessary to the expression and fulfillment of accountability.

ACCOUNTABILITY POINTS OF REFERENCE

☐ All roles exist in the organization with clearly identified expectations and outcomes enumerated in advance of performance.

☐ The success of a role is directly related to what happens as a result of having done the work rather than simply identifying the work process.

☐ Performance evaluation should be an indicator of accomplishment in what was achieved rather than simply an assessment of process and/or function.

☐ The functional content of a role is relatively fixed but not permanent; role functions change as demands change.

☐ A role is successful to the extent that it is flexible enough to respond to changing expectations for performance and outcomes.

☐ The content of a role is always negotiable and does not reflect the absolute control of leader, individual, or team.

☐ Accountability represents and demonstrates the requirement to create a goodness-of-fit between work processes and outcomes.

☐ Accountability is role specific and cannot be enforced by mandates, law, or external obligation because all accountability is internally generated.

☐ Accountability cannot be unilaterally defined: it represents the aggregate results of mutual ownership, obligation, and relationship and is the product of negotiations that lead to a common commitment.

☐ Accountability reflects the understanding that the most effective decision is that which is implemented in the same place it is decided.

☐ Accountability requires the full engagement in investment of all stakeholders and cannot be sustained unless that investment is tied to organizational demands.

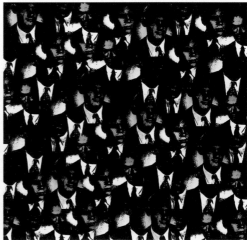

NECESSARY COMPONENTS FOR SUCCESSFUL ACCOUNTABILITY

☐ Team-based values and approaches are used as the work framework for organizations.

☐ Continual quality improvement processes are used as a basis for determining work and achieving outcomes.

☐ The majority of decisions are consistently made closest to the point of service or productivity where the work will be carried out.

☐ Each person's accountability is clearly aligned with the work expectations and performance outcomes to which that effort is directed.

☐ Individual performance evaluations should be replaced by team-driven performance definition, work processes, and outcome evaluations.

☐ As much as possible benefits and rewards should be directly related to performance outcomes in goal achievement.

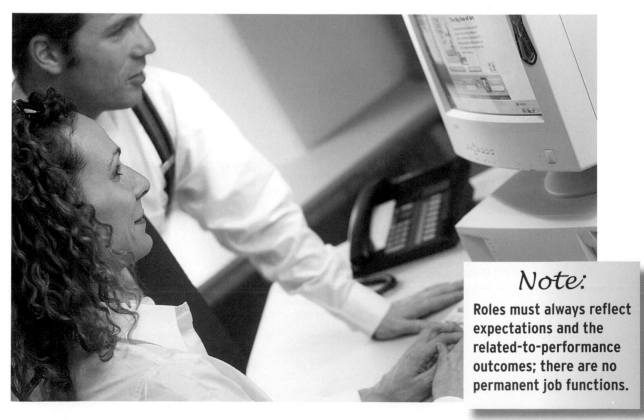

Note:

Roles must always reflect expectations and the related-to-performance outcomes; there are no permanent job functions.

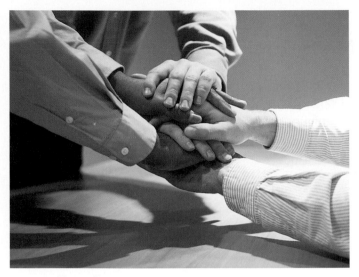

Ownership: The Central Requirement for Sustainability

During the entire history of work, superior-subordinate relationships have comprised the foundation of most work relationships. These relationships have often been expressed in terms of master-servant, employer-employee, parent-child, and superior-subordinate. Roles and relationships in work have historically been the subset of an owner-director command-and-control environment. Little value is placed in the contribution, communication, or personal ownership of work by the employees or subordinating workers. Data generated over the past 30 years have proven that such vertical, parental, and ownership notions of work and performance are simply not sustainable over the long term and ultimately affect productivity and organizational success.

This emerging reality has created a new approach to understanding work, the worker, and the relationship of each to the workplace. New age information has brought with it a deeper understanding of the value of individual work and the relationship of work to those who do it. In a more systems view of work, the understanding of the forces and effect of human capital and its contribution to value is a critical notion of both determining value and creating a sustainable framework for it.

Elements of Ownership

- Understanding the individual's value and contribution to defining work, meeting its obligations, and influencing its outcomes
- Creating the conditions and circumstances that embrace workers, engage them in decision making, and share in the generation of rewards
- Creating the conditions for innovation and creativity results in a milieu that is supportive of the value and contribution of workers
- Developing strong and competent leadership driven by worker involvement, team-based processes, effective communication, and sustainable relationships

> *Note:*
>
> **All work is owned by those who do it. Ownership is essential to accountability.**

LEADERSHIP AND TEAM SELF-MANAGEMENT ASSESSMENT

In order for teams to function effectively, they need good leadership. This is simply the basic inventory of leadership skills. For each of the points made, select the appropriate answer. The higher your score the greater your facilitation at team leadership. This should be looked at as a developmental assessment, not a leadership critique.

1. Almost never

2. Sometimes

3. Often

4. Regularly

	1	2	3	4
I believe that all team members should be encouraged to be self-directed.				
I try to establish the needs of the team members early in their relationship with each other.				
I encourage all members of the team toward self leadership.				
I make sure team and individual accountabilities are clear to members.				
I help the team identify hidden concerns or issues.				
Team members are always involved in decisions that affect their work.				

LEADERSHIP AND TEAM SELF-MANAGEMENT ASSESSMENT (CONT'D)

1. Almost never   3. Often
2. Sometimes   4. Regularly

	1	2	3	4
Problems of trust between team members are addressed as soon as identified.				
I develop and value strong interpersonal relationships between team members and myself as leader.				
There is a team process for accepting or declining process approaches or team methodology.				
I stimulate the team to undergo continuous process evaluation regarding their work.				
I develop opportunities for creative and innovative thinking and new methodologies for work.				
I develop opportunities for creative and innovative processes and new applications for work.				
I help the team identify good sources of information and ways of using it effectively.				
I encourage the team to develop informal mechanisms of support and socialization.				

| | 1. Almost never | 3. Often | | |
| 2. Sometimes | 4. Regularly | | |

	1	2	3	4
I stimulate the team to identify new ways of thinking and introduce new models of problem solving.				
I undertake with the team frequent assessments of progress and team effectiveness.				
I help the team to find their small successes in support of movement toward larger outcomes.				
When the team gets stuck I help them identify new approaches and paths of exploration.				
I help the team clarify conflicts in accountability and performance and methods for adjusting them.				
I am constantly "looking over the horizon" for new implications and information that will affect the work and direction of the team.				

Scores: 45-60   Excellent team leadership skills
30-44   Good leadership skills with some developmental needs
15-29   Some strong leadership skills that needs further team skill development
0-14   Basic skill development in team leadership with further reassessment

This small survey is simply a basic opportunity for self-assessment of fundamental skills related to team management. However, it serves as a reminder of the basic principles of team management and leadership that relates to the team processes and the elements of partnership, equity, accountability, and ownership—the basic subsets of effective team leadership.

References

Hackman, R. (2002). *Leading teams: Setting the stage for great performances*. Boston: Harvard Business School Press.

Lencioni, P. (2002). *The five dysfunctions of a team*. San Francisco: Jossey¬Bass.

Parker, G. M. (2003). *Cross-functional teams: Working with allies, enemies, and other strangers* (2nd ed.). San Francisco: Jossey-Bass.

Pedersen, A., & Easton, L. (1995). Teamwork: Bringing order out of chaos. *Nursing Management*, 26(6), 34-35.

Porter-O'Grady, T., & Krueger Wilson, C. (1998). *The healthcare teambook*. St. Louis: Mosby, Times Mirror.

Steckler, N. (1995). Building team leader effectiveness: A diagnostic tool. *Organizational Dynamics*, 23(2), 20-35.

Thompson, L., Aranda, E., & Robbins, S. (2002). *Tools for teams: Building effective teams in the workplace*. Boston: Pearson Custom Publishing.

Suggested Readings

Goleman, D. (1997). *Emotional intelligence*. New York: Bantam Books.

Goleman, D. (2000). *Working with emotional intelligence*. New York: Bantam Books, Inc.

Gottlieb, M. R. (2003). *Managing group process*. Westport, CT: Praeger.

Lewis, J. P. (2002). *Working together: Twelve principles for achieving excellence in managing projects, teams, and organizations*. New York: McGraw-Hill.

Peterson, R. S., Mannix, E. A. (2003). *Leading and managing people in the dynamic organization*. Mahwah, NJ: L. Erlbaum.

Porter-O'Grady, T., & Krueger Wilson, C. (1998). *The healthcare teambook*. St. Louis: Mosby, Times Mirror.

Willmore, J. (2003). *Managing virtual teams*. Rollingsford, NH: Spiro Press USA.

CHAPTER

2

MANAGING CONFLICT

To manage conflict well, the leader must understand the elements of conflict and see it as a normal expression of human relationship.

WHAT IS CONFLICT?

Conflict can be simply defined as interpersonal and intergroup differences resulting in opposition and confrontation when an individual or group impedes the values or action of another individual or group.

Understanding conflict requires the ability to actively look for it and to see the elements of conflict emerging in any given situation. The leader keeps a close eye on the communication dynamics going on in the workplace and seeks out all the places where potential conflict exists. The leader recognizes that conflict is always present in the workplace and is therefore continually aware of the potential for the emergence of conflict.

Note:

All conflict is normative. Conflict is simply the unresolved differences between people.

Sources of Conflict

- Differences
- Emotions and feelings
- Opposing views
- Acting on or out
- Tension
- Interpersonal
- Disagreeable

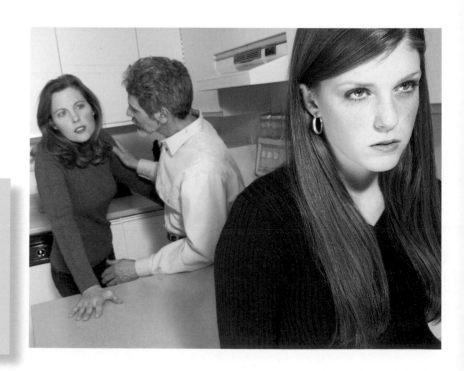

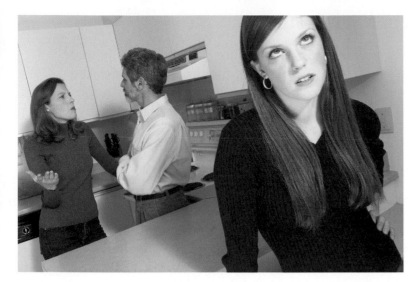

Note:

The leader makes it safe for people to express conflict and to share their experience off it, to develop a language for expression; in short, to make the experience of conflict normal.

Although all conflict is normal, it is not all acceptable. The leader must always look out for the inappropriate expression of sentiments and feelings generated that can lead to conflict. The creation of conflict directed to hurting another simply to get one's own needs met inappropriately must be guarded against by the leader. Creating conflict directed solely to hurt someone else is always inappropriate and must be dealt with quickly and clearly (Levine, 1998).

The Leader Looks for Signs

- Evidence of stress
- Indicators of pressure
- Snide comments
- Avoidance
- Inappropriate silence
- Anger statements
- Negative feelings
- Personal pain

Note:

The leader listens carefully in people's conversations with or about each other, always looking for the subtext or hidden message that might indicate the presence of the seeds of conflict.

Disagreement
Incompatibility
Values conflict

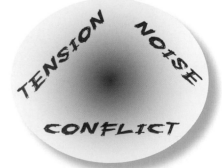

CONFLICT SITUATIONS

Every work situation provides an opportunity for stress and conflict. This is especially true in health care. Health care professionals frequently identify that their roles are fast-paced and exhibit high stress levels. The stress of work provides many opportunities for raising conflict that should stimulate a response from the manager. When individuals' needs are in conflict with the work and the environment, stressors are introduced; these stressors can be manifested in communication, relationships, interactions, or personal emotions. The manager should observe the signs of stress in its earliest stages in order to address it as soon as possible.

Signs of Stress

- Feelings of being overwhelmed
- More work than one can do
- Impatience with others
- Easy to anger
- Feelings of tearfulness
- Lost the focus
- Short temper
- Physical signs (headache, nervousness)

EMERGING CONFLICT

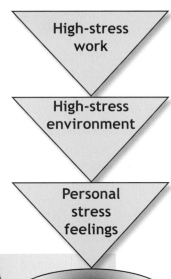

High-stress work

High-stress environment

Personal stress feelings

CONFLICT

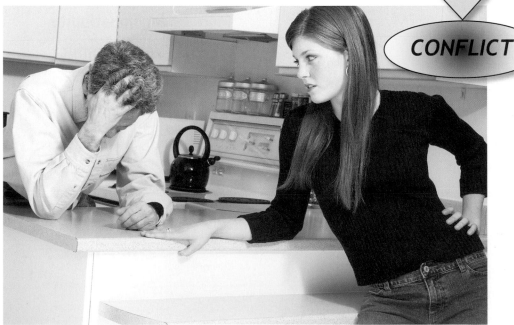

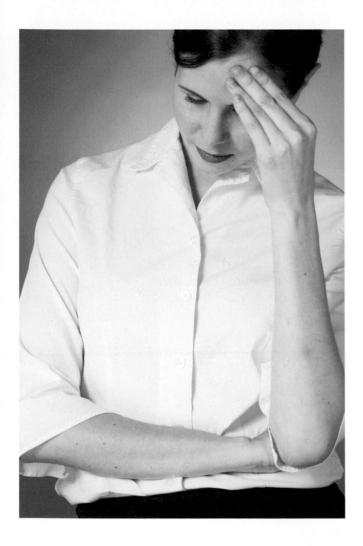

Early engagement of conflict

> Look for it.
> Recognize early signs.
> Address the symptoms.
> Make all feelings safe.
> Engage the person.

SCENARIO

SCENARIO

Nancy has been having trouble finding a babysitter for her daughter while Nancy is at work. Her frustration and concern over the situation are affecting her mood and relationship with other staff. It is also beginning to affect her focus in addressing the needs of patients.

As Nancy's manager, what is your first response to Nancy's situation?

Usually the greatest problem with conflict is avoiding it. The good leader, recognizing conflict is a normal response to any number of unusual circumstances, engages the conflict as early as possible. By directly addressing the individual experiencing the stressors that might lead to further conflict, the leader diminishes the impact and advances the possibility of resolution (LeBaron, 2003).

OPENNESS

The conflict effective manager creates an environment where staff members are comfortable with their own feelings and the ability to express them. An environment which is constraining, controlling, or highly formal creates structural barriers that make it difficult for individuals to either identify with their feelings or express them. The wise manager embraces feelings, regardless of their intensity. This leader is comfortable with the expression of feelings and has developed the skills necessary to address and respond to the context out of which they emerge. The leader needs to test her or his own "openness" quotient.

Q: Am I comfortable with my own feelings?

Q: Do I feel stress in the presence of conflict?

Q: Am I comfortable with other people's expression of feelings?

Q: Do I foster an environment of warmth and caring?

Q: Does the staff as a whole embrace each other's feelings?

Q: When there is anger or passion displayed, do I receive it or draw away from it?

Q: Am I physically warm and expressive with others' emotional responses?

Note:

Stressors are not always obvious. Sometimes the manager must look deeper for the subtle signs of potential conflict. Often small mood changes or distractions can be indicators that stress and conflict are in the wings. Ask about them the minute you see them.

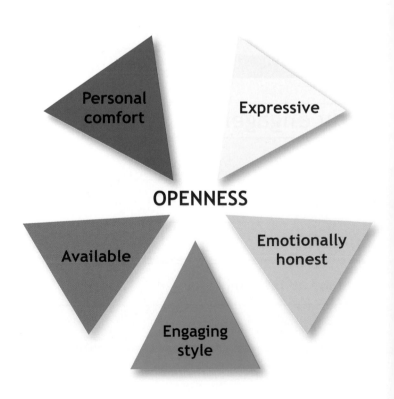

EMOTIONAL COMFORT WITH CONFLICT

A leader does not automatically become skilled at managing the stress of conflict. In our past social circumstances, much of the feelings and expression of conflict were considered unacceptable and inappropriate. Our best models of dealing with conflict are often our parents and our families. In family situations the effort was frequently to diminish, avoid, or eliminate conflict. In fact, conflict was often seen as a failure in the relationship and an inappropriate way to deal with personal and interacting family problems (LeBaron, 2003).

The family model for conflict is the one that often translates most frequently into the workplace. The leader, like the staff, brings a whole range of experiences, values, and past relationships to conflict in the workplace, along with all of the avoidance, ignoring, or inappropriate response to conflict that can accompany it.

It is important for the leader to recognize that managing conflicts is a skill that demands attention and development. It is not something that comes naturally, or is automatic, or should be ignored. In fact, the leader will need to learn the skills necessary to embrace conflict, manage it well, and use it as an opportunity for personal and organizational growth.

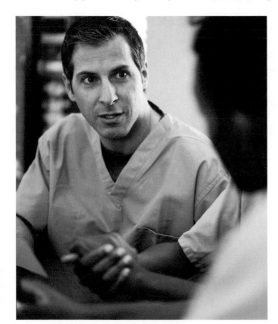

Personal Barriers to Engaging Conflict

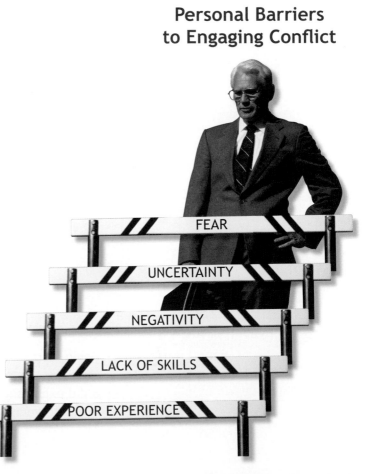

FEAR

UNCERTAINTY

NEGATIVITY

LACK OF SKILLS

POOR EXPERIENCE

Overcoming Personal Barriers to Engaging Conflict

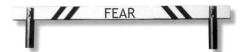

- First, confront it.
- Take three deep breaths.
- Examine what's going on inside you.
- Talk to someone else about your fear.
- Talk yourself through the experience.

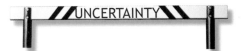

- Break the conflict down into parts.
- Identify which part has greatest impact.
- Stay in touch with feelings and reactions.
- Identify conflict as early as possible.
- Validate with others your identification skills.

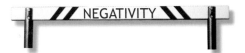

- Recall past experiences with conflict.
- Visualize yourself within a conflict.
- Observe family conflict dynamics.
- Talk with other family members.
- Write down and review your feelings.

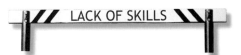

- Read about the conflict management process.
- Attend classes on conflict management.
- Do a role-play on conflict.
- Discuss conflicts process with others.
- Practice conflict scenarios.

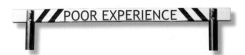

- Seek opportunities to practice.
- Begin mediating small conflicts.
- Have experts evaluate your progress.
- Build experience slowly.
- Evaluate your progress with peers.

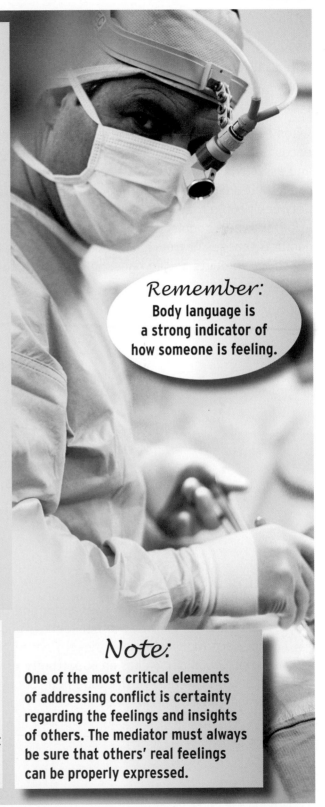

SCENARIO

Dr. Smith was particularly edgy today and appeared to be taking it out on everyone he met in the operating room. It wasn't as though he was this way often, but staff could never be sure exactly when Dr. Smith would be on the emotional edge. This made it especially hard in the surgical suite when people were already feeling stress about the surgery. Jane, the OR manager, was uncertain as to how to handle this situation. She knew that she could not let it go on unaddressed but was uncertain as to what the best approach would be.

Scenario questions

1. When is the best moment to address Dr. Smith's behavior?
2. Where is the best place that Jane could talk with him?
3. How does Jane deal with her own uncertainty?
4. What might be the best way to open the conversation with Dr. Smith?
5. Should Jane discuss her approach with her peers before beginning?
6. What expectations should Jane have of her conversation with Dr. Smith?

Remember:
Body language is a strong indicator of how someone is feeling.

Conflict management is a learned process. It gets better with time and experience. A leader should remember that practice and exposure enhance and advance the skills necessary to be successful in mediating conflicts. Therefore, seek out as much opportunity to mediate conflict as possible.

Note:
One of the most critical elements of addressing conflict is certainty regarding the feelings and insights of others. The mediator must always be sure that others' real feelings can be properly expressed.

Managing Conflict 31

HANDLING CONFLICT

Wherever people have the opportunity to make choices and to control their own lives, there is a potential for conflict. Everyone is different. These differences define us as individuals and make us unique. At the same time, they serve as fundamental sources of potential conflict when those differences run up against the differences of others (Wenger & Mackli, 2003).

When handled creatively and effectively, these differences can result in richer and deeper experiences between people. However, for this to happen, these differences must be handled creatively and assertively so they don't become or remain contentious. Unaddressed or ignored, differences can result in contention. This contention represents an emotional and psychological distance between people that can result in negative feelings, aggression, oppression, antagonism, and alienation between people. In most cases (about 90% of the time) mediators deal with interpersonal conflicts that result from a lack of understanding or perception of one for another. It is in anticipating these conflicts and in handling them that the leader will spend most of his or her time with mediation activities.

Note:

Making staff feel safe with regard to their feelings is the first step in managing conflict well. If people can express their feelings openly and honestly with each other with a sense of safety and confidence, often subsequent conflict can be avoided and individuals can feel stronger control over their experiences and relationships.

Creating a Safe Space:

- Move the parties away from each other and the place of conflict.
- Support each person in his or her feelings and emotions.
- Accept each individual's own perceptions of how her or she feels.
- Make sure each person has an opportunity to verbalize feelings.
- Don't attempt to resolve the issue before individuals express feelings.
- Be caring and supportive of each person experiencing the conflict.
- Accept whatever emotions are expressed in an appropriate place for it.

IDENTIFYING THE PROBLEM

The mediator's first task is to be able to get to the core issues that lie at the heart of a conflict situation. These core issues are identified by individuals as the "triggers" that hook into feelings of personal conflict. The good mediator seeks to find these central issues because they are the ones that most often hold people to their negative feelings. These issues do not have to be "right" or accurate, or even legitimate; they simply must be felt and expressed. Sorting through their legitimacy comes later in the process.

MAKE SURE ISSUES ARE EXPRESSED

It is important that the individuals expressing a conflict be clear and open about what is bothering them. If individuals experiencing conflict do not have the chance to fully express concerns and feelings, these feelings will emerge later in the process, causing it to slow or to begin all over again! Patience and thoroughness in the earliest stages of a conflict can often result in fewer problems in resolving it and a shorter time spent in processing it. The challenge for the mediator is to stay out of the way of expression and clarification. The mediator has no goal but helping others resolve their own issues.

Note:

The mediator does not own the problem and is not responsible for its resolution. The parties own it and are responsible for resolving it.

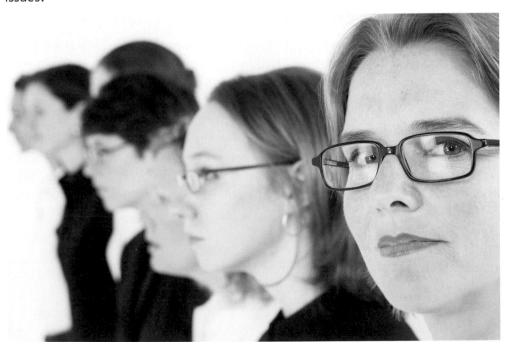

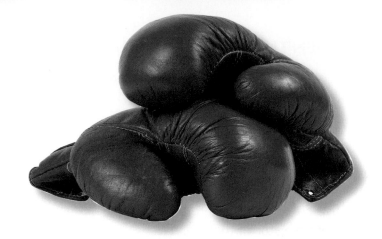

Kinds of Conflicts

- Relationship conflicts
- Information conflicts
- Interest conflicts
- Organizational conflicts
- Value-based conflicts

Causes of Relationship Conflicts

- ☐ Expression of strong feelings
- ☐ Altered perceptions
- ☐ Judgments
- ☐ Assumptions
- ☐ Poor communication
- ☐ Repeated patterns of behavior

Note:

Unaddressed feelings are the most common cause of lingering conflict. These feelings smolder just below the surface, building energy, igniting fuses, and ultimately resulting in a devastating explosion that is very difficult to recover from—for all parties!

SCENARIO
Relationship Challenging Situation

Rachel didn't know if she could stand one more negative comment from Michael. Ever since she had arrived on the nursing unit, Michael had virtually nothing positive to say to her. He seemed to track her every clinical move and knew exactly when she was overwhelmed or concerned and even when she was behind in her work. It was then that he seemed to comment about her pace, competence, and organization. Again this morning he started with the comments, even suggesting that she might not be able to keep up with the demands of the clinical work. His constant monitoring of her work and comments about her ability to keep up increased the stress level and made her even more tense in this new clinical situation than she would normally feel. Rachel didn't know what to do. If he didn't stop soon she would either blow up or just throw up her hands and leave.

Scenario questions

1. At this point in this scenario what should Rachel's first step be?
2. What kind of environment needs to be created to facilitate expressing conflict feelings?
3. What kind of a relationship conflict would you define this to be?
4. What kind of conflict is the most easily resolved?

Causes of Relationship Conflicts

- ☐ Powerful emotions
- ☐ Misperceptions
- ☐ Inadequate communications
- ☐ Negative behaviors
- ☐ Boundary issues
- ☐ Relationship history

Relationship Conflict Clarification

- ☐ Quality time together
- ☐ Raising children together
- ☐ Use of time
- ☐ Financial issues
- ☐ Patterns of behavior
- ☐ In-law issues
- ☐ Conflicts with the boss
- ☐ Coworker issues

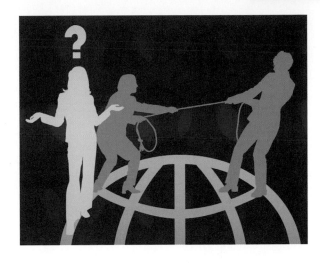

Note:

Relational conflicts usually begin as situational events. Left unaddressed, however, these primarily situational conflicts can become long-term sustaining relational conflicts that affect the integrity and the life of the relationship.

The most important first step in understanding relationship conflicts is being clear with regard to exactly how one feels and what the conflict might be. The worst kinds of relational conflicts are those that build on inaccurate perceptions, especially that which relates to either what was said or heard. Relationship conflicts are filled with emotional content. A part of the clarification process is providing time and expression for the emotional content so that mediation can take the individuals closer to the issues. Relationships are filled with meaning, and the feelings related to the significance of the meaning must be explored sufficiently before the parties can adequately translate them into language and communicate them effectively. However, dealing with feelings and dealing with issues must be separated at the outset so they are not handled in the same way. Each party must be given sufficient expression so the full range of sensitivities related to the conflict have expression and an opportunity to be recognized. In relationship conflicts, the greatest failure in their resolution is usually found in an inadequate allowance for the expression of feeling.

Causes of Information Conflict

☐ Missing information

☐ Inadequate information

☐ Not enough information

☐ Not the right information

☐ Inadequate interpretation

☐ Different views of the data

☐ Different information management

Note:

People think they have the right information without ever analyzing its source, the perspective it represents, the content, and the meaning it is attempting to project. A great deal of conflict can be avoided if people really thought carefully about the information influencing their actions.

THE RIGHT KIND OF INFORMATION

People make judgments based on their own perceptions, values, and management processes related to the kind of information they can access. Sometimes this information is inaccurate or inadequate. When combined with individual values and perceptions, it can become a potent mix for potential conflict. Available information itself demonstrates no bias until it is run through the perceptive and values filters of those who are reviewing it. Careful assessment and review of information is critical to any level of appropriate action. Before acting (that means drawing conclusions or making judgments), individuals should ask themselves the following questions:

1. Where does the information come from?
2. Is the information relevant to the topic or issue at hand?
3. Does the information correlate well with other sources of information?
4. Is the source of information credible? Is it complete?
5. Do I have enough information to draw any conclusion?
6. What are the possible views or perceptions related to interpreting the information?
7. What do I need to do to further clarify or verify information that is influencing my thinking?

Think:

☐ Am I making judgments before I have all the information I need?

☐ Have I clarified what is meant in the information before I draw conclusions about what I am going to do?

☐ Have I asked others about their perceptions and clarified my own reaction through the eyes and ears of others?

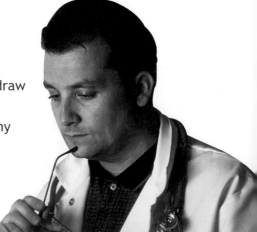

UNCLEAR INTEREST

It is important that clarity with regard to individuals' feelings and sensitivities related to the concerns at hand be established in the early stages of interest conflicts. Often the parties are unaware of the fact that they may share interests, there may be common ground with regard to their conflict related to the interests, or their perceptions about the conflict may actually have nothing to do with the interests. Many times in the arena of interest conflict, the challenge is not conflicting interests but is instead different insights and perceptions the parties bring to how they know the issue and how they have come to understand their role and relationship to it. Often what occurs in these cases is that the real interest is hidden within the expressed interest and the mediator must be able to get each party to the place where they are clear about what the underlying or hidden interest might be that may be truly generating the conflict. Of concern with interest-based conflict is the fact that the parties may not know what their genuine interests are; they maybe actually hiding genuine interest, perceptions may be obscuring the genuine interest, or they may even be unaware of what the real interest is. Here the mediator must often dig deeply to more clearly articulate the genuine interest and the real issues that may be associated with it (Constantino & Merchant, 1998).

Causes of Interest Conflict

- ☐ Conflict over the same interests
- ☐ Differing interests
- ☐ Differing perceptions of interests
- ☐ Process conflicts
- ☐ Procedural issues
- ☐ Emotional/psychological conflicts

Note:

Most interest conflicts have tremendous emotional and psychological attachment to the issue in conflict. The good mediator attempts to defuse the emotional and psychological passion in order to ensure the parties can get to a level of discourse that can lead to resolution.

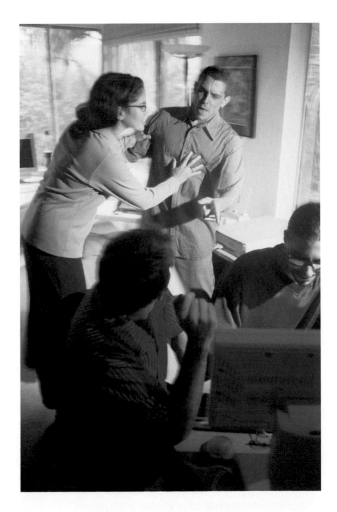

There are many sources of organizational conflict. Fundamentally, role differences can arise from any source significant enough to clearly identify differences between services and departments. Organizational conflicts can be resolved if sectional or unit goals can be disciplined by broad organizational goals and the commitment to owning and achieving the overall organizational agenda.

Causes of Organizational Conflicts

- ☐ Conflicting goals
- ☐ Conflicts between groups
- ☐ Intergroup competition
- ☐ Inadequate leadership
- ☐ Failure
- ☐ Compartmental departments

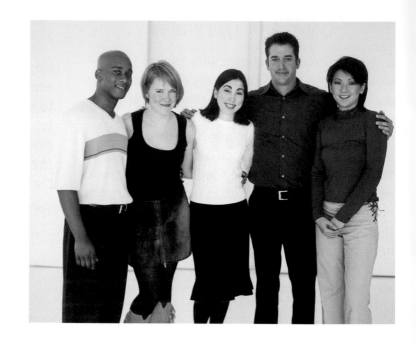

Note:

Organizational conflicts are best resolved when everyone in the organization is "singing off the same song sheet." When individuals and groups play out their own agenda at the expense of others or the whole organization, they create the frame for organizational conflict. To get past this or to ensure this does not happen, leaders must be sure that people see themselves as members of the larger organization committed to making it successful.

ASKING THE RIGHT QUESTIONS ABOUT ORGANIZATIONAL CONFLICT

Organizational conflict depends on the insight and caution of the leader. Carefully preventing groups to form for purposes not in direct relationship to the goals of the larger organization, reducing competition, eliminating elitism, and building cohesiveness help eliminate the potential for organizational conflict:

- How clear are the goals of the organization to everyone in the department?
- Does everyone in the department know how they contribute to organizational goals?
- Is competition directed toward advancing broader goals or serving a different agenda?
- Do performance measurements tell the story of the contribution to organizational goals?
- Does the leader encourage group competitiveness based on personal agendas?
- Are financial challenges in the organization putting people "on edge?"
- How does the leader tie individual work to the broader goals of the organization?

There are many sources of value conflict. Fundamentally, value differences can arise from any source significant enough to clearly identify differences between individuals and groups. Values conflicts are always very difficult to resolve because they relate generally and fundamentally to persons or groups with whom they identify themselves and their fundamental belief systems.

Causes of Values Conflicts

- Different cultures
- Different ethnic groups
- Different religious beliefs
- Different personal values
- Different political ideology
- Different economic, social status

Note:

Values conflicts can be resolved only when common ground can be established between the parties. There must be some element of belief and human experience with which the parties can mutually identify and through that experience find a route to building a stronger relationship upon which subsequent interaction can build.

ASKING THE RIGHT QUESTIONS ABOUT VALUES CONFLICTS

Values conflicts require a great deal of exploration and clarification. Understanding the parties' values point of origin is critical to getting at the source of conflict feelings and moving consciously to establishing common ground. Some clarifying questions are:

- Tell us what this feeling means to you.
- Tell us how your culture (religion, belief, value, practice, etc.) informs this value.
- What is your personal value or belief underpinning this issue?
- Tell us what you need us to understand about your value(s).
- What is unique or different about your value, of which we need to be aware?
- How do you need us to honor and respect that value in our dialog?
- What criteria related to your value do we need to consider in resolving this conflict?

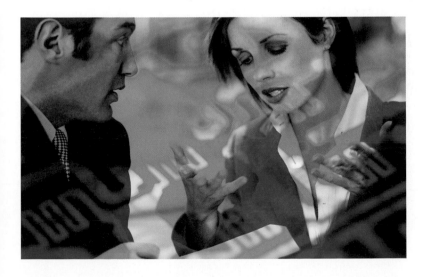

SEEING SIGNS OF CONFLICT

The effective leader sees signs of conflict constantly fomenting in people and in the organization. The conflicting interests and dynamic differences between people and cultures are always a rich source for conflict to percolate.

Leadership:

- Poor recognition of emerging conflict
- Inadequate conflict skills
- Highly competitive
- Seeks own agenda in spite of organizational goals
- Can't tie personal behavior to organizational expectations
- Actually likes conflict; pitting people against each other

Individuals:

- Problems with work competency
- Difficulty establishing relationships
- Personal anger
- Highly competitive
- Unclear about role expectations and goal requirements
- Unable to become a team player

Groups:

- Group relationship unformed or immature
- Groups aggressive or angry with other groups
- Unhealthy level of organizational competition
- Group goals incongruent with organizational goals
- Internally dysfunctional group dynamics
- Failure of the group to fulfill its obligations or achieve goals

SOME CONFLICT MANAGEMENT CUES

> Constantly develop skills.

> Conflict is always present; look for it.

> Listen between the lines; that's where conflict hides.

> Watch your people work and relate together.

> Keep an eye on your own feelings and reactions.

> Let people use their own words and expressions of anger.

> Don't rescue people from uncomfortable feelings.

> Keep an eye out for the quiet yet festering "wounds."

> Develop a staff-driven process for resolving conflicts.

> Allow personal emotions to be fully expressed.

> All conflict can be resolved.

A Brief Conflict Skills Assessment

In order for conflict to be properly handled the leader must have specific skills. This is simply the basic inventory of conflict skills. For each of the points made, select the appropriate answer. The higher your score the greater your conflict skills value. This assessment should be looked at as a developmental tool, not a test.

1. Almost never   3. Often
2. Sometimes   4. Regularly

	1	2	3	4
I have a good sense of the needs of the team at any given moment.				
I can anticipate important changes and alert the team before they directly experience the change.				
I work hard not to avoid conflicts.				
I undertake at least one developmental opportunity a year to refine conflict skills.				
I make it safe for people to identify and express conflicts at work.				
There is a staff-driven conflict resolution process in place on my work unit.				

A Brief Conflict Skills Assessment (cont'd)

	1	2	3	4
Staff have opportunities to test their mediation and conflict resolution skills.				
The environment is conducive to anyone expressing feelings of conflict.				
We have fewer conflict events on our service unit since implementing a conflict resolution process.				
There is a mechanism in place for following up on conflict resolution and ensuring it was effective.				
The trust level on my unit is consistently high.				
Staff are satisfied with the conflict process used on our unit.				
We regularly evaluate the conflict process on our unit and make changes to make it more effective.				

SCORING:

1-13   Need much work

14-27   Growing

28-40   Building well

References

Costantino, C., & Merchant, C. (1998). *Designing conflict management systems*. San Francisco: Jossey-Bass.

LeBaron, M. (2002). *Bridging troubled waters: Conflict resolution from the heart*. San Francisco: Jossey-Bass/Wiley (distributor).

LeBaron, M. (2003). *Bridging cultural conflicts: A new approach for a changing world*. San Francisco: Jossey-Bass.

Levine, S. (1998). *Getting to resolution*. San Francisco: Berrett-Koehler.

Porter-O'Grady, T., & Malloch, K. (2002). *Quantum leadership: A textbook of new leadership*. Boston: Jones and Bartlett.

Wenger, A., & Mockli, D. (2003). *Conflict prevention: The untapped potential of the business sector*. Boulder, CO: Lynne Rienner.

Suggested Readings

Blackard, K., & Gibson, J. W. (2002). *Capitalizing on conflict: Strategies and practices for turning conflict into synergy in organizations: A manager's handbook*. Palo Alto, CA: Davies-Black.

Kriesberg, L. (2003). *Constructive conflicts: From escalation to resolution* (2nd ed.). Lanham, MD: Rowman & Littlefield.

Kritek, P. B. (2002). *Negotiating at an uneven table: Developing moral courage in resolving our conflicts* (2nd ed.). San Francisco: Jossey-Bass.

Porter-O'Grady, T. (2004). Constructing a conflict resolution program for healthcare. *Healthcare Management Review*, 29(4), 278-283.

Porter-O'Grady, T. (2004). Embracing conflict: Building a healthy community. *Healthcare Management Review*, 29(3), 181-187.

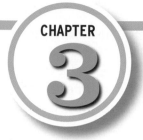

CHAPTER 3

TEAM PERFORMANCE: EVALUATING RESULTS

Teams are effective only to the extent that they are able to achieve the purposes and ultimately the outcomes to which they are directed.

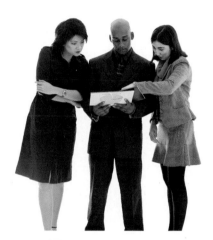

Note:

Evaluating the effectiveness of team performance is as essential as the work itself. Teams must always keep their focus on achieving their purposes and obtaining their outcomes.

TEAM-BASED PERFORMANCE EVALUATION

Everyone experiences, at some level, the components of performance evaluation. As people are employed, one of the first expectations they confront is the fact that they'll be evaluated at some time in their work experience. Performance evaluations have historically focused on the activities and functions of the individual worker. Job descriptions and work standards have often been used to enumerate and validate individual performance, as well as to measure it. Most performance evaluations reflect a very functionally oriented, activity-based, process-oriented set of criteria that simply indicate the relationship of individuals to the activities expected from them. This more functional orientation to evaluation looks at processes, tasks, skills, activities, and the specific relationships among them to determine the individual's effectiveness. As a result, historically, the focus of evaluation has been on the individual rather than the team, and the aggregated and collective value of the contribution of work has been overlooked. Therefore, the aggregated effort and impact of the collective work experience and its role in adding value and achieving outcomes are completely overlooked and frequently missed (Folger & Cropanzano, 1998).

The Problem with individual Evaluation

Although there certainly has been significant precedent for individual evaluation in the history of performance evaluation, there remains little evidence of its value. Most individual evaluations do look at individual skills, abilities, talents, functional proficiency, manual dexterity, and a few elements of the individual's relationship to the group. However, what is not measured is performance within the context of critical value. Because the notion of value depends on an outcome orientation and focuses on the effects of work, results become the focus of meaningful evaluation of performance. Results always reflect the outcome of the activities of performance and are the best source of evidence of value related to those activities, regardless of any other measure. The challenge with regard to results-oriented or outcomes-oriented performance evaluation is that very little of individual approaches to evaluation translates well into successful outcome evaluation processes.

Changing from Process to Outcome

The format for performance evaluation changes with the focus on outcome. Some tips on changing the mindset from process to outcome include the following:

☐ Remove the job descriptions as the sole basis for defining performance.

☐ Raise questions about the results of work rather than the processes of work.

☐ Build a foundation for team-based performance measurement.

☐ Look for value in action instead of simply task-based functions.

☐ Challenge staff members to question everything about what is being done to determine if it has value.

The Value Equation

In health settings the focus on value means measuring outcomes of care against cost of providing service, the value of the service provider's time with the quality expectations for care.

Quality/Cost x Time = Value

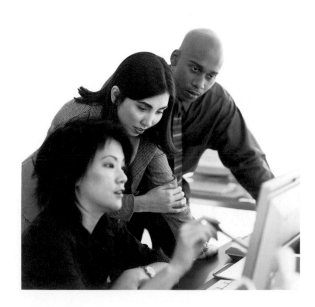

THE VALUE OF TEAMS

Although the organization should certainly look at individuals' relationship to performance outcomes, the notion that sustainable outcomes are the result of the integration of the activities of a number of individuals should take precedence. Sustainable and comprehensive outcomes depend on the relatedness, the interface, and the relative contiguousness of the full series of actions undertaken by a number of individuals comprising a team. Outcomes always drive the evaluation of performance. Value (the impact of outcome) must always be the foundation of performance evaluation. The evaluation mechanisms of themselves must look at both the individual and the team in relationship to each other. When integrated and aggregated, team and individual give evidence of comprehensiveness and the potential for sustainable outcomes. This level of understanding changes the whole focus and meaning of a performance evaluation and broadens its effect (Gibson & Cohen, 2003).

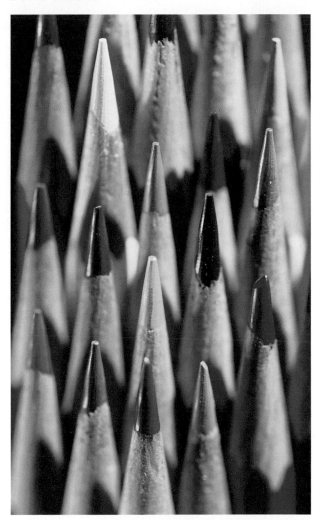

Common Myths about Teams

- Good teams don't need strong leaders.
- Teams can always be self-directed.
- Failure is a sign of an ineffective team.
- Good teams don't experience conflict.
- Teams should never experiment.
- individuals, not teams, are important.
- You cannot really evaluate teams.
- Left alone, teams get into trouble.
- Teams are always well supervised.
- Individuals perform better than teams.
- Team players are compliant and quiet.
- Teams who err are failures.

Note:

Value is evidence of the integration and aggregation of effort in a way that achieves and sustains performance expectations and their relationship to the continuous attainment of desired outcomes. Focus on either process or outcome without a clear understanding of the goodness-of fit between each with the other threatens the probability of ensuring the organization's sustainable health.

PERFORMANCE AND RELATIONSHIPS

No longer can performance evaluation simply be viewed in light of the efficiencies of work effort and work process, or the functional skills of individuals. Performance evaluation must now focus on the relationship between individuals, their activities with each other, and the aggregation of those common activities and their effect on sustainable outcomes and the creation of a product or the delivery of a service.

Increasingly, in all work environments, buyers and sellers, payers, providers, and consumers are looking carefully at the value of what they get for their dollar. Several issues are reflected in this condition or situation. First, is the need to control cost and be clear that what is paid for with regard to product or service is clearly reflected in the value one obtains from that product or service. Second, buyers, payers, providers, and consumers look at the quality of the product or the content of the service to ensure that the activities, functions, and processes associated with the product or service result in the best that can be obtained for the price that is paid. Third, there is a growing interest in the impact of service on an individual's life experience. Therefore, a broad frame of reference is required for clearly delineating the value of a service or a product and the relationship of the work that went into producing it, rather than looking at either element alone. Specific quality and service now no longer mean simply giving everyone the same level of quality. Instead, today, quality of a service or product depends upon how specific and unique it is in addressing the needs of the user. The tighter the fit between the demands and needs of those who buy a product or service, and the more specifically the product or service meets the needs of the individual, the higher the perceived level of quality (Stretch, 2003).

Mass-Customization

☐ Customization is individualized.

☐ Products and service are personalized.

☐ Work is individualized.

☐ Customers interact with designers and providers.

☐ Unique customer requirements drive the design.

☐ The "user" is the final determinant of quality.

☐ Interactive technologies drive customization.

☐ Work is flexible, quick, and responsive.

☐ Market is fragmented through economies of scope.

☐ Customization generates increasing demand.

☐ Products and services change constantly and often.

TEAM-BASED PERFORMANCE FACTORS

As teams become more frequently the basis of work performance in every sector, the method of performance evaluation radically shifts. Teams now become the basic unit of work and are therefore the foundation for the measurements of work, team performance, and outcome achievement. In team-based approaches, the organization is not interested simply in the activities, effectiveness, or function of the individual but rather the collective outcomes of the team as a whole. Indeed, teams are obligated to be concerned with the work of all involved individuals and the performance relationship that each individual has with other team members. As a result, two levels of evaluation operate: the team's internal evaluation of the relationship of each member to the other as well as the individual's contribution to the work of the whole team. The second focus exemplifies the team's performance within the context of expectations and outcomes.

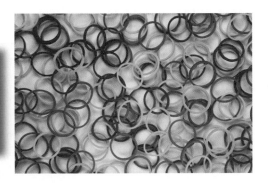

Note:

The quality of service is always determined by the user of that service.

Note:

The forces of change are continuous and endless.

Team-Based Evaluation Process

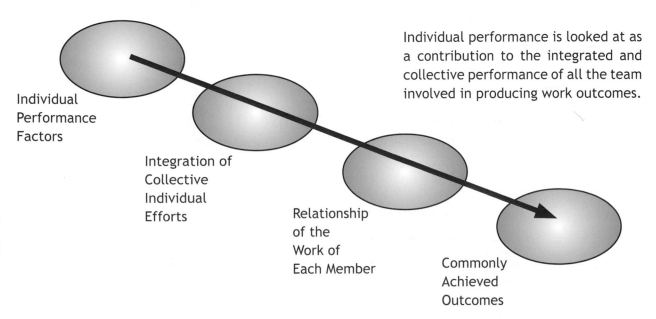

Individual performance is looked at as a contribution to the integrated and collective performance of all the team involved in producing work outcomes.

Individual Performance Factors

Integration of Collective Individual Efforts

Relationship of the Work of Each Member

Commonly Achieved Outcomes

TAKING CARE OF THE NEEDS OF THE INDIVIDUAL

Simply because teams are identified as the foundations of work, the central component of achieving successful outcomes does not diminish the value and the personal needs of every individual who makes up the team. The team is not some amorphous undefined entity. Teams are a collective of individuals who commit to gathering for a common purpose, rendering their unique talents and skills in a way that benefits the collective work outcomes that are reflected in the skills of each and every member of the team (Watkins & Rosegrant, 2001).

Performance evaluations are always a dynamic and controversial element of organizational life. Exactly what should be evaluated, how evaluation processes work, and how the evaluation dynamic itself should be constructed and conducted, along with the role of the individual in the organization and the team, are the topics of much discussion. Each of these issues individually affects the organization's perception and approaches to performance evaluation. The organization's culture supporting team-based approaches must also adequately address the needs of the individual as a member of the system and as an element of the team in the same way that addresses the needs of every member of the organization.

Every individual is intrinsically motivated by a composite of values and purpose that bring meaning to all of his or her endeavors. Extrinsically, the primary purpose of work for every individual is to ensure that the individual can earn a satisfactory living and can establish a satisfying quality of life. However, this extrinsic desire, although sufficient enough to keep people working, is clearly not enough to keep them continuously motivated. Therefore, personal motivation demands more than simply meeting the extrinsic demands that often keep people in the workplace.

Individual Recognition

Individual and personal recognition is the foundation upon which team-based relationships are constructed. Therefore, the following elements are critical for expressing the value of the individual:

☐ Team members have a mechanism that acknowledges the value of each member of the team.

☐ All members know and value the specific role they play in the team.

☐ Every member honors the unique character and content of the relationship of every team member.

☐ Each team member's contribution is clearly enumerated in relationship to its value with regard to sustainable outcomes.

INDIVIDUALS AND TEAM PERFORMANCE

Individuals are always valued within the context of the team. The primary source or origination of that value is located and constructed within each team. Evaluation of performance is a reflection of this construction.

Roles:

- Perform quality measures.
- Make work changes together.
- Negotiate relationships with each other.
- Correct errors and work problems.
- Set accountabilities, goals, and outcomes.
- Conduct group meetings.

Activities:

- Identify individual contributions.
- Find the interface between individual and team work.
- Articulate individual contribution to the whole.
- Identify individual performance with team goals.
- Enumerate accountabilities for specific performance.
- Note individual contribution to team effort.

Process:

- Role descriptions defined for all individuals.
- Clearly articulate process in the team charter.
- Individual accountability is clearly defined.
- Specific individual contributions to team goals enumerated.
- Team outcomes are clearly defined in advance.
- Team performance expectations measured against work outcomes.

VALUING DIFFERENCES

Good teams recognize the essential diversity that is a fundamental of their construct. Rather than attempt to eliminate it, smooth over, or minimize its impact, good team leaders recognize it, honor it, and use it as a sensual source of all innovation and creativity. The value of diversity requires specific and critical understanding with regard to its effect on team process (Porter-O'Grady, 2004a):

- ☐ Diversity recognizes the unique potential of every member of the team and expects that potential to be realized in personal contribution.

- ☐ The difference in team members is the source of solution to team problems and must be accessed effectively to ensure sustainable problem resolution.

- ☐ Cultural differences increase the variability and team process and create increased opportunity for creative effort.

- ☐ Personal skills and attributes that are highly differentiated create a mosaic of contributions to broaden the base of value and increase the opportunity for innovation.

- ☐ Individual uniqueness must be expressed and appreciated within the context of the team through frequent exposure and dialog, such that contribution can be clarified and valued.

- ☐ Team leaders must value differences and makes team members fully aware of the contribution of differences to the success of team effort and evaluate individuals within the context of their willingness to accept differences and to value the unique contributions of each team member.

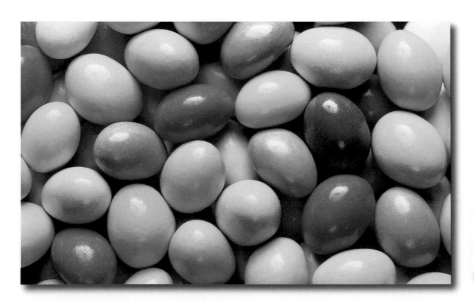

Note:
Homogeneity constrains access to the truth; diversity is essential to finding truth. Teams always will recognize the central diversity and essential differences that are necessary for a team's own creativity and sustenance.

CREATING A TEAM-BASED CULTURE

The organization's culture supporting team-based approaches must always address the needs of the individual as a member of the system, just as it addresses the needs of the team and its contribution to the outcomes of the work of the system.

The culture of a team is composed of the individual characteristics of each of the members. Teams are an aggregation of personalities and character. Clearly this difference can be either an asset or a deficit. The challenge is overcome when the common culture of the group emerges out of the integration of the individual and personal qualities of all members of the team. In this case, culture is built, person by person, working through differences to find in them the elements that interface with the essential common aspects of the team that will advance relationships and facilitate work outcomes.

It is important for each individual to be recognized within the context of the team through which he or she expresses membership in the organization. Rather than the organization focusing on the support, relationship, and rewards of individual work, these factors should originate and generate out of the team's own work and inform the work of the individual. The organization relates to the team, the team then relates to the individual. This construct is a foundation for building a team-based infrastructure that constructs the team as the basic unit of work and builds communication, expectation, and rewards within the context of team values.

The challenge in creating a culture of team values is in building a sufficient infrastructure and management performance culture that recognizes, operates, and rewards teams for their effort. Individual rewards are generated by team members, such that recognition, value, relationship, communication, and rewards are all generated within the context of team structure, process, and relationships. In this way the organization builds an infrastructure that is essentially team driven.

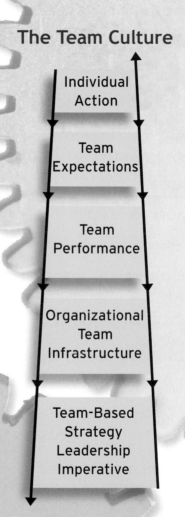

The Team Culture

- Individual Action
- Team Expectations
- Team Performance
- Organizational Team Infrastructure
- Team-Based Strategy Leadership Imperative

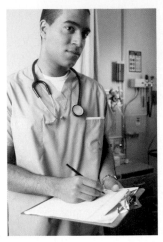

> **Note:**
> The team must be evaluated as a whole.
> Each team member is either contributing to
> the effectiveness of the team or affecting
> it negatively. It is the team's obligation to
> evaluate the effectiveness of its members.

ENSURING INDIVIDUAL MOTIVATION

The ability to keep people involved and invested in their work depends on the organization's ability to allow the worker to fully participate in decisions that affect what the worker does. Within this context the worker has a right to expect:

❖ A clear understanding regarding the expectations of the individual's work

❖ Freedom to fully participate in decisions related to the individual's work

❖ Involvement in all policy and procedural decisions affecting the individual's work

❖ The generation and self-management of specific information affecting individual work

❖ Openness and honesty regarding expectations, performance, and goals of the work

❖ Sufficient organizational support and resources to be successful in doing the work

ENSURING INDIVIDUAL AUTONOMY

Each worker needs to define a level of autonomy to be fully invested in his or her work. In order to effectively contribute to the goals and purposes of the system, the individual must be aware of and clearly articulate personal effort with the effort of the team. There are specific elements of autonomy and individual action that facilitate individual decision making:

☐ Each worker knows the parameters of his or her decision making.
☐ Each worker is expected to make accountable decisions.
☐ Each decision reflects related team decisions.
☐ Each individual has the skills necessary to make decisions.
☐ Each worker is evaluated on the competence and effectiveness of their decisions.

EVALUATING THE TEAM'S EFFECTIVENESS

Adherence to the Rules of Engagement

Each team must have a set of operating rules or terms of engagement that identify the parameters within which the team operates. These terms of reference become a framework that guides or disciplines the team's activities and functions as well as the team members' relationship with each other.

Some Rules of Engagement

- Regularly scheduled meeting times
- Participation reflecting the commitment of team members
- Timeliness of meetings and attendance
- A clear agenda, followed faithfully and appropriately
- Good team business process
- Adequate framework for dialog and participation
- Members consistently meeting their obligations
- The discipline of team rules applied equitably and consistently
- The chair's enforcement of team expectations and performance

Evaluating this step forms the first foundation in assessing whether the basics of team function are operating effectively; 90% of problems regarding teamwork and collective action can be related to issues reflecting rules of engagement (Porter-O'Grady, 2004b). Not consistently acting on the rules of engagement always creates impediments to successful team performance.

Foundational Team Rules

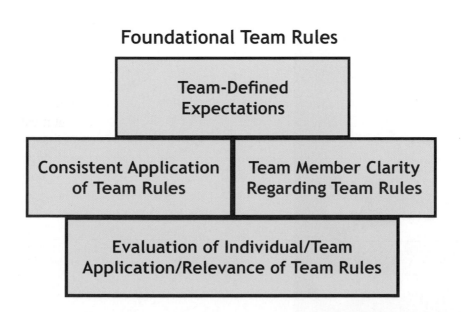

Team-Defined Expectations

Consistent Application of Team Rules

Team Member Clarity Regarding Team Rules

Evaluation of Individual/Team Application/Relevance of Team Rules

TEAM CLARITY REGARDING ITS ROLE

Following the initial formative and definitive stages of basic team function (the rules of engagement) are the processes associated with clarifying the functions, activities, relationships, and outcomes of the team. It is imperative that each team member know what his or her contribution is to the team, the team requirement for the member's role, and the aggregated expectations of the team for its own functions and activities, as well as the requirements that will be essential to ensure that the team acts effectively. Issues of team leadership, team responsibility, member accountability, communication, and the intersection of the team's work with the organizational system as well as with other teams is an important component of ensuring that the team is effective and its roles are applied consistently. Through this process of role and responsibility clarification the team is clear about what it expects of members, what its role is in the relationship to goals, and what is necessary for team success.

The Team Clarification Process Involves:

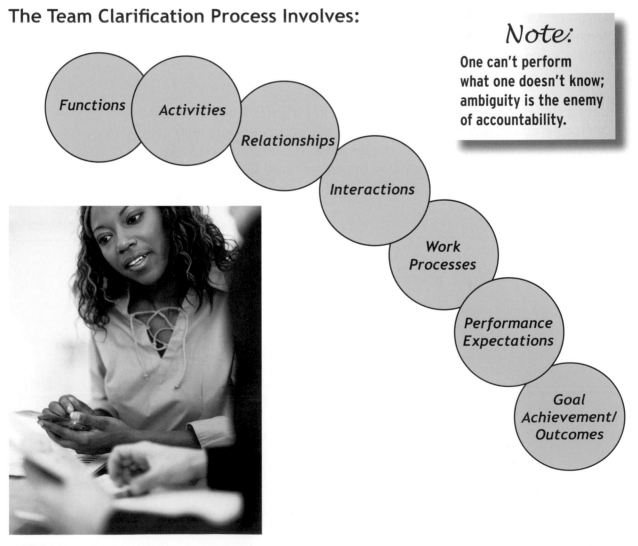

Functions

Activities

Relationships

Interactions

Work Processes

Performance Expectations

Goal Achievement/ Outcomes

Note:

One can't perform what one doesn't know; ambiguity is the enemy of accountability.

EVALUATING CLARITY OF ACCOUNTABILITY

In team-based work, accountability is a critical element of the team's viability and continuing function. Accountability is one of the central components of the whole process of integrated team-based organizational approaches. Accountability is a foundation of performance in every team. Unlike responsibility, which focuses on process effectiveness, accountability focuses on outcomes. The achievement of sustainable outcomes is the chief purpose and value of the work of the team and every member must be committed to that goal. As identified in other sections of this book, accountability is one of the four key principles crucial to the effectiveness, sustenance, and success of team effort.

Investing Team Members in Accountability

Involving all team members requires a methodology of inclusion and deliberation that is used throughout the work process:

1. The format for deliberation and involvement must make sense to each participant and advance the value of the whole team.
2. A consistent method that obtains broad-based involvement of each member is required to ensure that every member is aware of expectations and performance requirements.
3. Enumerate clearly at the conclusion of dialog and decision making the elements of the decision in a way that group consensus, understanding, and consistent application can result following the group's meeting.
4. Evaluate performance and progress against agreed-upon expectations and goals so that each member can see his or her relationship toward goal accomplishment.

The Three Stages of Accountability

Stage 1: Clarity: Each person must know how his or her own work relates to the goals of the team.

Stage 2: Specificity: No generalizations are acceptable; each role must be specifically enumerated in relationship to team functions.

Stage 3: Outcomes: All team members must know their unique contribution to the attainment of results.

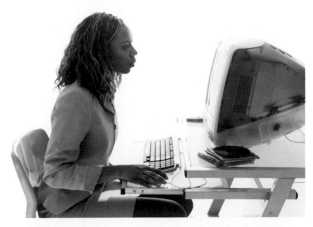

Evaluating Teamwork Effectiveness

Each of the phases of evaluation depends on successful achievement and performance of the previous phase. Clearly, an effective, operating, and functional team requires the formation of purpose and direction and work toward successful processes, structures, issue resolution, and challenge confrontation as required for the functional appropriateness of successful team process.

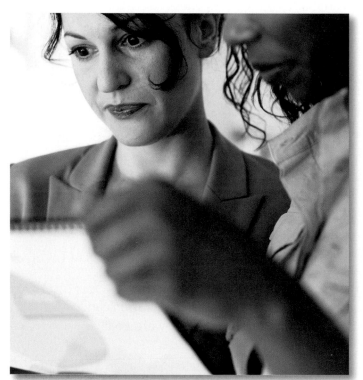

Good Peer-Work Relationships

1. The establishment of a good, clear working agenda
2. Clarification in the common understanding of the purposes, objectives, functions, and activities expected of the team
3. A consistent and clearly enumerated meeting methodology with regard to how the team effectively undertakes its work, applies its process, and meets goals
4. An evaluation process that reviews the framework, processes, expectations, performance, and goal achievement of the team

Required Team Evaluation Elements

- ☐ Clear statement of purpose
- ☐ Team-member understanding of goals
- ☐ Appropriate methodology for team process
- ☐ Clear accountability of team members
- ☐ Understanding of the role of each team member
- ☐ Level of commitment and trust between members
- ☐ Good problem solving and issue clarification
- ☐ Clear ability to resolve conflicts and challenges
- ☐ Good team leadership and facilitation
- ☐ Consistent and timely achievement of goals and outcomes

EVALUATING TEAM MEMBERS' OUTCOME ORIENTATION

A systematic approach needs to be used by the team in order to evaluate its effectiveness. There are a number of approaches that deal with team-based evaluation and tying team performance to outcomes. Perhaps the simplest, yet most effective best understood format for the evaluation process is the plan, do, check, act (PDCA) process. First utilized by Deming, the PDCA process has become increasingly valuable as a context or framework for evaluating and processing team action and goal achievement. The centerpiece is the focus on planning and acting on plans with a specific focus on achieving outcomes. In this process evaluation, this focus on outcomes requires that the team evaluate goals, work processes, performance expectations, causes, inputs, outputs, solutions, alternatives, indeed anything that has an effect on the team's effort to achieve the goals to which planning has been directed. The fundamental questions of evaluation for the team are:

❖ What are we doing?

❖ What are the specific components of our work activity?

❖ What are all of our process elements and stages?

❖ What are our expectations and outcomes?

Strategy and Goal Formation Process Framework

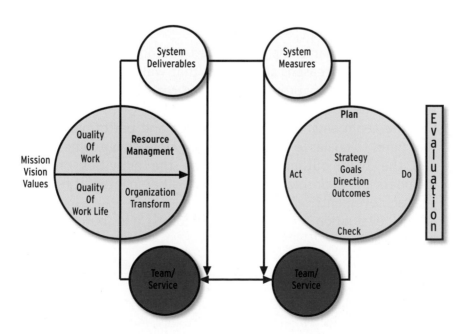

Evaluating Team Planning Effectiveness

Are All Members Thinking Outcome?

❖ Are team deliberations always identifying the anticipated expected outcome or impact at the outset?

❖ When describing work do staff members focus on the goals, expectations, and results of their effort rather than simply on the process?

❖ Do team members tie issues, problems, or concerns to the effect they have on goal achievement and outcomes?

❖ Ultimately, can team members tie all processes, work activities, and goals to the mission and purposes of the organization of which the team is a component?

❖ Do team members understand the grid and matrix of relationships and intersections between team effort, team relationships, organizational interfaces, and the common achievement of the systems goals through the convergence of the action of all teams in the organization?

Do Team Members Understand Their Role in Planning and Goal Achievement?

☐ Does the team name the anticipated outcome in advance and then "back into" the reasons and actions that will achieve it?

☐ Can a team identify present issues and realities that make achieving the outcome both possible and desirable?

☐ Can the team enumerate the behaviors and performance activities that need to coalesce around achieving defined outcomes?

☐ Can the team outline and coalesce the activities of individual members and their relationship to each other in integrating efforts for goal achievement?

☐ Is the evaluation of process, structure, and outcomes defined in advance?

Evaluating Individual Team Member Performance

a. Look carefully at the goodness-of-fit between the work activities and individual in the role expectations of the team.
b. How well does the individual understand the interface between his or her activity and those of the team?
c. Is each individual clear about personal contribution to team outcomes?
d. Are other conflicts between individual issues and team relationships worked out consistently?
e. Do individual team members adjust performance and behavior to act in concert with team expectations?

Looking at Team Process Effectiveness
How does the team handle:

- Conflict processes?
- Relationship issues?
- Process challenges?
- Quality issues?
- Team member relationships?
- Performance issues?
- Work variance and changes?
- Achievement/lack of outcomes?

Tools for Assessing Process Effectiveness

☐ Work process check sheets
☐ Experience or application logs
☐ Survey tool results
☐ Histograms of past team processes
☐ Team focus work or groups
☐ External and internal trend analysis
☐ Charts, tables, graphs

Note:
Evaluation of team performance is constant, consistent, and regular.

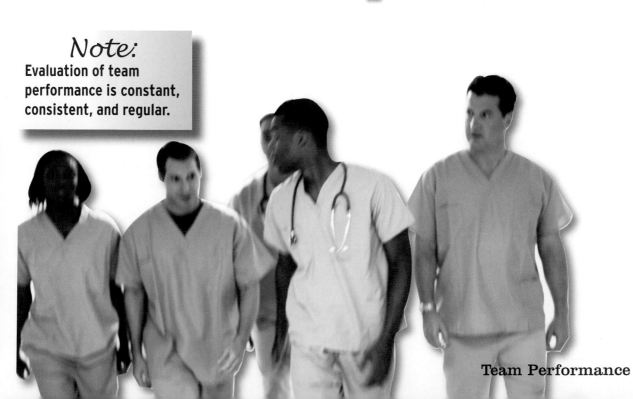

EVALUATING STANDARDS APPLICATIONS

Standards should serve as a basis for enumerating and evaluating the action of the team and the activities of individual members. Several standard components serve as key priority elements for the team:

1) Critical paths that establish specific work processes.
2) Accountability definitions and performance elements for each team member reflecting his or her contribution to the critical path.
3) Performance expectations that are defined for each member in conjunction with each member's contribution to the work goals of the team.
4) The specific outcome elucidated for each critical path or protocol to which the team processes are directed.
5) The process evaluation elements that indicate team members' adjustments or changes in critical path necessary to meet goal outcomes.
6) Assessment of the standards and protocols applied to the work process and used as a vehicle for evaluating the relationship between work and its outcomes.

Documentation

The process of documenting for evaluation purposes is no different from and requires no more detailed process than that which is used to document the team's progress towards goals. The evaluation of teams and their members is embedded in the goal achievement process and should not be separated from it. Individual performance evaluation should be tied to the team. The evaluation process is hooked together with measures of goal achievement. The team's effectiveness is disciplined by the quality of their work and the achievement of their goals. Performance evaluation separated from this reality has no value as a measure of team performance; therefore, all individual performance is a reflection of the achievement of team goals.

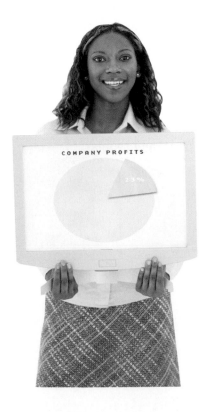

COMPANY PROFITS

GROUP PROCESS AND PERFORMANCE EVALUATION

All teams have a life cycle. The stages of team development have been identified earlier in this book derived from forming, storming, norming, and performing all the way through initiation to extinction. Every individual in a group affects the character and the life of that group. In fact, the group becomes whatever makes up the life of that group in each and all of its members. Group development, facilitation, leadership, and the movement of the group toward defined outcomes require an understanding of the relationship of each to the other in the group to all the process dynamics which make it successful. This performance cycle defines a framework within which the group's life proceeds. All the way from individual competencies through team member expectations, the criteria for the performance of the team, protocols or standards which measure progress, and the evaluation of performance against outcome are all included in the cycle of performance expectations for the team.

Team Performance Cycle

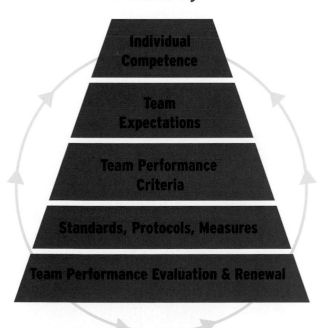

Individual Competence

Team Expectations

Team Performance Criteria

Standards, Protocols, Measures

Team Performance Evaluation & Renewal

Note:

The life and value of a team are directly related to its consistent achievement of sustainable outcomes.

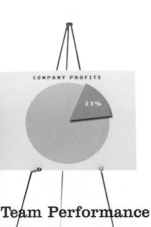

Team Performance 63

EVALUATING TEAM ADAPTATION/SUCCESS

The Building Blocks for Good Group Process

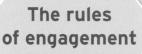

The rules of engagement

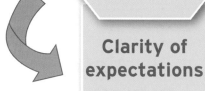

Clarity of expectations

Group leadership/ facilitation

Good group process

Team Adaptation

Charcteristics of each member

History of the group

Group maturity

Culture of group influencing performance

The successes of the group

References

Folger, R., & Cropanzano, R. (1998). *Organizational justice and human resource management*. Thousand Oaks, CA: Sage Publications.

Gibson, C. B., & Cohen, S. G. (2003). *Virtual teams that work creating conditions for virtual team effectiveness* (1st ed.). San Francisco: Jossey-Bass.

Porter-O'Grady, T. (2004a). Constructing a conflict resolution program for healthcare. *Healthcare Management Review, 29*(4), 278-283.

Porter-O'Grady, T. (2004b). Embracing conflict: Building a healthy community. *Healthcare Management Review, 29*(3), 181-187.

Stretch, J. J. (2003). *Practicing social justice*. New York: Haworth Press.

Watkins, M., & Rosegrant, S. (2001). *Breakthrough international negotiation: How great negotiators transformed the world's toughest post-cold war conflicts*. San Francisco: Jossey-Bass

Suggested Readings

De Feo, J. A., & Barnard, W. (2004). *Juran Institute's six sigma: Breakthrough and beyond: Quality performance breakthrough methods*. New York: McGraw-Hill.

Enos, D. D. (2000). *Performance improvement—making it happen*. Boca Raton, FL: St. Lucie Press.

Snee, R. D., & Hoerl, R. W. (2005). *Six sigma beyond the factory floor: Deployment strategies for financial services, health care, and the rest of the real economy*. Upper Saddle River, NJ: Pearson Prentice Hall.

Watson, G. H., Conti, T., Kondao, Y., & International Academy for Quality. (2003). *Quality into the 21st century: Perspectives on quality and competitiveness for sustained performance*. Milwaukee, WI: ASQ Quality Press.

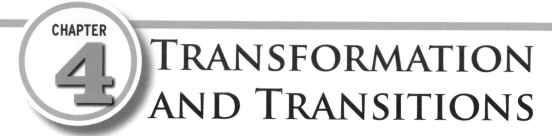

CHAPTER 4

TRANSFORMATION AND TRANSITIONS

To transform means to create and innovate; to change individuals and organizations in ways that they embrace their own futures.

WHAT IS TRANSFORMATION?

Transformation can be simply defined as a process of so fundamentally changing individuals and organizations that they more fully resonate with their own goals and the demands for a future, calling for a new set of expectations, behaviors, and organizational performance.

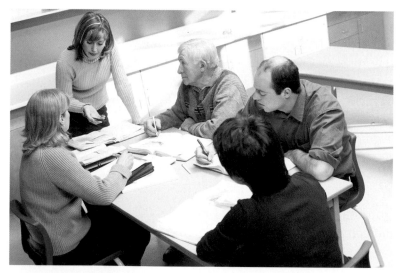

Elements of Transformation

- Creativity
- Innovation
- New behaviors
- New goals
- Deeper understanding
- Renewal
- Reenergized purpose

Transforming people and organizations requires that the leader be continually aware of the permanent and endless demands for a changing environment for human experience and for work. This leader is always aware that no change is permanent and that leadership requires an openness and availability for accelerating demands of personal growth and social complexity.

Note:

Personal transformation is always a requisite for organizational change.

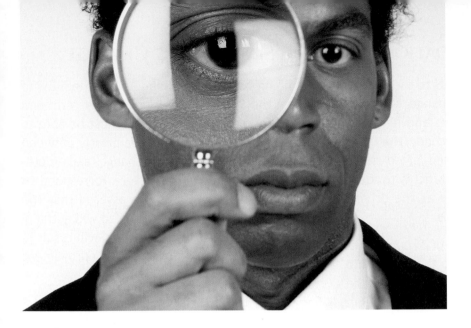

TRANSFORMATION NEVER WAITS FOR READINESS

People are always talking about whether organizations are ready for the changes that they must confront. Organizations are generally never ready for the kind of change they must make in order to be truly transformed. What often happens with organizations is that they find themselves in the midst of a major shift driven by external changes, economic shifts, or new technology and innovations. The good leader always keeps focus on the relationship between the external environment and the internal dynamics of the organization. Through this process, the leader is continually aware of the continual and dynamic interaction between the forces of change and the processes of the organization (Beer & Nohria, 2000).

Transformation calls for the leader to more clearly understand the critical forces that affect the specific changes having an impact on the organization and its people. This leader is always aware of the conditions and circumstances that affect the organization on the broader social and economic stage as well as in the competitive and operational environment of the organization. Keeping an eye on the horizon and incorporating the view of a changing world into the leadership process helps ensure both the leader and the organization that they are available to engage the changes that will invariably affect the life of both individual and organization.

The leader must become skilled at "wide spanning." This is the ability to have a broad view, drawing from a number of contexts and synthesizing the information obtained within the framework of both one's own experience and the work of the organization. Leaders should make no assumptions. Instead, the leader draws on a broad base of data, correlates that information, and makes decisions about what it indicates with regard to essential changes and organizational direction. The ability to scan and to synthesize relevant information ensures the leader as much readiness as can be accessed for the inevitable "moments of transformation."

BUILDING A FOUNDATION

There are two important elements to the change cycle. First, a great deal of change has happened over the past two decades and it is very difficult to sort through it; second, this very transforming change is composed of so much complexity that it has become difficult to identify the key elements that serve as the driving force for the subsequent changes.

The role of the leader in this set of circumstances is to translate the change to the staff, find meaning in the transformation, and obtain the necessary support and investment to begin change. The two key arenas for sustainable change are organizational form and individual behavior. Both need to be altered in order to implement effective change.

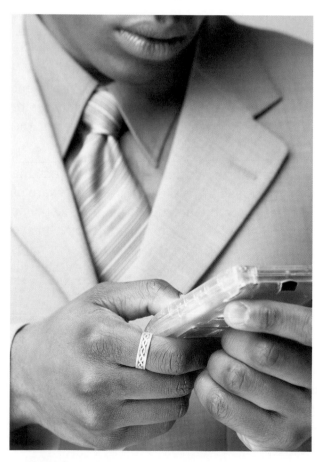

SUSTAINING CHANGE

A defining role for the leader is the ability to discern the difference between short-term and sustainable change. The leader must be able to manage work effort moving seamlessly between responding to appropriate change and implementing the necessary structure to respond to this change. Leaders must be assured that the path on which they have embarked will actually lead to a more desirable state, and will result in the enhancement of work and the improvement of work life.

For change to be clearly viewed, it is essential to have a proper frame of reference for it. In the framework of the changes currently being experienced, the context for change is not the same as past frames of reference. Current change represents a *paradigm shift*, which is a broader and deeper experience of change fundamentally altering our lived reality.

Note:

All change requires energy and commitment and is ignored at great personal expense. Accepting the reality of change is the first step to applying it successfully to our personal lives.

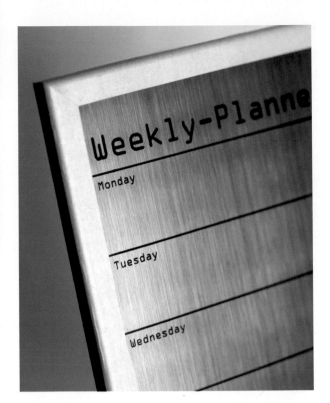

Meaningful Change

- Is sustainable
- Builds on previous changes
- Alters behavior
- Engages everyone
- Can't be ignored
- Must be embraced
- Is clear to all
- Is recognized as a journey
- Has no permanent point of arrival

A New Way of Seeing

Our experiences and our insights tell us about what we see and how it compares to those things we have seen in the past. Our experiences validate or challenge what we see and help us look for the meaning within. However, we frequently see those things for which our past experience makes it inadequate for us to translate. What we see is so significantly different from what we know that there is not sufficient context or framing to help us translate what we see with any clarity or meaning (Pearman, 1998). The result is a sense of chaos and uncertainty that remains as we sort through what we have seen and try to understand it with a template of our past. However, to be able to view the emerging change, we must change our orientation, understand the current context, and translate the change in the language that represents the contemporary or future frame from which the change is flowing.

Embracing Change

- Read the signposts accurately.
- Assess your own individual responses.
- Ask critical questions about what is happening to you.
- Watch the media, read journals, review newspapers.
- Talk the changes over with others; have group discussions.
- Get connected to other change seers and transformers.
- Identify your own challenges and facilitators with regard to change.
- Take care of yourself, get lots of rest, stay motivated

Toward a New Age

As we leave the industrial age and move toward this emerging socio-technical age, most of the characteristics of the time are still unclear to us, yet continue to inexorably unfold. Embedded in this new journey are some interesting yet uncertain circumstances we are not yet prepared to confront.

It is difficult to embrace an entire age of uncertainty. Such a change confronts our sensibilities and threatens our sense of stability. Our values, our way of knowing, our experiences, even our belief systems, reflect an age that is passing. Thus, the journey itself becomes threatening.

> ## Note:
>
> The experience of transformation is very much like leaving home and living on your own for the first time. The world remains the same but everything that tells you about the world is now different and requires a new response that no one else can provide for you. It's now all about how you adapt.

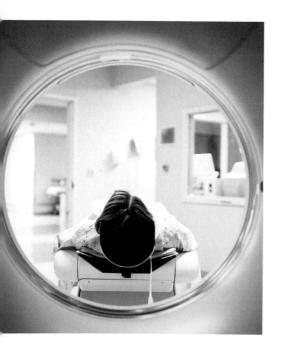

The Challenges of Change

Just imagine what it means to leave a home that you know well with all of the experiences of having grown up there. Imagine the environment, the recognizable and familiar, the friendly and supportive, all the things to which you have become accustomed. Consider all that you have learned, the intricacies, intimacies, and idiosyncrasies you have adapted over a lifetime. Then think about how it feels to leave this place and enter unfamiliar territory where your experiences are no longer validated, your history no longer supported, your values assaulted, your understanding challenged, and what you know considerably diminished. This is what it's like to enter into a new age, to undergo a paradigm shift, an adjustment in your reality where the territory is unfamiliar. That is what the shift from the old industrial and mechanistic framework for work means when reflected through the eyes of the new digital and highly technical age. This age is redefining our context, experience, frames of reference, indeed, the very way we live and work (Porter-O'Grady, 2003).

GETTING READY FOR THE JOURNEY

The challenge for most change is an individual's ability to engage personally in the processes of change. Engagement requires the ability to understand and to comprehend exactly what the changes are and how they directly confront us. Confronting change requires a level of willingness reflected in the energy we each bring to our own journey and adaptation to change.

In the midst of an age change, often many things no longer make sense. As we move from the industrial age into the digital age, many of the things that defined our way of life, our rituals and routines, and our habits and practices no longer appear to be relevant or effective. As a result, we become anxious and confused. We often find ourselves tense and uncertain, even tentative and nontrusting. It is important to recognize these behavioral characteristics as a part of the transformation process itself. It is natural to be unsettled and concerned as one watches dramatic changes occurring all around. What is not natural is to ignore them, fail to find meaning in them, refuse to engage their impact on our lives, or simply ignore them. We must see responding to these circumstances simply as the challenges of our time (Holman & Devane, 1998).

Indicators of a New Age

The wisest way to make change work for us is to know as much about it as we can. Our awareness can be heightened by noting all the indicators of change in the shifting circumstances that surround us and apply these changes within this context. There are new realities:

- Technology is altering the workplace.
- Communications systems have created the global community.
- National boundaries are meaning less every day.
- Information and the Internet are now the mediums of exchange.
- Creating the information infrastructure is the work of the new age.
- Human capital (people) must now become knowledge workers and are at the core critical value for the new age.

Note:

Change cannot be made without making noise. This noise is a sign of life in the organization and should never be silenced.

Signs of Healthy "Noise"

- Reacting
- Asking why
- Sorting
- Clarifying
- Exploring options
- Comparing with the past
- Sharing contrasting opinion
- Questioning authority
- Validating perceptions
- Contrasting ideas
- Challenging assumptions

Note:

The wise leader keeps an eye to the horizon, a ways prepared to confront and challenge past practices against new and emerging-realities.

The Essential Elements of "Loss Work"

- Name the changes as they occur.
- Identify the elements of work that will forever be lost.
- Get to individuals' meaning driving their work practices.
- Allow time for sharing individual and collective losses.
- Undertake symbolic acts, which celebrate the moment of loss.
- Allow individuals to give a voice to their sense of loss.
- Don't minimize the value of even the smallest elements of loss.
- Supplement individual loss with identification of collective loss.
- Allow emotional reaction; create a safe space for its expression.
- Bring closure to the loss so there is an endpoint for it.
- After enumerating and celebrating loss, move on.

THROUGH THE LOOKING-GLASS

In the midst of an age change there is as much to be lost as to be gained. As we leave the industrial age, there are many things that must be left behind. One of the challenges for the worker is in confronting rituals and routines practiced over a lifetime of work that now need to be assessed and evaluated with regard to their relevance. This may mean ceasing to perform particular tasks and functions in the future, leaving them forever behind.

The leader must remember that all of our conceptual, formative, developmental, and experiential activities unfolded in the age in which we are all now living. The challenge for the leader involves more than simply taking a journey into the new age. Indeed, much of how we perceive this journey, our personal experience of it, gives it the form and character it will take as we live it. And it will not be easy.

It is harder to let go of old concepts and practices than it is to take on new ones. Time spent in working creates habits and rituals that become associated with the very work we do (Matthews & Wacker, 2002). Leading work processes requires clear intention, a desire, to shift and change practices to reflect the new reality for work. Leaders must make it possible for these intentional processes to unfold. Because people seek to express their personal meaning through their work, taking on intentional shift in process means revisiting the meaning one has for doing work, restating it, making it possible for people to let old practices go and consider the possibility of new practices emerging. The leader makes sure that appropriate time is provided for this essential "loss work."

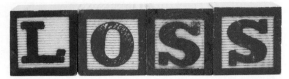

MAKING A SHIFT TOWARD NEW REALITIES

Much of what is emerging in this new age represents an entirely new way of thinking and knowing that differs considerably from our past experiences. As we now know, our greatest challenge is our ability to reflect the characteristics of the emerging age from the perspective of that new age, not from the perspective of our past experiences. We must now be willing, as well as able, to see and act within the context of the emerging reality. Leaders will need to adapt various strategies to this very important journey.

- We must recognize that our experiences coming out of the industrial age are no longer sufficient to the search for meaning in a new age.
- We must be available to embrace specific changes, not simply identify those changes. This means we must see the changes within their own context rather than through the mirror of our past experiences.
- Leaders must constantly reexamine their own perceptions as well as those of their staff, confronting preconceived notions and past biases as the increasing weight of evidence regarding the future calls us to a different place in order to live in it.
- Everyone must embrace the challenge that comes from the chaos in new thinking and the old models. People must know that they are constructing the journey as they travel and evaluating their progress in light of its relationship to emerging reality.
- Workers must disassociate themselves from past job content and processes. Work must be defined more clearly in relationship to new definitions and different measures of outcome.
- Leaders must engage stakeholders in a continual and dynamic dialog related to the changes, ensuring a collective commitment to the journey experience.

Note:

Leaders must be willing to engage their own loss first before expecting that others will be wiling to engage their losses.

Necessary Losses

- Old rituals
- Past routines
- Tasks
- Functions
- Jobs
- Roles
- Positions
- Security
- Fixed location

- Permanence
- Certainty
- Guarantees
- Protection
- Parenting (work)
- Old friends
- Stability
- Complaints

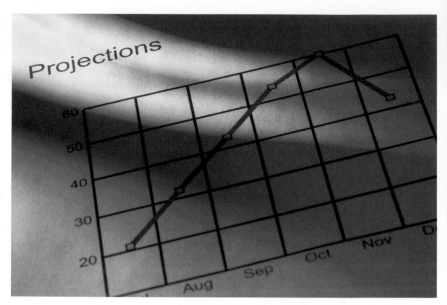

*Change is not a season;
it is, instead, a way of life.*

THE PROCESS OF LETTING GO

A shift such as that experienced in an age change cannot unfold without a great deal of conflict, uncertainty, and personal discomfort. On a daily basis we are bombarded with news that reflects the radical nature of our changes on the global, national, social, political, and business stage. We see shifts and losses with regard to jobs, mergers, economic and fiscal pressures, ethical and moral lapses in leadership, shifts in social mores, and increases and challenges with regard to cultural diversity, just to name a few.

Going to work certainly brings no relief; indeed the workplace often increases the level of stress. The uncertainties, anxieties, and fear that come from anticipating constant change in the workplace create a lack of confidence regarding competency and the security of work. In the past, confidence could be obtained from the consistency and security of work. No longer. With mergers, downsizing, redesign, restructuring, and reconfiguring work, there appears to be more challenges than can be tolerated by most individual workers. And yet, this is just the beginning.

Leaders must spend considerable time with staff in helping them understand the meaning and value in the changes they are confronting (Hagal, 2002). As much as possible the leader must help followers anticipate the stages of change in the elements of transformation. Furthermore, leaders must give staff the opportunity to speak out, to react, and to give a language to their personal journey, yet keep them focused and moving in a way that is relevant and appropriate to the demand for change.

Shifting to a New Reality

Much of what is occurring reflects a fundamental realityshift. Through the chaos and the vortex of change (in an age change) the leader constantly sorts the superfluous from the valuable. These chaotic events, while not comforting, are necessary elements of the journey. This chaos exists in the paradigmatic moments between old and new. These chaotic moments serve to unbundle our attachment to the reality that we are leaving by making it untenable, noisy, nonsense, and no longer successful for us. In many ways this chaotic moment forces us to confront our essential need for change and our individual response to it. These moments of chaos challenge us to look inward, to assess the conflicts between what we were and what we are becoming, and ultimately, to make some decisions that will keep us moving positively toward the new reality. Sustainability depends on the goodness-of-fit between the demand for change and our response to it.

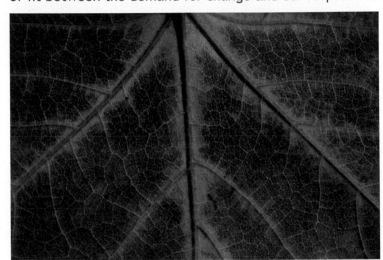

Note:

The leader must keep others from getting stuck in their losses in a way that cripples their ability to engage and continue the essential journey of change.

Helping People Move On

It is natural for people to hold on to what they know and what provides security and confidence in their own lives. Although leaders must allow staff and themselves the time and space necessary to honor past practices and to mourn their loss, they must not tarry in that place. It is not healthy to mourn forever. One of the worst things that can happen in the workplace is to become stuck at the point of mourning and be captured by looking backward in such a way that one cannot see the changes that have an effect on one's own life. The leader must formalize the process of mourning and of loss management such that it is structured and incorporated into the experience of change and movement. By doing this, the leader formalizes loss and incorporates the mourning process into the dynamics of change. In this way, a place is provided in the journey of change for those elements that relate to loss management. Failing to mourn will have an effect on subsequent adaptation to change. Spending too much time in the mourning process delays the engagement of change and cripples people's ability to experience and embrace the creation of their future.

Making Sense
of an Uncertain Future

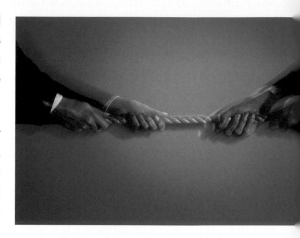

People are willing to make change if they understand what the change means to them personally. Meaning is critical to understanding and implementing change in a way that is specific to the work being done. Leaders often suggest how great change is for the workplace, even how it improves the products of work. However, people work because it provides value and meaning for them and they need to be able to translate the work they do at some level of personal value. Getting to this personal value means that the leader must understand the needs for meaning at the individual level, recognizing that everyone works for a different reason.

In order to engage stakeholders in changes with which they must actively participate, the leader must be able to translate the elements of the desired change into both language and practices that make sense to those who will do the work. Getting engagement and sustaining it will require continual and effective personal identification with the changes undertaken. Most important for the leader is to be able to describe well the characteristics of the "journey' of work. Here, the leader translates the work experience into a broader context, identifying where change will take the worker, how work will be different, and why it is better to engage and embrace the suggested changes.

It is imperative for the leader to understand that those involved in making change need to clearly understand the reason for the change, the shift in function and activities necessary to represent the change, the purposes of the change (in a way that advances and improves the work circumstances of the individual), the timeline for the change, and the anticipated impact on the outcomes of work. Here again, the leader needs to make this understanding as straightforward as possible to the needs and concerns of those involved. Wise leaders more easily determine the effectiveness of the change process by having those who must implement change restate, identify, and operationalize the change in their own words. Effective change agents use tools that relate specifically to the application of change from the perspective of the individual. In this way, the leader goes full circle, identifying the change and its elements, process and outcome implications, impact on individual behavior and work values, worker engagement, and improvement in the quality of service or product.

Battling Ritual and Routine

- Alter work patterns.
- Observe changing circumstances.
- Watch how others work.
- Keep knowledge current.
- Test competence frequently.
- Process impact of work.
- Keep focused on outcomes.

DISCERNING CHANGE

Collective insight is essential to effectively identify the characteristics and elements of any given change. To capitalize on appropriate indicators of change, leaders must acknowledge that a unilateral viewpoint is not sufficient. Individuals can have accurate insights with regard to the conditions and circumstances influencing an unfolding future. Still, good insight is informed by collective wisdom; that wisdom that reflects the diversity of views with regard to any given change. Diversity of information sources broadens insight and creates a deeper frame of reference for understanding it.

Collective wisdom is rarely given its due by senior leaders in many organizations. The notion of positional authority often predominates with regard to the value, importance, or effectiveness of information, which influences strategic and tactical choices. The truth is, however, that the broader the information base and the more diverse the insights related to it, the better the chances are that the information discerned and discussed here accurately reflects the conditions and circumstances of change. Of course, the context for such dialog must respect differences, reflect openness and clarity, be inclusive of a wide variety of disparate insights, and allow exploration of the unusual and uncertain.

Collective relationships based on trust and shared commitment are essential constituents of this kind of open dialog and collective wisdom. The good leader makes sure that people can express their views openly and confidently. Creating a contextual framework that is inclusive, trusting, and dynamic is critical to the accuracy of the insights and information shared and used for critical decision making.

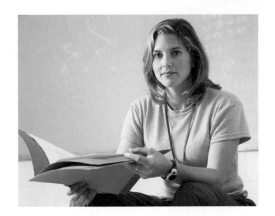

Note:

Change doesn't just happen, it requires making choices. The good leader understands that purposeful and strategic change is a reflection and application of good information, thorough dialog, and effective decision making.

Change Dialog

1. Lacks ambiguity
2. Is inclusive
3. Embraces differences
4. Is value based
5. Advances the organization

THE LEADER'S COMMITMENT TO TRANSFORMATION

A part of the role of the leader is to help the organization keep up with and, if possible, ahead of the changes that will have an effect on the organization's ability to do its work and to thrive in its own marketplace. Because of the rapid changes and shifts in the technologies and mechanisms of work, this demand for keeping ahead of the cycle of change has become a critical element of the manager's role.

In order to be effective, leaders must help the organization learn new ways of doing business. Creativity with regard to the styles of work process, mechanisms for responding to changes in technology, new knowledge management, and helping the organization with innovation and creativity are essential elements of the leader's role. The quality of doing business is as important as the quality of the service or the product. The way of working and of being present in the marketplace is now as important as what an organization does there.

Translating Change

- Avoid ambiguity.
- Use simple language.
- Apply people's experiences.
- Paint a picture.
- Tell a story of the change.
- Identify clearly what's different.
- Indicate individual expectations.
- Create scenarios.
- Communicate change decisions.

Leaders must exemplify in their personal behavior and understanding the need to incorporate an innovative mental model, a commitment to creativity, and an openness to exploration. This must become "the way" for most organizations rather than the exception to past rituals of doing business. Leaders therefore must be excited about the future, expressing a transformational orientation in everything they do with others in the organization. People must see in a leader this commitment to a more fluid and flexible expression of role and work such that it serves to influence and encourage others to embrace and live within the same creative frame of reference.

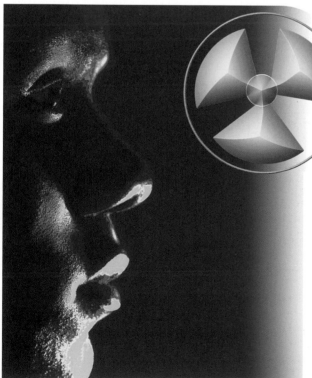

EVIDENCE OF REAL CHANGE

So many leaders look at numerical indicators of success and of change that they fail to recognize that success is really obtained by looking at broader indicators. Managers who express changes in the context of short-term thinking, and immediate numerical changes, specific dollar outcomes, failed to identify clearly the broader-based elements of effective change.

Transformation requires that an organization see itself differently from the perspective of those it serves and the services it provides. The wise leader sees these changes from a more global perspective, looking at the organization within the context of its broader set of relationships and intersections, attempting to express a clearer and more accurate notion of those circumstances and indicators that determine its long¬term viability (Duck, 2001).

A misguided or dislocated notion of the organization and its goodness-of-fit with the broader frame of reference within which it lives limits an organization's long-term viability and isolates its perspective from its real-time set of circumstances. Leaders step to the balcony frequently to develop a broader view of the organization's fit in the culture, society, and community. From this perspective a more accurate insight with regard to the demands of transformation can be better obtained.

Note:

The change agent must always be well informed, looking for information in unusual places, and bringing it back to share with stakeholders.

Standing on the Balcony

- Reading professional journals
- Reviewing technical advertisements
- Scanning national newspapers or business journals
- Assessing innovative businesses and their models
- Critiquing new approaches to service delivery and customer quality

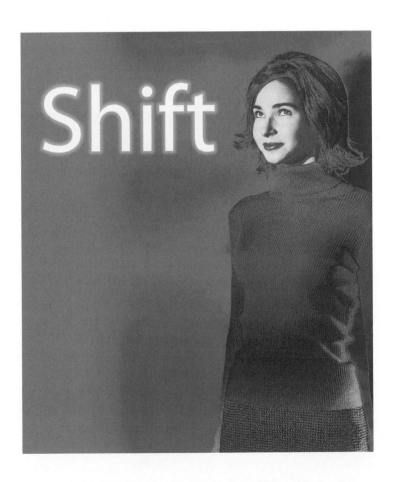

SCENARIO
Jack's Team-Based Learning

Jack Smith believed that it was important to incorporate staff in the process of discerning and defining changes that would affect the organization. Jack believed that it was important for everybody in his department to be involved in the process.

Jack recognized that all the professionals in his department were knowledge workers and therefore needed to be incorporated into the process of discernment and planning. He committed to the workers in his department the following values:

- The team must always be clear about its mission and purposes.
- Each team member must know what his or her work is.
- Every team member knows the contribution each makes to the team.
- Staff is involved in all decisions that affect the department's future.
- New knowledge/technology is shared continually in the team.
- The teams hold regular discussions regarding new information.
- No change in work occurs without team involvement.
- All team members are expected to participate in change dialog.
- Planning for change and implementing is driven by staff.
- Evaluation of effectiveness is always included in any change.

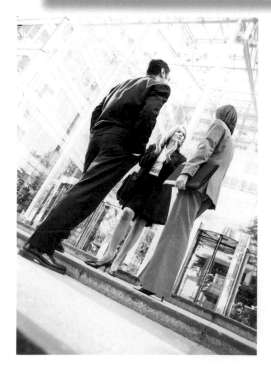

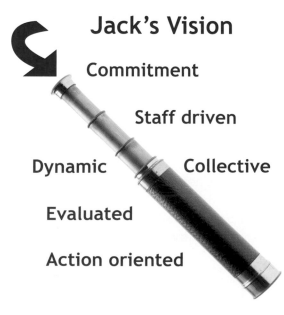

Jack's Vision

Commitment

Staff driven

Dynamic   Collective

Evaluated

Action oriented

Faith in the Vision

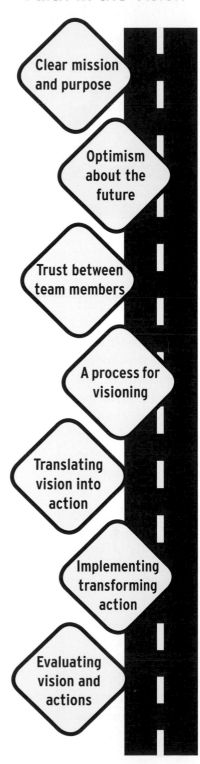

Clear mission and purpose

Optimism about the future

Trust between team members

A process for visioning

Translating vision into action

Implementing transforming action

Evaluating vision and actions

BELIEVING IN THE JOURNEY

Leaders often don't realize that they are also storytellers. The stories they tell, however, are not mythologies or fairytales, but instead images and scenarios that reflect a future state. The stories are the aggregation of the signposts, indicators, and dialog related to specific conditions or circumstances that identify or characterize appropriate responses to future demands.

Good leaders recognize that the stories they tell and the scenarios they create provide a context for those they lead. This frame of reference frames the dialog and discussions between team members related to the conditions that articulate a future state and provide a framework for the staff's discernment regarding appropriate action and response.

The visioning process is simply a glimpse over the horizon. It is an attempt to realistically assess the characteristics of the journey and translate them into language of experience and application. This process gives the staff an opportunity to participate in identifying those processes and activities that will change the work they do. Furthermore, this process builds a foundation, a faith if you will. There is a confidence in the "truth" of the journey and the goodness-of-fit between the actions leaders and staff take and a realistic future state within which they must live.

The engagement of the team in this collective enterprise creates a foundation in trust, a confidence in the choices that are made, a cohesiveness between and among team members around their own journey of change, and an effective model team members can use for engaging the demand for change. This process also creates a mechanism for embracing and translating specific changes into new ways of being and doing.

Transformation and Transitions 81

ABANDONING THE PAST

Many leaders, like their staff, have difficulty letting go of past practices. Leaders must lead the way in helping people abandon attachment to past practices and processes. This means a willingness to put an end to all kinds of past practices, products, processes, and ways of doing business. Whether one actually has to redo all work processes is subject to the vagaries and conditions of what the leader confronts when looking into the future. The leader will always need to ask "What do we do now?" The response to that determines the work activities. If that means some of those already performed must continue, the question is responded to in light of emerging realities rather than past practices (Christensen et al, 2000).

In abandoning past practices the leader must be able to ask a new set of questions. An important question relates to whether the realities that are emerging lead the leader and the team to undertake things in the same way as they have approached them traditionally. And leaders must make this questioning a relatively formal process, one that has regularity and is incorporated into the normal act of doing business.

Incorporating the process of abandonment into the ongoing leadership work represents a commitment to continuous and endless improvement. As the conditions and circumstances for work shift and change, so also must the insights with regard to how the work is performed, what actions take priority, and what processes need to emerge reflecting a newer reality for the work.

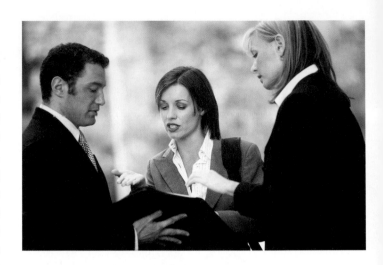

Yes But...

The staff may frequently object to the abandonment of past practices. The leader must make it safe for staff to confront directly the challenges, noise, and demands embedded in shifting from process fixation to the continuum of change. The leader must make these activities an ongoing part of the work of the team, such that the discernment of changes can be anticipated before they have to be implemented. In this way the leader is constantly preparing the staff for the very next change and making the change work. Innovation and creativity are not accidental. They require that the leader undertake systematic approaches to raising questions and changing behaviors. This dynamic challenges the organization and invests each team member in the process of sustainable change.

Complacency Checkup

- Does the leader exemplify engagement of change?
- Is the staff addicted to rituals and routines?
- Is there a general feeling of directionlessness in the team?
- Is there a focus on the short term rather than the long term?
- Does the leader set aside time for dialog regarding change?
- Do organized mechanisms exist for reviewing emerging technology?
- What journals and innovative information sources are available to staff?
- Do staff have access to experts regarding specific transformations?
- Are there opportunities to be imaginative and creative?
- Do executive leaders exemplify the engagement of change in themselves?
- Is the environment safe to explore new ideas in different directions?

Intangible Change Assets

A good leader uses every option, asset, and opportunity to facilitate and advance change. The skills and talents of the staff, access to experts, availability of the information infrastructure, the web, and collateral sources of information constitute intangible assets. The leader not only has awareness of these sources of information but also uses them at every opportunity to extend the knowledge base, deepen information, and make resources available to the staff in a way that facilitates their own knowledge and skill-changing journey. Access to sources of information and innovation helps the team remain agile, creative, responsive, intuitive, and constantly available to the sources facilitating viable change. The leader is always scouting for opportunities to broaden the frame of access for knowledge and information in a way that facilitates the staffs own change journey.

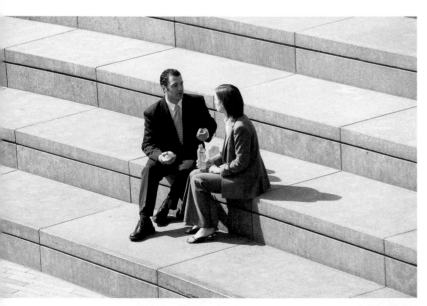

Note:

Crisis is often seen as a threat, not as an encouragement for change. The wise leader doesn't wait for crisis to initiate action. Instead, the good leader makes change a fundamental part of the work.

The Leader Is Always Challenging:

- The prevailing wisdom
- The management mindset
- Any past practice
- The validity and viability of information
- Rituals and routines
- The opinions and views of "experts"
- The leader's own views and opinions
- Long-held beliefs and strategies
- All work practices and processes

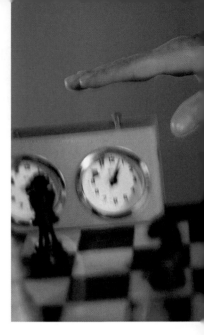

IT'S NOT ABOUT DOING MORE WITH LESS

So often leaders hear the words (and even hear themselves saying these words) "you must learn to do more with less." This is just not an appropriate model for helping the team engage and confront the vagaries and demands of transformation. In the history of work there's never been a continuous flow of adequate resources over a long enough time to meet the perceived needs of those doing the work. Resource availability is always highly variable. The issue isn't whether sufficient resources will ever be available, but how well the resources available are used to meet specific demands.

Leaders must always make good use of scarce resources. It is the awareness of the scarcity of resources yet the availability to them that is important to the leader. Each leader must know that he or she can never be in enough places, with enough time, or exposed to enough resources at any given time to meet the ever-growing demand for response. Still, the good leader creates a strong network and a series of linkages that allows this individual to access what is available and to make use of others in an effective way. In this way, resources are stretched and the network is used to provide what access that can be obtained in ways the individual could not sufficiently address alone.

Also, the leader must make good use of the wide variety of resources to which he or she is directly related. The field of experts within the department, staff with special skills, individuals with unique insights, all are a source of creative and innovative connections that can extend the leader's own skills in visualizing and anticipating transformational processes or events. Using both external and internal networks increases the option that the leader will be available to new insights.

IT DOESN'T ALWAYS WORK THE WAY YOU PLANNED

One of the first things leaders will come to know is that the best laid plans of women and men do not always work out as originally planned. There are always a number of reasons why plans don't work out as anticipated. The vagaries of change, new considerations, shifts in the environment, crisis created by a destructive or innovative technology, or even inadequate planning or visioning can lead to a strategic dead-end. When this occurs the leader undertakes a number of different responsive strategies:

- Reassess the information obtained.
- Adjust to changing realities.
- Look for new sources of information.
- Quickly change course and related actions.
- Adjust the strategic process to compensate.
- Seek new models for assessing the future.
- Review specific response processes and actions.
- Engage the staff in assessing the change in direction.
- Talk with different experts.
- Evaluate the impact of the failure on cost and process.
- Determine the actions and time frame for turnaround.
- Renew commitment for accurate information.
- Create scenarios reflecting the change.
- Initiate new change processes.
- Evaluate the effectiveness of response.

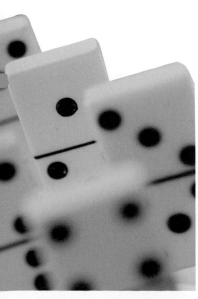

It's a Journey, Not an Event

It is important for the manager to know that the journey of transformation is a continual and dynamic one. It does not end. This means that the leader is always aware that change is the work of all organizations. Change is the one constant that is always present in the course of lived experience and the only reality that can be depended upon with absolute certitude. The leader harnesses this understanding and incorporates it into the ongoing way of doing business in the organization.

Learning leadership is also a journey. The leadership learning process is an endless dynamic that itself is constantly shifting and adjusting to the vagaries and realities of the journey. As technologies and ways of doing business unfold, new models of leadership and transformation also grow and develop. The good, effective leader keeps this in mind while developing the skills necessary to remain competent and effective. Leadership is an endless journey.

Transformation and Transitions 85

References

Beer, M., & Nohria, N. (2000). *Breaking the code of change*. Boston: Harvard Business School Publishing.

Christensen, C., Bohmer, R., & Kenagy, J. (2000). Will disruptive innovations cure healthcare? *Harvard Business Review*, 78(5), 102-112.

Duck, J. D. (2001). *The change monster: The human forces that fuel or foil corporate transformation and change*. New York: Crown Business.

Hagal III, H. (2002). *Out of the box*. Boston: Harvard Business School Press.

Holman, P., & Devane, T. (1998). *The change handbook*. San Francisco: Berreft¬Koehler.

Mathews, R., & Wacker, W. (2002). *The deviant's advantage*. New York: Crown Business Books.

Pearman, R. (1998). *Hard wired leadership*. New York: Davies-Black.

Porter-O'Grady, T. (2003). Of hubris and hope: Transforming nursing for a new age. *Nursing Economic$*, 21(2), 59-64.

Suggested Readings

Cashman, K., & Forem, J. (2003). *Awakening the leader within a story of transformation*. Hoboken, NJ: John Wiley & Sons.

Hesselbein, F. (2002). *Hesselbein on leadership*. San Francisco: Jossey Bass.

Peters, T. J. (2003). *Re-imagine! [business excellence in a disruptive age]*. London: Dorling Kindersley.

Riggio, R. E., & Orr, S. S. (2004). *Improving leadership in nonprofit organizations*. San Francisco: Jossey-Bass.

Trompenaars, A, & Hampden-Turner, C. (2002). *21 leaders for the 21st century: How innovative leaders manage in the digital age*. New York: McGraw-Hill.

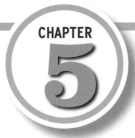

5 Transforming Te[
For Decisions

The major work of the team is to transform individual work into a collective enterprise representing the commitment of every player to the good of the whole.

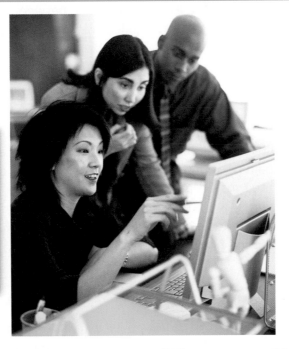

Teams are the form in which people work together for a common goal, adding value to each other and to the organization.

Note:

Teams are the most effective way of doing work. They are the means through which work is aggregated and best value is achieved from each member and for the organization.

TRANSFORMING THE WORLD OF WORK

As the world moves inexorably through the transitions and transformations necessary to exist in a new reality (the 21st century), people must also change. That means changing the way they do work and relate to each other. As work becomes more fluid and flexible, relationship becomes more critical. One would assume as work becomes increasingly virtual and mobility based, relationship would be less important. Nothing could be further from the truth. What really occurs is the need for a goodness-of-fit between all of the stages, elements, and components of work regardless of where they may be performed. Because there are multiple locations and teams working on anyone aggregated project, and these activities may be performed in a whole host of different places, ultimately, the work must come together to produce an integrated product or service. This linkage and integration are the common seeds of effectiveness in a highly decentralized work process. It is only through teams, tightly bound together, that this kind of work is possible.

Transforming Teams for Decisions 87

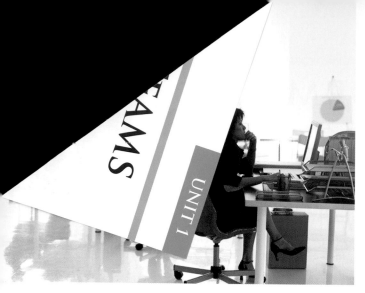

TEAMS ARE THE BASIC UNIT OF WORK

Much of the research in the past 30 years has informed leadership with regard to teams being the basic unit of work. Of course, individuals are always important to the process of doing work. The outcomes of work reflect the integration and activities of many people linked together in a common purpose and an integrated set of activities that produce sustainable work results. This interaction between people in undertaking the collective activities necessary to fulfilling the purposes of that work are increasingly critical to the viability and enduring outcomes of work (Porter O'Grady & Krueger Wilson, 1998).

Although the idea of organizing work within the context of team-based approaches is relatively new in human history, it is evident as far back as pyramid building in ancient Egypt. Still, research and study regarding the centrality of teams to effectiveness is relatively recent. Recent research on the concepts of empowerment, team relationships, personal involvement, ownership, and stakeholder investment have been generated in the past few decades with strong evidence of the need for addressing all of these in enduring work environments. These "communities of work" create the conditions and circumstances that allow an organization to be innovative and adaptive in ways that meet the ever-changing demand for creativity and innovation.

Teams: The Foundation of Work

The basic unit of work for the foreseeable future will be team-based activities. This is a shift from focus on the values of individual work. The team is a more accurate foundation of work because:

- Outcomes depend on collective contribution.
- The relatedness of work defines the distribution of work activities.
- Integration of work activities is necessary to sustainability.

Note:

Work can no longer be permanently compartmentalized. Segregating work from all the elements necessary to link and integrate it with the work of others in the digital age is no longer a method that leads to effectiveness or sustainability.

Changing the Control System

Movement to teams demands change from vertical and hierarchical control systems to horizontal and team-based models. Some historic requirements that must now be discarded include:

- Centralized control systems
- Hierarchical management approaches
- Limited information support systems
- Standardized human resource practices
- Command-and-control governance and administrative processes

Systems Insights

Team-based approaches are based on an understanding of how systems interact and relate with regard to activities and movement toward goals and values. There needs to be a fuller understanding of:

- The needs of teams
- The way teams work
- The relationships for team effectiveness
- Leadership skills and managing teams
- Leadership skills and managing teams
- The unique way teams communicate
- The process of collective problem solving
- Understanding the personality of teams
- Merging individual performance with teams
- Increasing the value of personal ownership
- Implementing collective decisions
- Linking the efforts of teams together
- Evaluating work effectiveness
- Adapting or adjusting and performance

TEAM OWNERSHIP

To most, it sounds rational and appropriate to recognize the value and the contribution of people to each other and to work. But this is easier said than done. Whereas team-based approaches are certainly rational, the historic design of the workplace has been based on a set of different work principles. The belief was that the locus of control for work rests in the hands of those who own the means of work. In truth, the means, activities, and values of work are spread equitably between and among the various stakeholders: those who finance operations, those who manage, and those who produce the outcomes and products of work. Each plays a role in the delicate balance between all the factors necessary to ensure effective outcomes and to create sustainability for all stakeholders. Forgetting this "value equation" puts the organization at risk and creates conditions for failure (Harshman & Phillips, 1994).

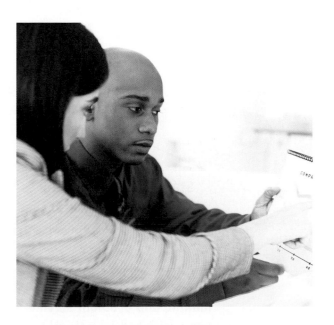

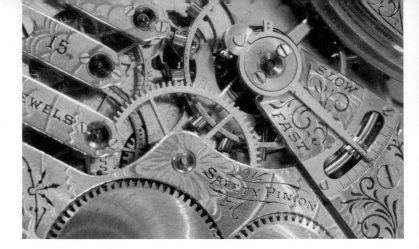

CREATING TEAM INFRASTRUCTURE

For teams to be successful they must be a way of doing business and a part of the continuous dynamic of the organization from top to bottom.

Teams are a strategic imperative.

Senior management supports the team approach.

All leaders operate within the context of team processes and are skilled in team management.

Staff operating in teams is the expectation of the organization and is supported through continual team learning.

Team processes are used for all decision making and problem solving and are evaluated for effectiveness.

Leadership commits to changing from the vertical and hierarchical control systems to more horizontal and team-based models of leading others. Some of the past models of behavior that must be discarded are:

- Centralized control systems
- Hierarchical management approaches
- Limited information support structures
- Standardized human resource practices
- Command-and-control management processes
- Parental patterns of management behavior
- Passive staff decision roles
- Punitive control measures

Note:

Team-based approaches require a more detailed understanding of group process from team leaders. These leaders must be involved in a continual, dynamic, and endless continuum of team learning.

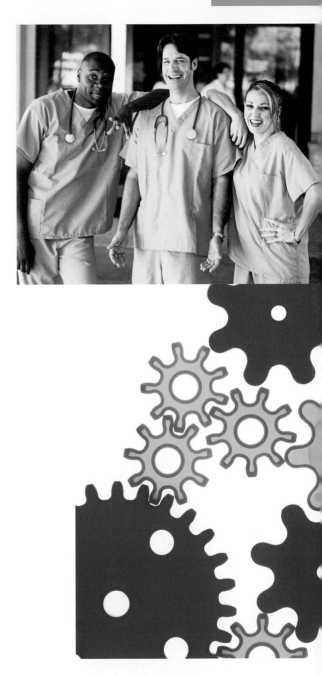

Working "in between" Two Systems

The journey to team-based decision-making and operating processes is not short, or easy. Good leaders recognize that they are going from one kind of management infrastructure to another. This requires the ability to transition between two extremely different approaches to leadership and to "doing business." The staff must be carefully led away from traditional hierarchical and parental processes into more adult-to-adult approaches to decision making, relationship building, and self-management. For some, the journey will be positive and personally rewarding and freeing. For others, the movement away from parental, protected, and passive roles may be more dramatic and involve more personal challenges. The wise leader recognizes the differentiation in people's adjustment to team-based approaches, and individualizes responses based on individual needs and growth patterns of team members. What isn't negotiable, however, is the movement toward team-based approaches as an organizational imperative, and all team members should be fully aware of that.

Transforming Teams for Decisions   91

The Whole System is a Team

It is important for leaders to recognize that the team approach must be embedded in every aspect of the system's work processes. In fact the whole system must operate within the context of team management. It is inappropriate for senior leaders to behave in a highly individual way and then expect all other aspects of the organization to operate within the team framework. Team-based approaches must be inculcated throughout the organization and must operate at all levels as the organization's way of doing business. The value of team-based approaches is extended by the willingness of senior leaders to model in their own behavior the growth, adaptation, and adjustment to group process for decision making, undertaking work processes, and evaluating the effectiveness of work outcomes.

In order to facilitate this dynamic, it is important that problems and issues in relationship, productivity, communication, and interaction between and among all team members at every level of the organization be addressed within the team format. In order to avoid the "us/them" behavioral pattern, the organization must operate at all levels within the same team-based pattern of function. If team-based behaviors are to emerge and be sustained, team constructs across the system must apply a set of beliefs and a pattern of processes in a way that ensures team-based practices are undertaken in all places in the organization (Hackman, 2002).

To ensure success of team-based approaches, all members of the organization, regardless of their role, must see themselves as part of a team. In effective team-based organizations no one member, regardless of role, can act unilaterally out of context of his or her relationship to membership in the team. This requires an organizational discipline in individuals and members as a way of interpreting and applying the team strategic imperative throughout the organization. In this way, a personal discipline is applied to the behavior, role, and expression of each member as work processes in a way that is consistent across the system.

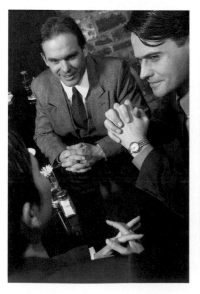

Committing to Team Change

In the course of doing all work, management and staff members must be prepared to do the following differently from the past:

- Integrate the decisions each person makes with the goals and processes of the team.

- Incorporate the strategic requirements, goals, and expectations of the system into the priorities and activities associated with all team processes.

TEAM LIFE STAGES

Some Considerations for Team Effectiveness

As the teams move through their specific stages of development, the team leader, working at the periphery, is constantly monitoring and measuring effectiveness of interactions, relationships, problem solving, and work processing. The team leader recognizes that resolving issues in any of these arenas early creates a frame for team effectiveness and success that can operate over the long term. Creating a culture of openness to issues of concern with regard to problem solving, work processes, and relationship building establishes a frame of reference for the team that is positive, disclosing, and safe. Through this early engagement of issues, the leader sets up a foundation upon which subsequent problem solving can build and team success can be ensured.

Forming
Initial stage of team development in which rules are uncertain and team expectations, rules, and roles are unclear

Storming
The formative stage of group process, filled with conflict as the group begins to establish roles, relationships, and rules around purposes and work of the team

Norming
Work processes are established, rules are agreed to, systems are set up, and creative work patterns emerge in ways that more clearly define the team

Performing
The team now begins to work well together, undertake processes, work through difficulties, achieve objectives, and measure result

Evaluation and Retooling
The team assesses internal and external dynamics, makes decisions about more effective processes, and refines this team's work rules, roles, and relationships

OUTCOMES DRIVES EVERYTHING

Team leaders must be aware of the fact that the work of the team must be directed toward achieving meaningful results. Often teams get so focused on their work and activity processes that they forget that the purpose of the team is to fulfill the expectations that their work is directed to fulfill Teams are formed around purpose and performance expectations and the team leader must always keep these realities before the awareness of team members (Hambrick et al, 1998).

Occasionally team leaders must intersect the work processes to undertake both an analysis and synthesis between the work, its purposes, and the achievement of outcomes. The leader always keeps before team members the awareness of their role and relationship in light of the goal to which their work is directed. This evaluation continually ensures that work and outcomes are always linked.

Note:

All teams experience conflict. All conflict has value. The good team leader who looks at conflict as a normal part of team effectiveness simply looks to engaging conflict early and often.

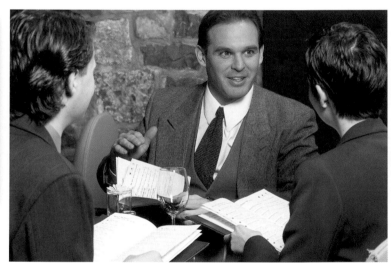

Team Leader's Checklist:

• Make sure all the elements of the team and team performance are acting congruently.
• Maintain a consistent leadership style that best fits the character and content of teamwork.
• Make sure the team adheres to all the rules of engagement that they have developed and corrective action is undertaken early when there are breeches.
• Manage team error and conflict early and well, establishing processes that address these issues calmly as a normal part of team process.
• Watch for individual behavior that acts in opposition to the synthesis and effectiveness of team performance.
• Meet frequently with individuals and full team to assess progress, confront issues, undertake learning, and measure goal achievement.

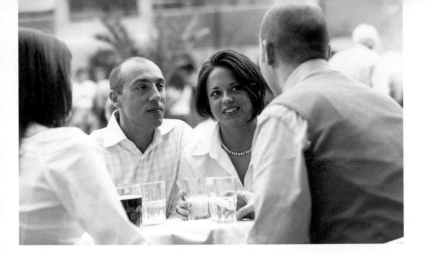

Note:

In the presence of team conflict, the team leader always recognizes that the leader role is neutral, simply facilitating the conflict process.

SCENARIO

Sam is the team leader of a relatively new hospital first response team. The team is finishing the first stage of development (storming) and is developing rules of engagement, performance expectations, and common goals between and among team members. The team has been making good progress with regard to its formation activities; however, it is having some difficulty dealing with conflict emerging between two strong nurses. Sam sees this conflict coming fairly early in the process, but is a little concerned about how to properly address it. Two other nurses on the team are becoming aware of the conflict between the two strong personalities and both have come to Sam mentioning their concerns that this problem may be growing and is beginning to have an effect on team cohesiveness as well as their team processes.

Sam wants to take care of this problem as quickly as possible. In the past, Sam has always taken care of these issues in a one-to-one exchange, exerting his personal leadership. He realizes, however, that this is a team issue and should be addressed within the context of the team. He knows that the team must own its relationships between team members and work to resolve this conflict as soon as possible. Furthermore, Sam knows that, as team leader, he must facilitate the processes that will lead to confronting this issue, ultimately creating a framework for the team's ability to work together and achieve outcome. Sam feels struck and needs some insight and assistance. He's come to you for guidance.

Exploratory questions

- What are the elements of the conflict resolution process that Sam must be aware of as he walks through the stages of addressing the conflict between these two individuals?

- How does Sam engage the team in owning and investing in this conflict resolution process?

- How does Sam keep the environment safe yet push for resolution among team members as well as ensure a successful conflict resolution process?

- How does Sam evaluate the effectiveness of the process and whether it made any difference?

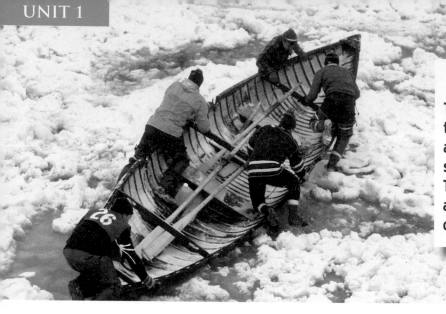

Note:

The leader always acts within the context of the team for all decision-making, problem-solving, and work processes. The wise team leader never acts unilaterally or out of concert with team members.

Empowering the Team

For teams to be effective they must recognize that they have accountability for performing their role in exercising their functions. Teams must have a clear understanding that they are free to make decisions, undertake their work, evaluate their effectiveness, and make corrective adjustments. The role of the leadership of the organization is to make it possible for teams to feel their own empowerment and to express their own accountability. Some elements evidencing an empowered team environment are:

- A clear definition of the power the team has to make decisions, undertake action, and evaluate performance
- A clear definition or team charter outlining the purpose, meaning, and value of the team as a way of defining its mission and direction
- A clear set of parameters that identify the roles of team members, the parameters of behavior, the consequences of noncompliance, and the rewards of performance
- A clear delineation of work expectations and performance processes through which each member of the team works with others to achieve team objectives
- A simple and precise understanding of the group accountability including a delineation of the group's authority to act in framework for decision making
- A broad understanding of the autonomy or rights of the group to decide, perform, and reconfigure work in a way that ensures more effective outcomes
- A clear and continual dynamic process of learning and development that ensures team members have an opportunity to advance their knowledge, understanding, and, ultimately, their performance
- Mechanisms for conflict resolution and problem solving that identify both the roles and processes of team members in a way that ensures resolution of team concerns
- A methodology for identifying the intrinsic and extrinsic rewards that relate directly to team performance and goal achievement in a way that is fair and equitable and focuses on team outcomes rather than simply individual performance factors

SPECIAL CONSIDERATIONS FOR THE TEAM LEADER

Frequently the quality of the team depends on the character of the team leader These individuals have a special obligation to help the team work well together, deal with their critical issues, and succeed in achieving their outcomes. Often whether a team is working well is directly related to the quality and effectiveness of its leadership. Good team leaders help the team focus on its purpose and goals and build all processes, relationships, and communication strategies in a way that facilitates goal achievement. Furthermore, the leader helps the team keep its focus, avoiding distractions and undertaking corrective action when errors or missteps affect the work of the team or interfere with goal achievement. To determine a team's effectiveness, the leader needs simply to observe the action and interaction of the team.

Critical Elements for Good Team Leadership

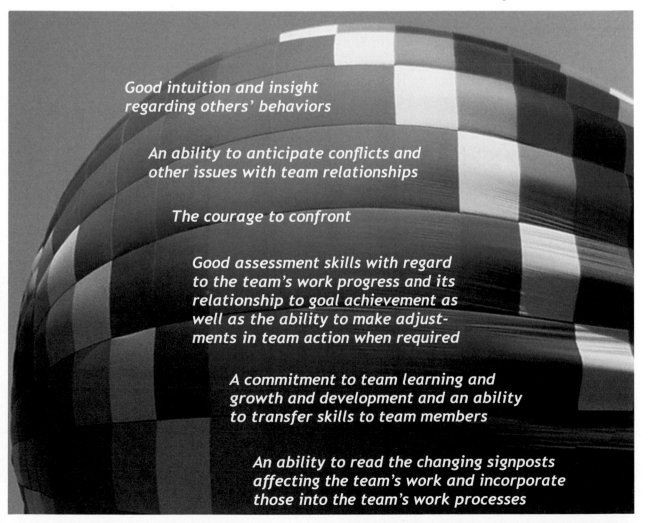

Good intuition and insight regarding others' behaviors

An ability to anticipate conflicts and other issues with team relationships

The courage to confront

Good assessment skills with regard to the team's work progress and its relationship to goal achievement as well as the ability to make adjustments in team action when required

A commitment to team learning and growth and development and an ability to transfer skills to team members

An ability to read the changing signposts affecting the team's work and incorporate those into the team's work processes

Some Do's and Don'ts of Team Leadership

Do's:

- Give the team the information it needs to work well.

- Help the team with skill building in relationship to its work.

- Build effective communication mechanisms between and among team members.

- Undertake corrective action potentially impeding teamwork as early as possible.

- Evaluate the effectiveness of the team as you go—do not wait.

- Confront conflict early and assess often.

- Review goals and progress toward them with team members regularly.

- Reward and encourage team members' successes frequently and well.

- Assess external and internal impediments to team effectiveness and remove ASAP.

- Celebrate team successes frequently.

Don'ts:

- Oversupervise the team and control the team processes.

- Criticize or punish team members in the presence of others.

- Personally own the work of team members as though it belonged to you.

- Ignore internal or external dynamics with the potential to impact team effectiveness.

- Let the team get tangled up in peripheral and nonessential issues that impede their work progress.

- Let the team forget that their work serves a purpose and has value.

- Take all the credit for the team's work and identify them as "my" people.

- Overwork the team without providing ample time for relationship building, social interaction, and celebrating successes.

- Limit information or access to resources that might affect team goal achievement.

HONORING TEAM CREATIVITY AND INNOVATION

Team leaders need to be aware that coalescing team action increases the potential for creativity and innovation. Ritual and routine are the enemy of creativity and often work to impede, even kill, the dynamics necessary for the creativity to be conceived and, ultimately, to emerge. The leader must be constantly aware of the potential power of ritual and routine and how it numbs the mind and insulates both the individual and collective effort of the team from exposure to the opportunities for the unique and unusual. It is the role of the team leader to encourage breaks from the routine; develop mechanisms and methods that encourage the team to think differently, analyze their work processes, and deliberate on issues that might affect efficiency, effectiveness, or the value and quality of the service or product.

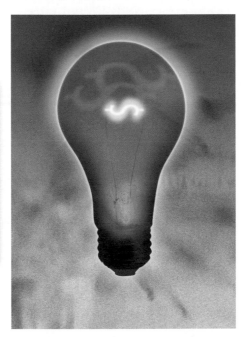

Note:

Everyone is creative if the right influences and forces facilitate expression-creativity needs only freedom and opportunity to be translated from an idea to reality.

Note:

Creativity and innovation are not unique and special; they are in every human being, seeking an oportunity to be expressed and to take form.

Innovation calls for a way of thinking that breaks from the usual and ordinary course of working or doing business. The innovative mind recognizes that knowledge and thinking merge to create opportunities for seeing a new way and attempting different approaches. The leader must make it possible for this kind of processing to emerge within the context of the team. Team members must be permitted to experiment and explore options in the course of undertaking work. The leader must encourage, even reward, attempts at looking at the work differently and assessing work processes and relationships with an eye to improving, even changing, work in a way that is either more effective or produces better results. The leader recognizes an innovative team is one that is skilled at managing knowledge, work processes, and activities in a way that can advance value. Innovation always has the potential for improvement or enhancement, even dramatic change. The solid creative leader is one that recognizes the dynamic of innovation and the opportunities for emergence of the innovative moment and whose leadership continually makes it possible for a sustainable innovation to take shape.

KEEPING THE TEAM FOCUSED

> > Make sure the team is always aware of its mission.

> > Know who has what accountability for what decisions.

> > Make sure planning is thorough and done ahead of work.

> > Ensure that each team member is aware of his or her role and individual contribution to the team's work.

> > Do frequent consensus testing to make sure that every individual's understanding of the work matches the understanding of the team as a whole.

> > Clarify misunderstandings, misperceptions, or conflicts in role and performance early to minimize impact on the team's work.

> > Evaluate team's process, relationship, and progress frequently.

> > Integrate the efforts of the team and evaluate their interface in order to ensure that each team member's effort is synthesized with the work of the team as a whole.

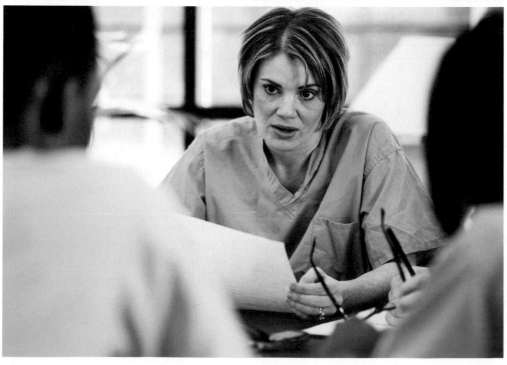

RESOLVING TEAM PROBLEMS

Identifying the problem—All teams have the potential for difficulty and for challenge. In the context of all human relationships the potential for conflict always exists. The leader knows this, anticipates it, and is constantly prepared to deal with it. The leader, therefore, always has a focus on the potential for problems, helping the team with the awareness of that potential and in identifying those problems as soon as possible. Problems left too long or dealt with too late have the potential for greater impediment to accomplishing the work than those addressed early.

Creating individual awareness and ownership of problems—Once the problem or concern is identified by the leader, it is vital that it be shared with individuals or a collective body of team members. The leader must always remember that team members possess their own problems. The team leader never makes the problem her or his own. When this occurs, a transfer in the locus of control for its resolution also occurs. The solution is always operating within the context of the team members and in the process of their work. The leader facilitates dialogue, discernment, and problem solving with the appropriate owners of the problem.

> *Note:*
> **The leader helps the team with reality-testing as a way of making sure that the team's perception and its work requirements are congruent in a way that continuously advances the team effort toward team goals.**

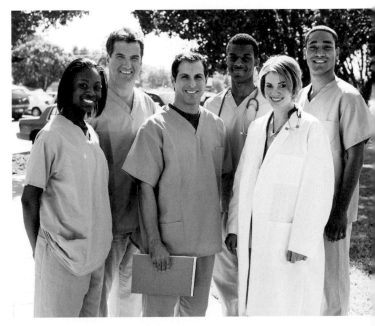

Moving the group to resolution—Resolution is more a journey than a destination. The leader is helping the team assess the most appropriate responses to problems or concerns and the identification of the best strategy for addressing the problem in a particular time frame or within the context of a particular circumstance or process. Here the team leader is always concerned about techniques and methodologies that might be applied to problem solving as a set of tools for the team members in creating an objective format for problem solving. The team leader draws from these objective processes, helping the team focus these techniques in a way that can address the issue, find the solution for the problem, and help the team to move toward its goal.

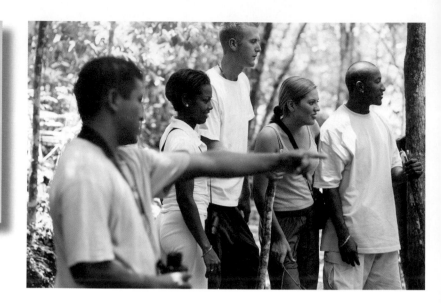

MAKING EFFECTIVE TEAM DECISIONS

All decision making requires a formal process that has implications for the long-term effectiveness of decisions made by the team. The kinds of decisions the team makes influences the process selected for it. For example, if decision making focuses on efficiency and effectiveness, decision making should be more formal, structured, and process oriented. However, if the decision relates to an incremental or incidental activity or function of the team, the process can be more situational and informal. At any rate, there is series of processes that the team must engage in order to ensure effective decision making occurs:

- Identify the issue and those involved in addressing it.
- Gather a comprehensive database of information influencing the issue.
- Analyze the information with regard to what it is telling you about the decision.
- Search for the options embedded in the relevant collected data.
- Evaluate the options and their implications:

☐ Are they consistent with goals?
☐ What are their possible implications?
☐ How do they inform the action that we will need to take?

Decisions must always influence action and therefore must ultimately be directed toward taking action. Therefore, the ultimate role of data, assessment, and looking at the influences and implications of external and internal issues affecting decision making ultimately must lead to actually making decisions. Data must lead to taking action related to good decisions, and evaluating the effectiveness of the decision based on the action and the outcome. This dynamic between information, preparation, and decision making is always evidenced with regard to its effectiveness in the quality in the viability of the outcome.

TEAM-BASED DECISION-MAKING PROCESS

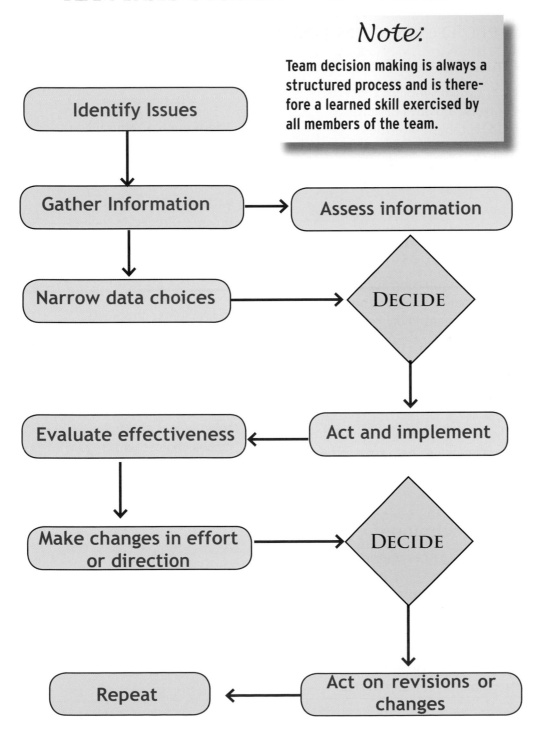

Note:

Team decision making is always a structured process and is therefore a learned skill exercised by all members of the team.

Identify Issues

Gather Information → Assess information

Narrow data choices → DECIDE

Evaluate effectiveness ← Act and implement

Make changes in effort or direction → DECIDE

Repeat ← Act on revisions or changes

Sample Techniques for Team Decision Making

Nominal Group Technique

- Useful when time is a concern
- Controls for issues of power
- Helps establish priorities
- Can aggregate ideas
- Builds group acceptance
- Is transparent

Affinity Groups

- Build consensus and acceptance
- Use a smaller group for process
- Let participant know how broadly the idea is supported
- Also offset power
- Effectively use time
- Value and support individual and group ideas
- Take more time than nominal group
- Use one idea to help spark others

Delphi Technique

- Can use to gather information from outside team
- Good for brainstorming
- Key ideas are identified and related ideas are drawn
- Good for gathering much information from a broad group
- Participants feel safe to share

Finding the Best Technique

There are a whole range of approaches to disciplining decision making and incorporating the team within the decision-making process. Processes such as flowcharts, workflow diagrams, Pareto charts, cause-and-effect diagrams, matrices and stratification instruments, checklists, scatter diagrams, brain-storming, and multi-voting are just a few of the tools that teams can use in making good decisions. The team leader carefully makes choices with regard to what decisions need to be made in the processes that support decision efforts.

SOME THOUGHTS ON CONSENSUS

Voting on issues is never the most effective way of making decisions. Group agreement on what the right or best decision is, generally, is the most appropriate approach to making decisions. Not everyone can agree with all decisions. Agreement about decisions is not nearly as important as the determination of what actions can be taken that are most appropriate to the circumstances in any given time. For some participants that approach may not necessarily lead to their personal decision being advanced. However, in team-based processes, if members are faithful to the process, the right decision and appropriate outcome can most frequently be attained. Continual assessment and reevaluation of the process and the decision and its implementation help guarantee the right decision will always be achieved.

Consensus is simply finding the best approach acceptable enough, under the circumstances, to team members that it can be tested, experimented with, or supported in the process of implementation. Consensus is not necessarily a unanimous vote; it may not be every member's priority. However, through the active participation and involvement of all group members, through adequate generation of appropriate data, through good group dynamics and conflict resolution, discussion, and facilitation, a consensus-based decision generally indicates a direction for the decision that would not be as clearly indicated through any other choice (Goleman, 1997). Reaching consensus requires that every team member participates fully in the process of decision making. This may mean several rounds of dialog and discourse around a disciplined process. Good consensus is always evident in the thoroughness of the process, the consideration given to members involved in the dialog, and support for the most commonly evident basis upon which a decision can be made.

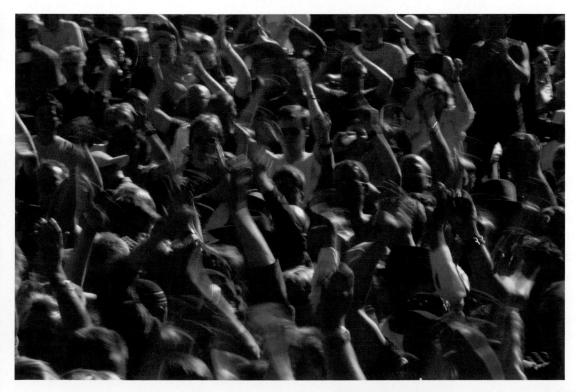

THE TEAM LEADER AND QUALITY DECISION MAKING

Team Leader Is Always Focused on Quality

Team leaders are interested in outcome as much as they are concerned about process. The most common problem in management is the failure to understand that leaders must always focus on results. Although quality is often focused on improving processes, ultimately the fundamental work of quality must be the impact it has on the mission, purposes, and values of the organization. The good team leader helps keep the focus of the team's work on its achievement of defined expectations and sustainable outcomes (Gotlieb, 2003). This is a quality focus that requires the following elements:

- Emphasizing outcomes through working on creating good process is critical to effective goal attainment. Problems, issues, and processes are most effective when they are transparent, constantly studied and improving so that the final product of the work represents a good fit between work effort and commitment to goals.

- The role of the team leader is to continually build excellence into every aspect of the team's work. Leadership around quality focuses consistently on encouraging team members to focus individual work effort and the collective integration of effort on the achievement of common goals to which all team members have committed.

- Using objective and scientific processes must become a pervasive part of the team's effort. Each element of the disciplined work process, assessment mechanisms, action steps, and evaluation processes must be subjected to rigorous review and constant adjustment. In good team process, variation is constantly assessed, translated, and adjusted so that effective outcomes are sustained.

- Improvement is a continual process. The team represents its commitment to excellence and quality by producing products and services of ever-growing value while reducing errors, resource use, and inefficiencies in work processes and relationships.

Note:
Quality team outcomes are always a reflection of quality team processes, relationships, and dynamics. The effective team leader recognizes the essential relationship between all of these elements and achieving sustainable outcomes.

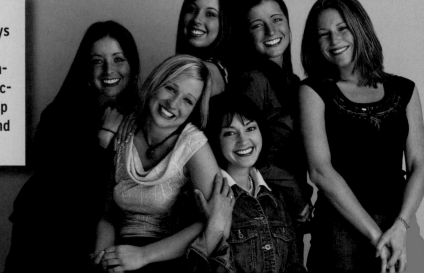

References

Goleman, D. (1997). *Emotional intelligence*. New York: Bantam Books.

Gottlieb, M. R. (2003). *Managing group process*. Westport, CT: Praeger.

Hackman, R. (2002). *Leading teams: Setting the stage for great performances*. Boston: Harvard Business School Press.

Hambrick, D. C., Nadler, D., & Tushman, M. (1998). *Navigating change: How CEOs, top teams, and boards steer transformation*. Boston: Harvard Business School Press.

Harshman, C. L., & Phillips, S. L. (1994). *Teaming up: Achieving organizational transformation*. Amsterdam; San Diego: Pfeiffer & Co.

Porter-O'Grady, T., & Krueger Wilson, C. (1998). *The healthcare teambook*. St. Louis: Mosby, Times Mirror.

Suggested Readings

Belbin, R. M. (2004). *Management teams: Why they succeed or fail* (2nd ed.). Oxford: Elsevier/Butterworth-Heinemann.

DuBrin, A. J. (1995). *The breakthrough team player: Becoming the M.V.P. on your workplace team*. New York: Amacom.

Fisher, K. (2000). *Leading self-directed work teams: A guide to developing new team leadership skills* (rev. and expand ed.). New York: McGraw-Hill

Graen, G. B. (2004). *New frontiers of leadership*. Greenwich, CT: Information Age Pub.

Harris, C. (2003). *Building innovative teams: Strategies and tools for developing and integrating high performance innovative groups*. New York: Palgrave Macmillan.

UNIT 2: BUILDING DECISION-MAKING SKILLS

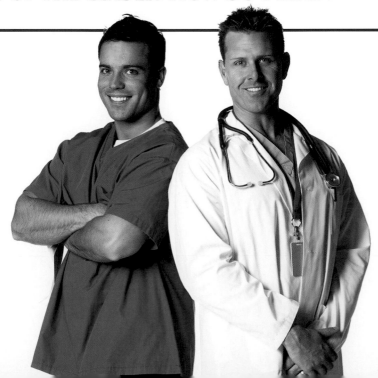

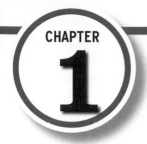

MAKING EFFECTIVE DECISIONS

Decisions are not automatically good because the individual is skilled. Good decisions reflect the collective wisdom of the right stakeholders committed to mutually beneficial outcomes.

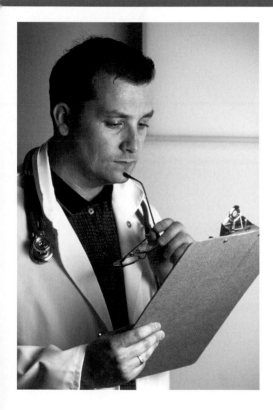

MAKING GOOD DECISIONS

Decisions are even more important than action. Effective action is informed by great decision making (Russo & Schoemaker, 2001). There is much evidence of people having taken action based on ineffective or poor decision making. In leaders, the ability to facilitate good decisions is critical to effective action and great leadership. Where decisions are made and how they are constructed and by whom are critical and basic elements of leadership and great teamwork. The leader not only exemplifies great teamwork, but also expects in it every facet of team performance.

The Core of Good Decisions

Several elements or factors affect good decisions:

- Amount of information available to the decision maker
- Skills and abilities of the decision makers
- The environment within which decisions are made
- The tools available for making decisions
- The time frame within which decisions are made
- The complexity of the issues affecting decision making
- The goals to which decisions are directed
- The mechanisms in place for evaluating the quality of decisions

INFORMATION AND DECISIONS

Good decisions are informed decisions. A decision can only be as good as the data that supports it. A critical failure in good decision-making occurs when the information the decision maker has is not adequate to address the content of the decision. But no amount of information will be fully adequate to all decisions, meaning that there will always be some level of information deficit in all decisions. Still the decision maker wants to make sure that as much of the right kind of information is available as possible.

Information Supports Good Decisions

- Valuable information is up-to-date information.

- Good information for decisions comes in a usable format.

- Too much information is as bad as too little.

- Good information tells you what you need to know, not just what you want to know.

- Information does not represent values or judgment.

- It's just data—don't look for what isn't there.

INFORMATION IS A RIVER, NOT A THING

Information generation and management is a dynamic that is endless and continuous. Good management information relates directly to those things the organization values and uses to affect the products of its work. Information is a tool that must always be available in the right form, giving data to those who need it in a form they can use and at a time that has the greatest impact. There is nothing worse than the right information at the wrong time or the wrong information at the right time. Good information systems have data continually available to users in a way that they can readily access it based on timing and their need for it (see below).

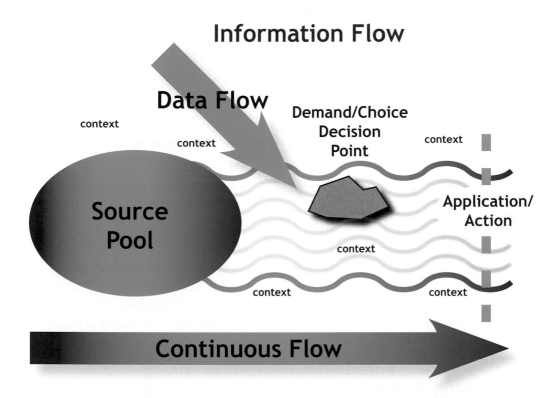

Flow and Application of Information

- Information is gathered and mixes in a source repository.
- Data link and integrate to provide a frame for information demand.
- Need for information takes form and a demand is made for it.
- Data are generated in a format that can be used and applied.
- The context or work translates meaning/value from the data.
- Action taken is based on the utility and application of data.

BUILDING DECISIONS ON GOOD INFORMATION

The leader knows how to draw out specific and applicable data in such a way that it can be used clearly and specifically to inform the work and evaluate its effectiveness and value.

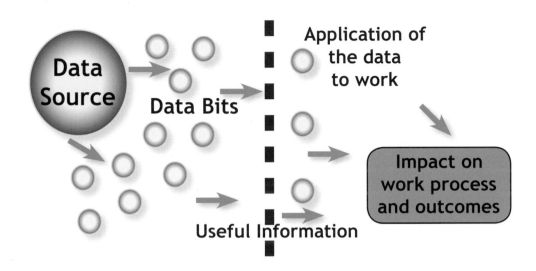

Decisions Reflect the Value of the Information

Information is a tool—no more. The leader recognizes the value of information and works to create a good fit between the information gathered and the work activities and purposes of the team. The wise leader never gathers or generates information that doesn't directly inform or support the actions of the team, for fear of making it irrelevant or overwhelming the worker with data that have no value. Information should always support good decisions. A leader should always ask:

- Is the information relevant?
- Is the information necessary?
- Can the information be understood?
- Is the information useful to the user?
- Is the information in a form that can be readily used?
- Is there too much information?
- Is the information arranged in a form that makes sense to the user?
- Is the information specific and applicable to the issue at hand?
- Is the information timely and current?
- Are the information sources reliable and dependable?
- Can the team apply the information and affect process or outcome?
- When evaluating information can it be directly related to the outcomes?
- Is information flexible and fluid, changing when demand for it shifts?

What are the Skills of the Decision Makers?

Good decisions cannot come from people who are not adequately prepared to make them (Sanders, 1999). Good information is certainly a great tool for good decisions, but information will have no value if the individual does not know what to do with it. Both the leader and the team must be capable of making effective decisions. This is reflected in their mutual ability to think and act in a way that advances the work and achieves its outcomes. Of course, the skills of decision making must be in the hands of those who do the work. This means that the leader must be good at transferring skills to others and helping them apply the skills.

Skill-Sets for Good Decision Making

Leader Decision Role

1. Build a frame for good information gathering and use.
2. Transfer skills for reading and translating information into useful data.
3. Build skills for applying data to decision processes.
4. Apply the processes of effective decision making.
5. Identify skill deficits in decision making and undertake corrective learning.
6. Raise the bar when decision skills grow in the staff.
7. Evaluate effect of decisions and adjust processes as needed.

Staff Decision Role

1. Develop skills in information gathering and management.
2. Apply good decision techniques to work processes.
3. Exercise skills in interpreting and applying data to work.
4. Supplement skills in data based decision making.
5. Assess individual and team skill levels in decision processes and construct a developmental plan.
6. Evaluate level of excellence in achieving outcomes.
7. Experiment with new approaches to information and decisions.

THE LEADER'S ROLE IN DECISION MANAGEMENT

It should be clear that in team-based approaches, the leader makes few decisions. The team based approach to work is different than any other model. Leaders recognize in team-based frameworks that decisions must be located as close to the point-of-service as possible. The good leader works hard to make sure that there is little transfer of accountability from the staff to the leader when it comes to accountable decision making. As much as possible, the leader attempts to make few decisions (belonging to the staff) and certainly no decisions that extend outside of creating a supportive context for staff ownership of decision making. The leader sees her or his role as creating a good context for effective decisions rather than making those decisions himself or herself (Kaye, 2002).

Decision Leadership

> The leader teaches others how to make good decision.

> The leader transfers insights and skills to the team.

> The leader monitors the skill level of the team and addresses learning needs of the team.

> When new information becomes available, the leader generates it to the team to use.

> The leader is always looking for opportunity for the team grow and continually participates in developing them.

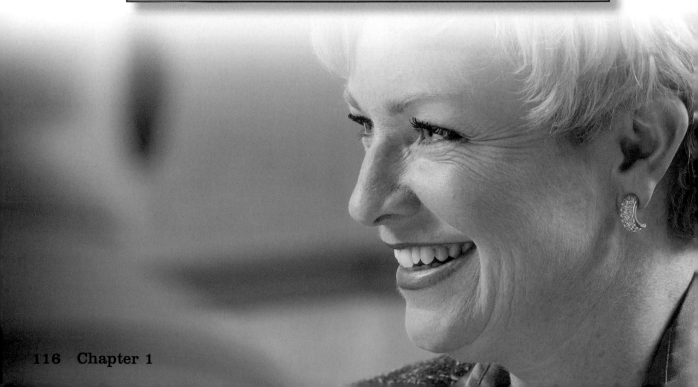

UNDERSTANDING ACCOUNTABILITY

Accountability is the most overused and misunderstood element of leadership today. It is often mistakenly connected with responsibility, to which it has only an indirect relationship. Accountability assumes that an individual knows the value and contribution of his or her work. Accountability requires that the work have an impact, in short, make a difference. In this scenario, the professional knows the value of the work, determines the anticipated contribution it will make, and evaluates the work against the outcomes to ensure it actually accomplishes what it is intended to do (Stack & Burlington, 2002).

Accountability requires that there is a direct relationship among decision, action, and outcome. In many clinical processes there is a lack of specificity and clarity regarding the direct relationship between action and result. There is precious little evidence that this relationship is well established in clinical practice. The dynamics and processes associated with evidence-based practice come closest to addressing this issue. Effective foundations for good decision processes are built on establishing the relationship between clinical decisions, actions, and results. The leader facilitates the formation of a framework that supports this kind of clinical action and encourages staff ownership of the decision process and its effect on action and outcomes.

UNDERSTANDING SHARED DECISIONS

Locus of control is important to the understanding of good decisions (Porter-O'Grady, 2004). Effective decisions are made by those who will have accountability for implementing them. Making decisions close to the place those decisions will be acted upon assures the likelihood they will be effective. Sustainable effectiveness in decision-making and action depends on the direct relationship between the ownership of the action and the person of the decision maker. Too often, those who make critical or strategic decisions rarely implement them. Often those who carry out the action of decision making are never involved in making the decisions. One can only wonder why there is so little ownership of work or its products when those who define the work are frequently not those who will execute it. Effectiveness of decisions is enhanced to the extent that both the maker and executor of decisions are the same person. This inclusiveness of the planners and actors together in the process of planning and deciding is a central theme of shared governance and shared leadership. Shared decision making reflects the partnership and equity necessary to ownership and execution of decisions. Effective decisions are directly related to successful process and outcomes; in fact, good decisions are validated by good process and satisfactory and exemplary outcomes. These levels of excellence cannot be sustained without the strong ownership by the purveyors of excellence in both the decisions that drove them and good action that achieved them. Furthermore, the strength of the relationship between individual and ownership of decisions is the best indicator of subsequent good practice.

DECISIONS AND ACCESS SKILLS

In the digital age, access is a critical skill. The ability to access information in a form that can be used and applied quickly and effectively is important in today's work processes. Time is a major concern in meeting the needs of work and the service needs of others. Because of the impact of technology, it is possible to adjust and alter work processes quickly and to change the effect of decisions in a moment's time. The team must be able to quickly access information and just as quickly make decisions because the frame or reference for their work adjusts and changes quickly.

The leader must role model this level of flexibility and fluidity with regard to decision making and change in the work flow. If the leader cannot use the tools of modern technology or demonstrate access skills and a willingness to continue personal growth in these areas, she or he should not expect the staff to do so either. Remember, the leader creates the context for work. Staff cannot go where the leader has not been.

Developing Access Skills

Leaders create the context and provide the opportunity for staff to acquire access skills:

- The latest technology for information management exists in a form that can be learned and used by team members.
- Leaders see that teaching and transferring access skills are a fundamental part of the role in the 21st century workplace.
- Real-time decisions require current and viable information that can be managed and added to with information about its application and value as well as its effect on subsequent work activities.
- The leader evaluates the technology available and the skills of the team and adjusts demand with the team's capacity to use the tools.

Note:

Increasingly, access skills are an important part of the talent base of the team. Leaders who understand this are one step ahead in their readiness to achieve and sustain team goals.

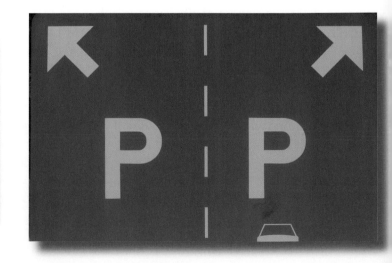

TEAM DECISION-MAKING EFFECTIVENESS

Work decisions belong to the team. Leaders have to make sure that the processes and skills necessary to good decisions are available to team members. Effective decisions require specific skills.

Decision Challenges

1. Being bombarded by data that are not valuable
2. Team member bias with regard to what is right
3. Lack of consensus related to the correctness of a decision
4. Interpersonal disagreements about right course of action
5. Poor problem-solving or conflict-resolving skills
6. Confusion related to who is accountable for what in the decision process
7. Unwillingness to change or grow as the informatin requires a shift in work

Decision Facilitators

1. Good mechanisms for sorting through data
2. Team member open to confronting disparity between data and personal views
3. Lack of consensus related between data and to the correctness of a personal views
3. Good consensus skills
4. Accountability for response clearly determined in the team
5. Problems are confronted quickly and effectively
6. Accountability is well defined between team members
7. Fluidity and flexibility are built into team processes and change management

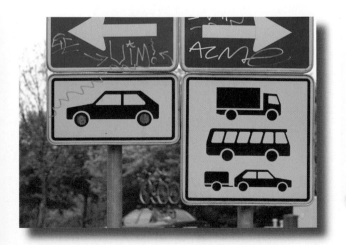

Note:

The team's readiness to respond to the challenges of shifting data and work demands keep it fresh, open, and available to new opportunities for success.

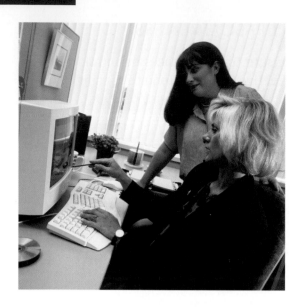

Elements of a Good Decision

- Clear and understandable
- Can be implemented
- Relates directly to the outcome
- Links team work efforts together well
- Is not cast in stone (cannot be changed)
- Is always action oriented
- Is based on the right course
- Is fully implemented by the team

Team-Based Decision Process Flow

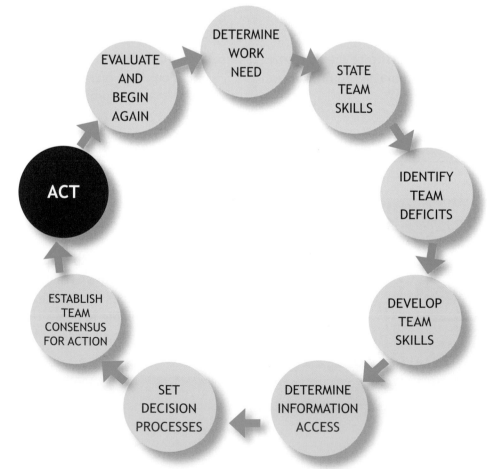

Point-of-Service Decision Rules

> Staff are always accountable for work rules and roles.

> The leader develops staff decisions and never makes decisions for them.

> The decision-making skill level of the team reflects the aggregated skills of individual members.

> A broken place in any one part of the team means brokenness in the whole team.

> Interpersonal differences or personality conflicts must always be confronted or else they poison the team's work.

> Decision competence is not static; skills must be refined and continuing development is a requisite of effectiveness.

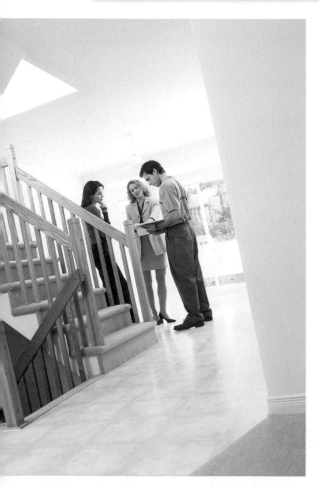

Effective Team Decisions

- Equal understanding of data
- Good consensus around data response
- Ability to stop and question
- Mutual positive movement to goals
- Ability to evaluate and change
- Good problem-solving skills
- Able to change course quickly if needed

Managing the Timing of Good Decisions

Good strategy demands the consideration of the timing of actions as much as it pays attention to the activities resulting from decisions. The effective leader knows the value of timing in decisions and plans action accordingly.

This leader always ensures that:

1. Time is an element of all decisions and its importance is a part of the dialog with regard to making good decisions.
2. Implementing a decision includes timing it so that it has the greatest impact on work and related processes.
3. Leaders recognize the value of time in considering resource allocation and the variances around when more or less of them will be needed in the process of doing work.
4. All work takes time. It is important to include the time values necessary to complete work in the planning stage. After all, time IS money.
5. Changes in time factors and/or variables must be communicated to all stakeholders so the effect of such changes can be incorporated into the work process.

TIMING DECISIONS

Nothing is more important than the right decision at the right time. History is full of stories of bad timing and how opportunity or strategy was affected because of missing the time "mark" by moments. Nothing is more critical for constraining or facilitating decisions than good timing.

Values of Good Time Management of Decisions

- Affects the pace of work
- Influences the cost of work
- Sets parameters for the results
- Disciplines the process of work
- Defines expectations for completion
- Sets schedule for staging work

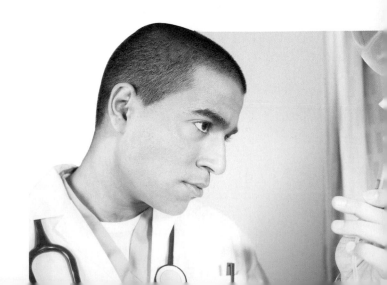

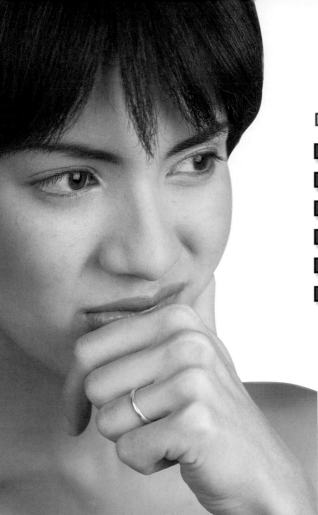

Decision Capacity

- ■ Situational need
- ■ The nature of the team's work
- ■ The method of the team for decisions
- ■ Combined talent of team members
- ■ The right tools and information
- ■ Evidence of successful decisions

Characteristics of Good Decisions

All necessary skills are available to the decision.

The correct information supports the decision.

The team is willing to make the decision.

The decision leads directly to expected outcomes.

The decision ultimately raises team performance.

OVERCOMING INDIVIDUAL DECISION DEFICITS

1. Deal with a lack of willingness by relating the decision to the content of the work. Remind the participating staff that they will ultimately be affected by decisions that relate to their work. This should help them become aware of their own response to it.
2. Address a lack of skill by tying the type of decision to the skill that the situation requires. Make sure the staff can act with the right level and kind of skills needed by the situation.
3. Help individuals design a developmental plan for decision effectiveness that addresses explicit skill needs and provide the opportunities to learn the necessary skills.

Overcoming Team Decision Deficits

1. Identify the team practices that constrain good shared decision making and work to develop and refine them.
2. Clarify individual actions that constrain the team-based approach to problem solving and successfully seeking solutions.
3. Have the team evaluate particular scenarios in which decision making was required—assess the dynamics and work to identify where problems exist and what would help resolve them.
4. Have the team role-play the more difficult situation or challenges. Watch experts role-play and have the team members mirror the behaviors as practice.
5. Have the team evaluate the decision process regularly to update and improve its skill.

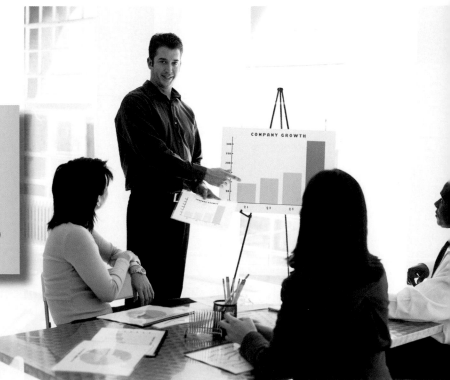

Note:

The leader is constantly monitoring both individual and team to identify decision skill needs and connects the team to the resources necessary to keep decisions effective.

Constructing an Effective
Decision-Making Process

**BACKDROP FOR
DECISION MAKING**

- Environment
- Capacity
- Skills

**SUSTAINABLE
OUTCOMES**

**PROCESS OF DECISION
MAKING**

Process Factors

· Work Model
· Team Effectiveness
· Work Goals
· Performance Measures

Decision making requires a discipline that can be replicated over time. Leaders must ensure that the process of decision making is relevant to the issues at hand and leads to sustainable results.

The process should always:

■ Be systematic and applied consistently in order to ensure its value over time.

■ Have defined steps that can be learned and applied in such a way that evaluation of them shows viability.

■ Be sure each step has a mechanism for assessment in order to pinpoint issues and problems as quickly as possible.

■ Have a mechanism for quickly adjusting and changing decisions when evidence suggests a need to change.

■ Exhibit techniques by tying processes to obtaining outcomes, ensuring the best decisions result in the best outcomes.

Making the Right Decisions

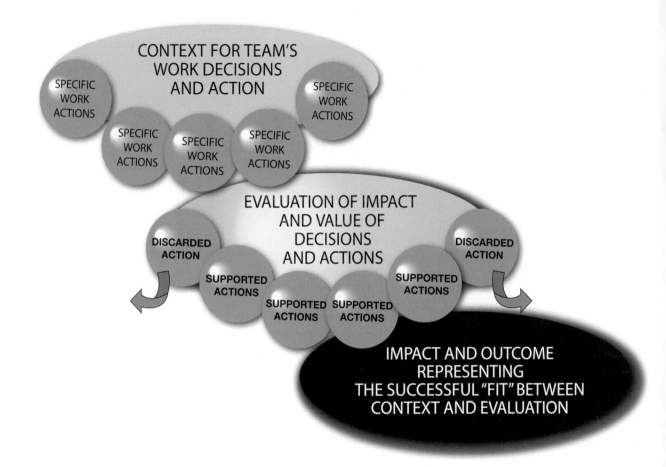

CONTEXT FOR TEAM'S WORK DECISIONS AND ACTION

SPECIFIC WORK ACTIONS

SPECIFIC WORK ACTIONS

SPECIFIC WORK ACTIONS

SPECIFIC WORK ACTIONS

SPECIFIC WORK ACTIONS

EVALUATION OF IMPACT AND VALUE OF DECISIONS AND ACTIONS

DISCARDED ACTION

DISCARDED ACTION

SUPPORTED ACTIONS

SUPPORTED ACTIONS

SUPPORTED ACTIONS

SUPPORTED ACTIONS

IMPACT AND OUTCOME REPRESENTING THE SUCCESSFUL "FIT" BETWEEN CONTEXT AND EVALUATION

ENSURING GOODNESS-OF-FIT

All decisions should be represented in the good fit between excellent process and desirable outcomes. The leader has a primary role in assuring this "fit" by creating the conditions that make it happen:

- Good information and foundation for decision
- Full engagement of team in decision and action
- Faithfulness to the agreed-upon process steps (see above)
- Adjustments in steps and work process
- Evaluating stages and fit of process to results

How Do You Know It's a Good Decision?

Making Good Decisions

- The information tools are consistent and dependable for all members of the team and the information is actually used.
- The information is in a form that is understandable and has meaning for the team members.
- Team members act in concert, each applying his or her own skills in a way that aggregates in the best interest of the work of all members.
- Agreement with regard to approach and application is clear and well understood so that each team member is contributing to actually achieving results.
- Adjustments in patterns of behavior and action can occur in "real time" and can be incorporated into the work flow seamlessly.
- Retooling a decision does not "destroy" the energy or commitment of team; instead, it is a normal part of the work process.
- New data call for new decisions and new actions.
- Evaluation strengthens the decision process with teams discarding what doesn't work and affirming what does work well and renewing the energy to perform with high levels of excellence (Stone, 2004).

Leader's Role in Decision Evaluation

- Make it safe to stop and look at action.
- The latest evaluation tools are available.
- Staff have time to review work progress.
- Corrective action is a positive process.
- It is safe to discard irrelevant practices.
- Leader introduces new methods carefully.
- Staff have time to change behaviors.
- Error does not result in punishment.
- Decisions are always team driven.

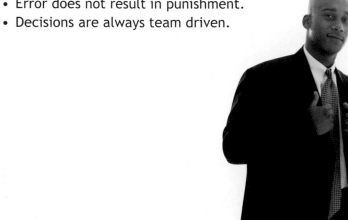
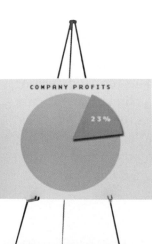

COMPANY PROFITS

23%

Making Effective Decisions   127

THE LEADER'S DECISIONAL COMPETENCE

Although it is clear that leaders should not be making practice decisions (these belong to the staff), it is also apparent that the ability to understand the decision-making process (including staff skills) is critical to the exercise of the leader role. The leader must always anticipate the need for decisions, the information necessary to make good decisions, the processes important for success, and the mechanics involved in particular decisions. It is the obligation of the leader to keep the team focused on its work and the efforts necessary to coordinate the team to achieve the outcomes to which the team's energy is directed (Sample, 2001).

The vagaries of human dynamics always affect the progress of the team. Would that it were true that everything worked well and progressed precisely as it should. The good leader knows that the vagaries of life are not simple or even straightforward and that almost anything can negatively influence the process, causing work flow to be interrupted or even stop altogether (Argyris, 2000). The intuitive leader anticipates this dynamic as a part of the journey of work. She or he does not see it as an aberrant process but a normative condition in all human dynamic processes. When it occurs the leader always:

- Recognizes the demand for adjustment as a part of the dynamic of decision making and calmly helps the team adjust to its presence.
- Keeps up with the latest decision-related information, generating it to the team in a way that can influence their choices and their work.
- When raising the question, puts it in proper context so the team can deal with the issue in a way that directly depends on their own experience.
- Helps the team define and incorporate evaluation mechanisms into the process of work so that corrective processes can occur immediately in small increments of change rather than later in large chunks of change.
- Enumerates what has worked and what has not, giving the team permission to discard what doesn't work so that they can safely explore a change in practice and incorporate that which is effective in their work process.

The Leader's Decision Check-Off

- Staff own decisions.
- Staff have skills for good decisions.
- Learning is a normative work state.
- Punishment is removed from work.
- Experimentation/exploration is good.
- Change is an acceptable reality.
- Decisions always improve.

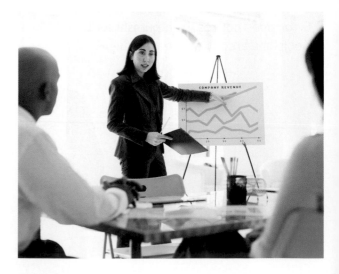

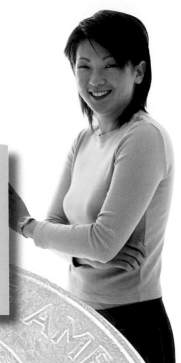

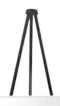

Note:

Decisions are not inherently good or bad. They are good to the extent that they are well informed, are accurate, are relevant, are well applied, and make a difference; they are bad when they are not.

EXCELLENT DECISIONS

1. Well informed
2. Competent
3. Skilled
4. Shared
5. Relevant
6. Practical
7. Valued
8. Consensus based
9. Flexible
10. Outcome driven

POOR DECISIONS

1. Poorly informed
2. Random and variable
3. Unformed
4. Unilateral
5. Ritualized
6. Impractical
7. No commitment
8. Nonaligned
9. Rigid
10. Process driven

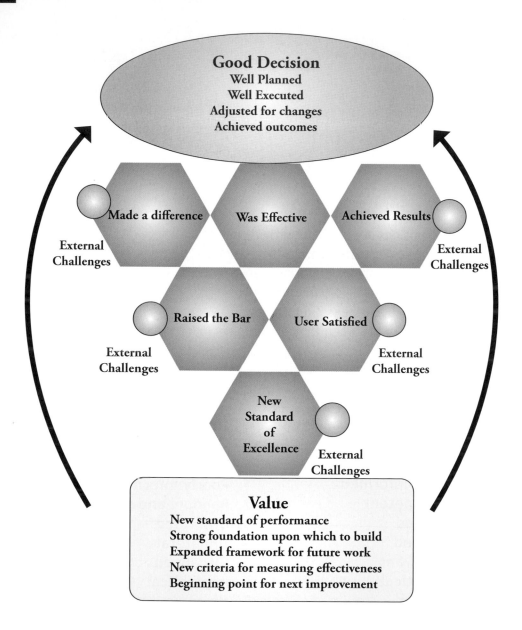

Evaluation is a cyclical process (see above) that is continual and dynamic. It never ceases to be a part of the work process. The effective leader always incorporates the evaluation process into every activity of work. Leaders are forever attempting to make sure that the standard is continually challenged and the practices are forever improved in order to ensure the continuing effort at improvement bears results and makes a difference for both workers and customers.

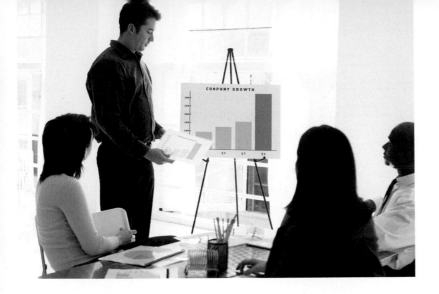

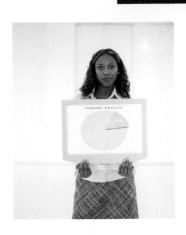

Effective Decisions and Sustained Excellence

- ■ Clearly defined decision-making process
- ■ Committed team members reaching for results
- ■ Good communication processes among team members
- ■ Great evaluation and corrective action strategies
- ■ A process for team learning and development
- ■ Problem solving within the process of implementation
- ■ Evaluating process and progress
- ■ Changing directions when necessary
- ■ Innovation and creativity are normative
- ■ The team celebrates its success; moves to higher level of performance

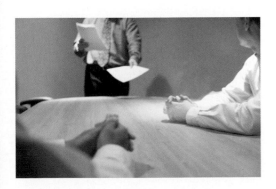

Note:

The team is always "in process" and never is at the highest level of its own performance. Teamwork is a work in progress and all of its decisions drive it to the next level of excellence. Decisions are always precursors to action—making a difference is the product of the team's efforts and the reward for good decisions and excellent work.

References

Argyris, C. (2000). *Escaping the management trap*. Oxford, UK: Oxford University Press.

Kaye, B. (2002). *Up is not the only way*. New York: Consulting Psychologists Press, Inc.

Porter-O'Grady, T. (2004, January-February, 2004). Accountability and action. *Health Progress*, 44-48.

Russo, E., & Schoemaker, P. (2001). *Winning decisions: Getting it right the first time*. New York: Currency-Doubleday Books.

Sample, S. (2001). *The contrarian's guide to leadership*. San Francisco: Jossey-Bass Publishers.

Sanders, R. (1999). *The executive decision-making process: Identifying problems and assessing outcomes*. Westport, CT: Quorum.

Stack, J., & Burlington, B. (2002). *A stake in the outcome*. New York: Currency Doubleday.

Stone, F. M. (2004). *The essential new manager's kit*. Chicago: Dearborn Trade Pub.

Suggested Readings

Deming, P. (2001). *The invisible future*. New York: McGraw-Hill Publishers.

Goad, T. W. (2002). *Information literacy and workplace performance*. Westport, CT: Quorum Books.

Porter-O'Grady, T. (2001). Profound change: 21st century nursing. *Nursing Outlook*, 49(1), 182-186.

Porter-O'Grady, T., & Malloch, K. (2002). *Quantum leadership: A textbook of new leadership*. Sudbury, MA: Jones and Bartlett.

Rheingold, H. (2002). *Smart mobs*. New York: Perseus Books.

CHAPTER 2

LEADING THE ADULT-TO-ADULT WORKPLACE: WHO AM I LEADING?

Moving out of a superior-subordinate or parent-child relationship at work is the first step to ensuring ownership and engagement.

LEADING ADULTS

Perhaps one of the most difficult arenas of leadership is related to the leaders' styles. Many approaches to leadership and work reflect a more parent-child set of values and processes than good leadership foundations. The challenge for leaders in the workplace is to recognize that they are one among peers. It is not the role of leaders to direct people into their will or agenda. Instead, a good leader helps people understand the contribution they can make, the value of that contribution, and the role they play in the life of the organization.

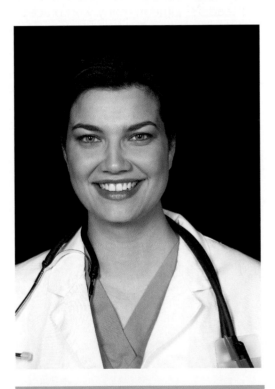

Adult-to-Adult Approaches

- Providing sufficient information
- Raising the right questions
- Giving others tools
- Helping others with problem solving
- Evaluating progress
- Focusing on goals
- Supporting others' decisions
- Helping others set dierction

Parent-Child Approaches

- Supervising and managing
- Controlling and managing
- Discipline and punishing
- Telling and stating
- Focusing on details
- Micro management
- Directing and correcting

LEADING THE ADULT EMPLOYEE

It is difficult to imagine that much of management reflects parent-child dynamics at work. The real challenge for the leader is to be able to provide leadership and maintain adult relationships in every aspect of its application. Accountability in the workplace cannot be achieved if the fundamental relationship that describes what goes on there between people is not based on solid adult-to-adult principles.

Much of leaders' time in many workplaces is spent taking care of problems, issues, concerns, relationships, and a whole host of other variables that operate in an organization that has primarily parent-child constructs for the manager's work. A simple review of management job descriptions can often demonstrate the parental role priorities identified in the workplace. Much of the expectation of the supervisor is to see to it that the staff are compliant, controlled, directed, and closely managed to make sure that they fulfill the mandates and obligations of the organization. Notions such as partnership, accountability, agreement, joint goals, sharing, and interaction are frequently

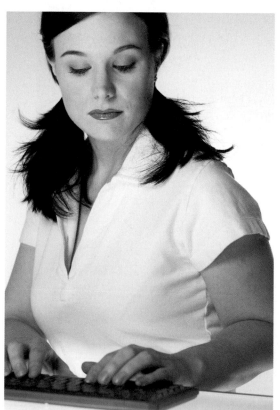

not found in the script that represents what we expect managers to do (Porter-O'Grady & Wilson, 1999).

In an effective adult-to-adult work environment the notion of partnership, engagement, and investment predominates. This workplace recognizes the unique contribution that each member of the work community contributes to the fulfillment of the goals of the organization and contributes to the quality of relationships there. In an adult workplace it is recognized that nothing can be sustained unless there is a mutual agreement and investment of all the stakeholders in achieving goals and advancing the values of the organization. This effort requires partnership, ownership, and systems of accountability if an adult-to-adult environment is to be built and sustained. In this scenario, the leader is predominantly a partner, sharing the same goals and commitments as any other participant in the organization's life. This leader recognizes that everyone is a stakeholder in the organization's work and that engagement must be mutual in order for the purposes and goals of the organization to be met and the life of the organization to be advanced.

ACCOUNTABILITY: THE CORE OF ADULT LEADERSHIP

Adult-to-adult work relationships depend on the presence of a specific frame of reference for expressing those behaviors in the workplace. The most effective framework for expressing adult to adult relationships is the principle of accountability (Malloch & Porter-O'Grady, 2005). Different from responsibility, accountability calls for partnership, equity, and ownership on the part of all stakeholders. This represents a mutual commitment on the part of all participants in an organization to the purposes and goals of the organization as expressed through its work. The effect of workplace transmits and translates this understanding to all workers from the moment of their inception into the workplace and throughout the very dynamics of everyone's work. All work requires some level of accountability in order for outcomes to be achieved and sustained over time. The elements of accountability are:

- Every worker is seen as a partner in the enterprise.
- It is expected that every individual is fully engaged in the life of the workplace.
- Workers are part of a membership community, not simply employees of the entity.
- Expectations with regard to partnership are made clear at the outset of the relationship.
- Stakeholders fully own their work and its contribution to the purposes of the workplace.
- All members recognize that their role is interdependent, requiring interaction with other stakeholders.
- All participants in the membership community have value; that value must be clearly enumerated for all to understand its contribution.
- Each member in the work community must demonstrate his or her value and its contribution in enhancing and advancing the value of the oranization.

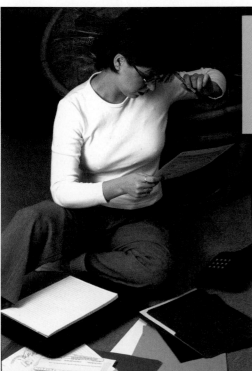

Three Elements of Accountability

- Autonomy—the right to act
- Authority—the power to act
- Competence—the knowledge to act

Accountability and Value

Every member of the work community has value. It is a requisite of work that the value contribute to the aggregate value of the work of all members of the organization. It is only through the collective value of each participant in the work life of the organization that the organization's purposes and values are sustained throughout the life of the organization. A failure to clearly enumerate and articulate value ultimately contributes to the failure of the organization to fulfill its purposes and achieve long-term goals.

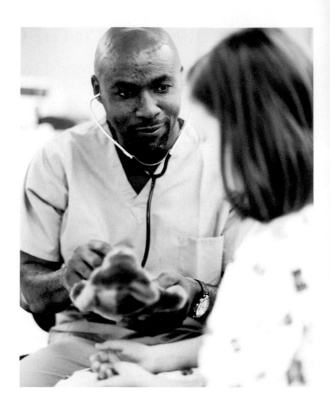

Elements of Value in the Effective Workplace

- Everyone has value to the extent of their ability to contribute to the goals and purposes of the organization.
- Each member of the work community is expected to fully express competence and values in all their work efforts.
- Every leader understands the individual and unique values of each worker and successfully aggregates the individual values to advance collective goals.
- Each member's value to the organization is clearly enumerated and expressed within the context of the goals of the organization so that all members are aware of the contribution of each member.
- Value is continually enhanced by providing opportunity for learning new approaches, enhancing skills, and advancing innovation for each member of the work community.
- All members must know that value returned to them in the form of benefits and rewards is, in part, recognition of their own personal commitment to the organization's goals and its long-term success.
- Leaders recognize the unique talent and skills of each member of the work community and seek to recognize, honor, and use those skills in ways that advance the quality of work of the organization.
- The leader honors and celebrates the value and contribution of each worker in regularly scheduled acts of celebration and recognition.

AUTONOMY: THE RIGHT TO ACT

Autonomy recognizes the essential independence of individuals to live and act on their own, and to ultimately take full responsibility and ownership for their own acts. This fundamental right does not change in the context of work. Individuals are still individuals and have full right of ownership over their actions and contributions. This is an important concept within the consideration of the skills and talents of leadership. Leaders must recognize that they not only acknowledge the fundamental autonomy of the individual but also incorporate that understanding into the life and relationship of the organization that they lead. Failing to honor the individual uniqueness and the autonomy of people ultimately costs the work and the workplace through the reaction to the diminished valuing of the individual. In an environment of diminished value or objectification, the individual will lose interest, investment, and ownership in his or her own work effort. The product of this circumstance is minimal effort, little commitment, and passive-aggressive relationships at work. The wise leader understands the following elements in the exercise of her or his role:

1. Individuals have a right to be respected and honored for their uniqueness, not simply for their contribution to the work.
2. Autonomy recognizes the separateness of individuals, requiring the leader to honor each person's unique characteristics and contribution.
3. The leader assesses and integrates the unique characteristics and contribution of individuals, aggregating them and assessing the product of their mix and its value to the work effort.
4. Each leader has a right to expect from the individual a full commitment to the contribution of the unique skills to the work effort of the whole, lending value to the pursuit of work goals.

Note:

Autonomy suggests that all individuals have a right to their uniqueness and should expect that it will be honored and validated in the workplace, not homogenized and diminished in a context driven by sameness, ritual, and routine. The death of individuality at work, ultimately extinguishes the value of a person's unique contribution.

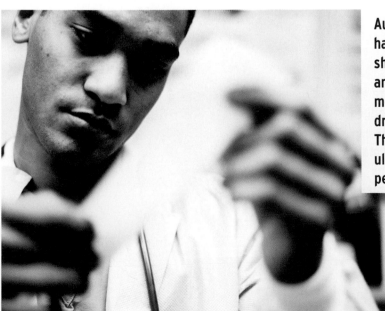

AUTHORITY: THE POWER TO ACT

People may have the right to act and still not act. In order to legitimize the right to act, individuals need to be clear about what power they have to act and influence others to act. Power is sim ply the ability to act and cause others to act in concert. The ability to create the "concert" is the expression of the power to act. If there were no coordinating and consolidating capacity in a community of people, chaos would reign and lives would be endangered. Power creates order and integrity around action and generates a frame for integrating action around a common purpose or goal. This agreement character of positive power is the glue that holds people together within a common set of values and a community-supported set of parameters. In the positive application of power, the community empowers certain individuals and groups to make decisions about the viability of the relationship and action of the group. This is why power is so important in the exercise of accountability.

Elements of Distributive Power

- The expression of power is legitimized by the consent of those upon whom it acts.
- There is a clearly delineated definition of the characteristics and limits of power.
- Power relates to creating a cohesive response to a common purpose or value.
- The exercise of power is judicious and carefully applied.
- Power is never exercised beyond the need for it and only at the level of the least amount needed to sustain concerted action.
- Individuals never apply concerted power over the authority of groups to act, nor do groups control the authority of the individual to act. Clarity regarding this issue of locus of control must be available to all who are affected by the exercise of power.

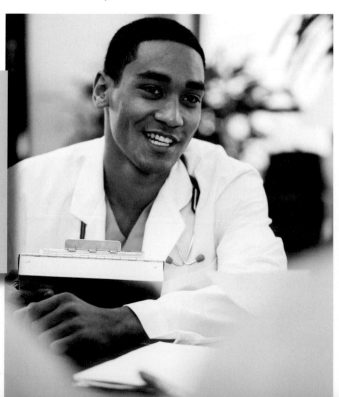

Note:

Accountability requires the appropriate exercise of power in a way that acknowledges the role of individuals and groups in its expression. Failure to have the power to make decisions and to ensure these decisions are acted upon limits the ability to achieve results and to ensure a good fit between purpose, workers, work, and its outcomes.

COMPETENCE: THE ABILITY TO ACT

Accountability cannot be ensured if the competence necessary to both decide and act are not present. Everyone has seen a set of circumstances in which individuals holding leadership roles may have the autonomy and the authority to act but lack the competence to act correctly because of a lack of knowledge or inappropriate application of the leadership role not congruent with the circumstances or expectations of others. Leaders and staff, in the expression of their defined accountabilities, must be aware of the need to be competent in their expression or suffer the loss of confidence and support of others. It is this issue of lack of necessary competence that has the most critical effect on the expression of accountability (Porter-O'Grady & Malloch, 2002).

Elements of Accountability-Based Competence

- There is an effective skill level related to the decisions over which the individual or group is accountable.
- Competencies related to the group process necessary to integrate thinking around specific decisions are present in the individual of the group.
- The critical factors that relate to providing information and support to decision making are available to all accountable participants.
- Developmental opportunities are available for continuing competence development in individual and team-based decision making.
- Opportunities for undertaking corrective action related to past decision making are available to participants in a non-punitive manner.

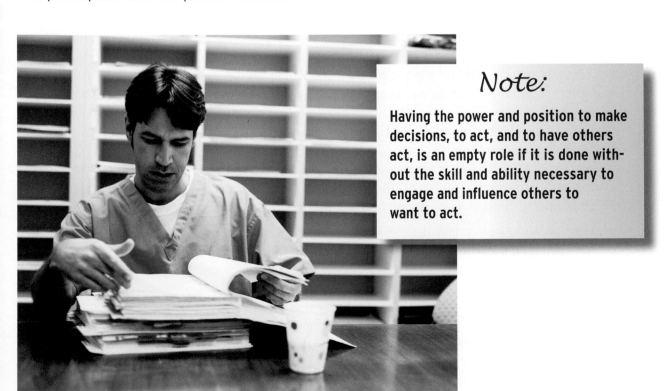

Note:

Having the power and position to make decisions, to act, and to have others act, is an empty role if it is done without the skill and ability necessary to engage and influence others to want to act.

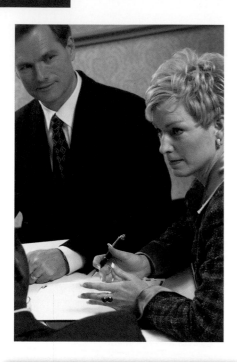

CLARIFYING ACCOUNTABILITIES

◼ They are specific, clear, and understood.
◼ They relate specifically to work outcomes, not work processes.
◼ Performance expectations reflect agreed-upon goals and/or performance outcomes.
◼ Work expectations, performance, and results reflect defined role accountabilities.
◼ Performance evaluation includes the goodness-of-fit of the alignment between accountabilities and work outcomes.

The Accountable Leader

Leadership is clearly a behavior. However, it is the role most directed to create a context of accountability, a place where individuals can fully express and contribute to the goals of the organization from the perspective of their unique contribution. Leaders create context This is no less true with regard to providing a framework where accountability is the expectation for performance and is the behavioral expectation of all members of the work team. The leader makes this possible by establishing the priority of accountability in defining roles, performance expectations, and outcomes. In accountability-based environment the leader focuses on clarifying expectations, as well as, the obligations for work. This leader attempts to create a goodness-of-fit between the skills and talents of the worker and the outcomes to which those talents are directed. After clarifying expectations, the leader focuses on performance factors and helps individuals tie their specific work effort to the expectations for results. It is from this perspective of orientation to results that the leader's relationship to the staff, and the staffs relationship to their work is enumerated. Therefore, the accountable leader always:

• Ensures that each worker knows their specific expectations and contributions to outcomes before undertaking the work effort directed to achieving them.
• Assists each participant in defining and evaluating performance and progress against specified work objectives.
• Builds in environments that stimulate positive and productive relationships between team members in a way that commits their common energies to the fulfillment of work objectives.
• Encourages self-evaluation and self-correction in performance related to expectations and outcomes.

Creativity and Innovation in the Leader

The leader must emulate for others the commitment to the journey of change and transformation. The leader cannot expect that anyone else will be excited about the opportunities of change if the leader does not represent this excitement in her or his own role. Leaders are always asking others to be accountable for the changes that affect their lives. What is critical is the understanding that the leader creates the context for others' enthusiasm and commitment. It the leader does not represent this enthusiasm within the role, it cannot be expected that others will demonstrate it in their roles. In order to engage others, the leader must have a "compact" with innovation that includes the following (Campbell & Burnaby, 2001):

- A willingness to risk and confront the vagaries of change everyday
- An ability to demonstrate in her or his own role the tolerance for chaos and complexity as the "window" to the future
- A clear expectation that all will be involved in the journey to transformation and contribute to the construction of the appropriate response to it
- The ability to translate the signposts of change in the language of the staff in a way that excites and engages them in its application
- Rewarding innovation and creativity with support and encouragement and challenging others to further development

Signposts of Innovation

- **New technology**
- **Emerging work processes**
- **Failure of old processes**
- **Changing priorities**
- **Shift in expectations**
- **Altered outcomes**

Personal Creativity

- **Openness to the new**
- **Continuous learning**
- **Hunger for information**
- **Use of the media**
- **Experimental attitude**
- **Willingness to risk**

CO-CREATION

Wise leaders recognize that innovation cannot be unilaterally driven. Ultimately, the creative act is a collective one and requires an ability to excite others and get them on board. No one person is responsible for creating the future, even if the idea was generated out of the thinking and reflecting of an individual. To translate ideas into action requires the concerted effort of a number of committed people in the dynamic act of co-creating—the transformation of an idea into reality (Albrecht, 2003).

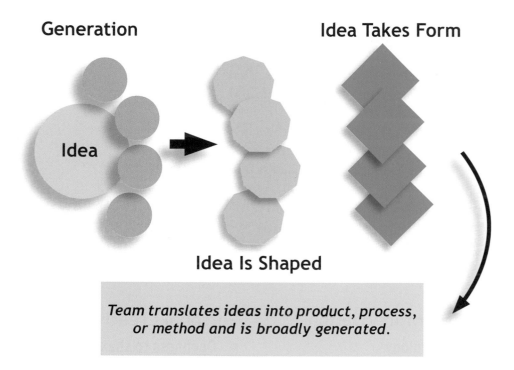

Generation

Idea

Idea Takes Form

Idea Is Shaped

Team translates ideas into product, process, or method and is broadly generated.

Creativity Demands Engagement

- Creativity can generate from individuals or teams but must be shared in order to be translated into something of value.

- The leader gathers the creative team together to feed their insight with dialog, challenge, new thinking, and willingness to explore further.

- The leader can identify in the creative person the unique expression of creativity and make it possible to be nurtured and expressed.

- Creativity within must be regularly nourished by new thinking and exposure to other creative people or it dies.

ADULT-TO-ADULT COMMUNICATION

Leaders have to end the dependency on parent-child relationships at work. So often much of the crippling nature of the relationship between managers and staff is driven by this vertical and controlling interaction. In the contemporary age, where accountability is so essential to the values and outcomes of work, this kind of relationship simply cannot be sustained. Yet because of the years of such behaviors on the part of managers and staff, it is difficult to imagine how these entrenched actions can be overcome.

Change begins with expectations. Leaders and managers must change the expectations staff have with regard to their role. The controlling parental character of the interaction must be replaced with a more partnership-based approach that represents a basis in equity. Each must understand and value the unique relationship to achieve outcomes. The manager provides the context for work; the worker provides the content. When these accountabilities are forgotten or misaligned or confused between the roles, respect and legitimate contribution from them gets lost. It is in honoring and living the distinct accountabilities each has to their role (and to each other) that value can be obtained from both (Bolman & Deal, 2003).

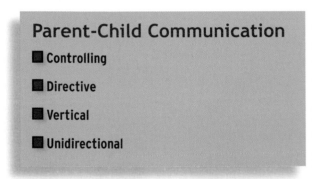

Parent-Child Communication

- ■ **Controlling**
- ■ **Directive**
- ■ **Vertical**
- ■ **Unidirectional**

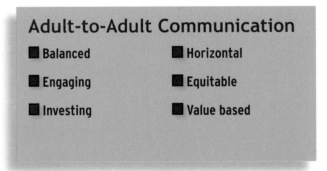

Adult-to-Adult Communication

- ■ **Balanced**
- ■ **Engaging**
- ■ **Investing**
- ■ **Horizontal**
- ■ **Equitable**
- ■ **Value based**

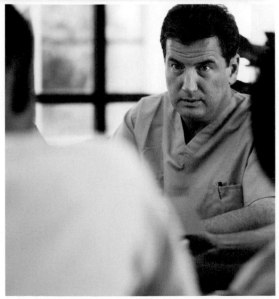

Note:

Managers must stop parenting the staff and staff must stop childish behaviors and relational dependencies. In a parent-child environment, the behaviors become dysfunctional and develop into a conflicted codependency that diminishes the respect each has for the other and ensures that no sustainable value and outcome can ever be achieved. Productive and healthy workplaces require an adult-to-adult relationship.

Ovecoming Parent-child Behaviors

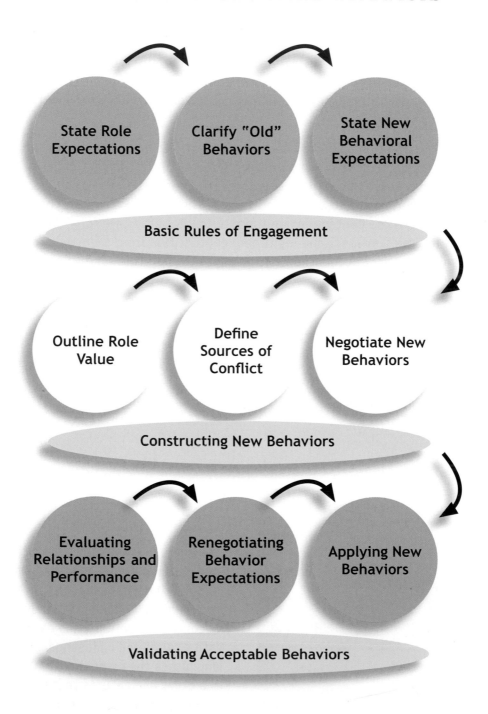

State Role Expectations

Clarify "Old" Behaviors

State New Behavioral Expectations

Basic Rules of Engagement

Outline Role Value

Define Sources of Conflict

Negotiate New Behaviors

Constructing New Behaviors

Evaluating Relationships and Performance

Renegotiating Behavior Expectations

Applying New Behaviors

Validating Acceptable Behaviors

Extinguishing Parental Behaviors in the Leader

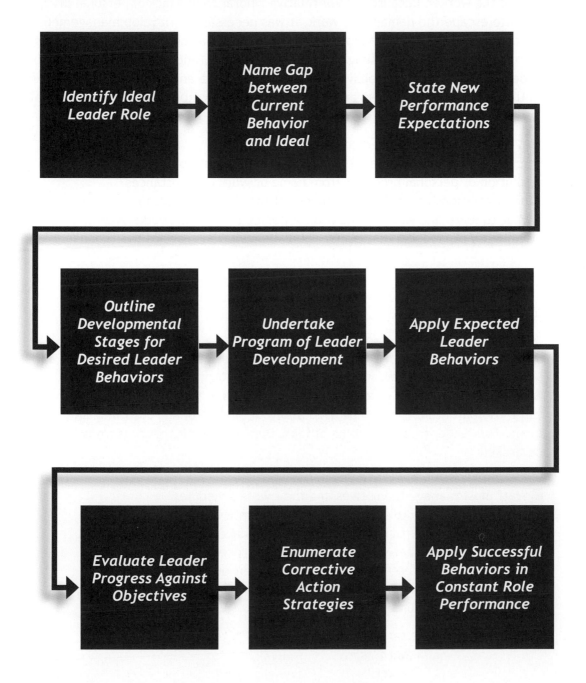

CONFRONTING CHILDLIKE BEHAVIORS IN THE STAFF

For years the staff have been positioned as the "children" of the organization. Much of the control mechanisms in the organization were directed to controlling the otherwise undisciplined and misdirected energies of the worker. Because of their relative ignorance and lack of personal discipline and their willingness to escape the demands of work, it was necessary to develop management-derived control mechanisms to provide the frame for acceptable behaviors. Interestingly enough, such mechanisms proved to be a self-fulfilling prophesy for leaders, and the staff ended up behaving exactly as expected. Indeed, such behaviors have now become entrenched within the American workplace on the part of both managers and staff. The staff now represent the following pattern of behavior:

- No control over their own work schedules
- No full participation in the assignment of work tasks and responsibilities
- External resolution of personal problems from home or work circumstances
- Nonresolution of relationship conflicts arising out of the work relationship
- Being told what to learn and what is required for personal continuing education
- Parental disciplinary procedures that punish "bad" behavior and reward the "good"

Pushing the "Children" into Adulthood

Leaders must stop the parental patterns of behavior in their tracks if there is to be any meaningful accountability and ownership in the staff. No longer can those parental behaviors be used as a tool of control and staff management. The leader must undertake at least the following if that pattern is to be broken:

- ■ "Mama" doesn't work here anymore.
- ■ Staff must manage themselves and their work schedules.
- ■ Staff must be able to problem solve their own issues.
- ■ Staff must fully participate in setting work goals and processes.
- ■ Evaluation of competence is always a staff process.
- ■ Staff must be competent enough to solve their own problems.
- ■ Team-based approaches must be used to set direction, undertake work, and evaluate outcomes.

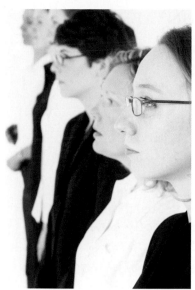

Note:

Staff cannot be accountable for what the leader demands. Leaders must enable the staff to set their own agendas and meet performance objectives. Although leaders may define the "what" and "why" of work, staff defines the "how."

CREATING STAFF OWNERSHIP

Leaders cannot get from the staff what they do not own. One of the basic tenets of professionalism is the commitment to the accountability of the individual, which depends on personal ownership of role and obligation for its full expression. The leader must allow this dynamic to operate everywhere in the organization:

1. Never allow staff to transfer issues and problems to the leader to resolve.

2. Be clear about the elements of accountability that differentiate the role of the leader from that of the staff.

3. Develop decisional skills and group process talent within the staff.

4. Give staff the tools and information they need to make good decisions.

5. Supplement staff decisions with resources that enable them to succeed.

6. Evaluate staff skills and develop individual where deficits exist-never step in and exercise the skill yourself.

7. Celebrate success and reward accomplishments.

8. Provide opportunities to be creative and innovative in work planning.

9. Advise staff when parameters change or new information emerges.

10. Lose the "dead wood" and the naysayers, ASAP.

RESPONSIBILITY VS. ACCOUNTABILITY

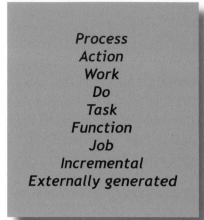

Process
Action
Work
Do
Task
Function
Job
Incremental
Externally generated

Product
Result
Outcome
Accomplish
Difference
Fit
Role
Sustainable
Internally generated

Distinguishing Responsibility from Accountability

Staff often get the concepts of responsibility and accountability confused and treat them as though they were one and the same. As indicated here, they are not the same and need to be operationalized more fully. It is the role of the leader to keep them from being connected in ways that address neither responsibility nor accountability and provide no real framework for individual effort. The leader must focus the staff.

■ Keep eyes on the results and work backward to process work. Processes change, accountability rarely does.

■ Staff must define their own contribution to outcomes and sustain them over time.

■ The conditions of accountability, autonomy, authority, and competence are a part of developing maturity and should be evaluated regularly.

■ The leader supplies the tools; the staff provide the applications.

■ Staff must assess current levels of accountability and change based on what the results yield.

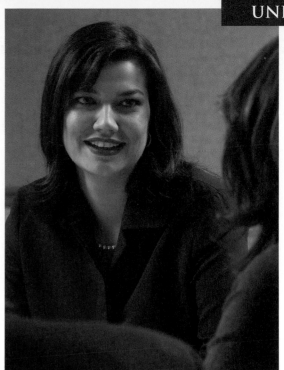

> ## Note:
>
> No one should expect to be invited to the full expression of partnership in the work of the organization. That invitation occurred when one accepted the opportunity to work. Everyone has the right to expect the full engagement of their work colleagues and the commitment necessary to make that successful.

EXPECTATION, NOT INVITATION

In the adult workplace, all participants are expected to play the role they consented to. There are no participants who do not express an obligation to the role they occupy. Indeed, there are no invited guests to the experience of life. One either owns the role played or the role is not occupied. This seems strange at first glance, but on deeper reflection, it is an extremely important tenet of the adult-to-adult workplace (Argyris, 1999).

Invitation to play the full role and partnership in meeting the organization's obligations is not a subset of membership in the work community. One is engaged in work precisely to make a contribution within the skill-set defined for the role. It is anticipated that the individual will commit all energies to the exercise of the role without encouragement or coercion. That commitment is a clear element of the expression of the role. Anyone not aware of that expectation as they begin the role isn't going to be expressive of it, even if invited to further commit to the behaviors or expectations for the role.

In the adult-to-adult equation, it is anticipated that all players are equally on board. This notion of equity is a primary centerpiece of the valuing of each role and the expression of its relationship and impact on the roles of others. The aggregated effort of all roles is necessary for the effective interface of energy in a way that ensures good outcomes and work products. Anyone shirking any part of the role will have a clear effect on the work of others and, ultimately affect the achievement of good outcomes. In such a circumstance, the effect is a negative one and reduces the net value of the work of all and pulls energy away from the collective effort to add value and produce good outcomes.

EXPECTATIONS FOR FULL ENGAGEMENT

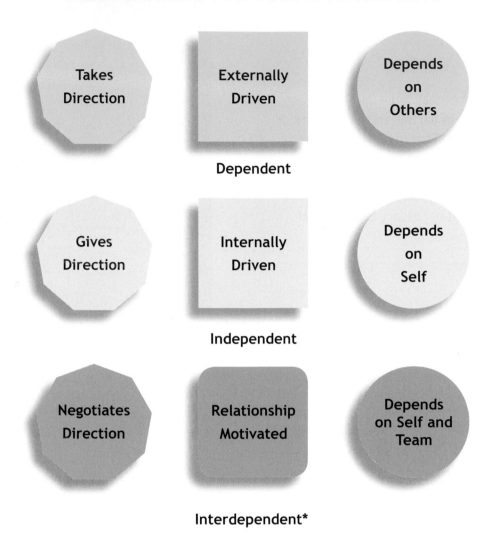

Takes Direction

Externally Driven

Depends on Others

Dependent

Gives Direction

Internally Driven

Depends on Self

Independent

Negotiates Direction

Relationship Motivated

Depends on Self and Team

Interdependent*

*The most adult pattern of behavior because it reflects a healthy interaction between the self and others and facilitates the collective contribution of all team members to the integrated effort necessary to sustain positive work outcomes.

ADULT-TO-ADULT WORK BEHAVIORS

Personal Components

- Strong self-awareness
- Knows own skill contributions well
- Is clear about relationship to others
- Is able to fully commit to the work team
- Open and available to other's evaluation and input

Relationships Components

- Can interact well with others
- Takes criticism with concern and willingness to hear
- Contributes to the work effort of others
- Knows the skill-fit of self to the work of others
- Can commit to the consensus goals of the team

Team Components

- Pulls own weight with regard to team effort
- Expresses contribution within the context of the team
- Recalibrates effort when team dynamics change
- Is a positive force within the team's relationship framework
- Celebrates success within the team
- Deals well with the conflict of creativity and diversity

Rules of Good Leadership

1. Do not assume the accountability that belongs to the team and to individuals.

2. Make sure all team members know their contribution to the collective work efforts of the team.

3. The team's goals and purposes must always be precise and clear to the members before expectations can be defined.

4. You are not a parent; make sure the team members can identify and resolve their own issues with resources you make available to them.

5. Ensure that the team has the right information to make decisions that affects their work—do not overload them with extraneous data.

6. Assess the potential for conflict early so that it can be resolved before it becomes war and impedes the team's ability to overcome it.

7. Help the team evaluate its dynamics and progress in the effort to improve and advance both work outcomes and relationships.

Note:

The wise leader never assumes the parental role and does not allow any one else to either. Staff must be self-directed and engaged in the full partnership of work relationships if sustainable outcomes are to be achieved.

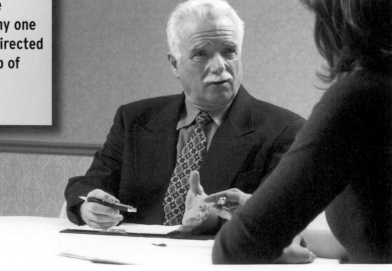

References

Albrecht, K. (2003). *The power of minds at work: Organizational intelligence in action.* New York: AMACOM.

Argyris, C. (1999). *On organizational learning.* New York: Blackwell Publishers.

Bolm an, L. G., & Deal, T. E. (2003). *Reframing organizations: Artistry, choice, and leadership* (3rd ed.). San Francisco: Jossey-Bass.

Campbell, P., & Burnaby, B. (2001). *Participatory practices in adult education.* Mahwah, NJ; London: Lawrence Erlbaum Associates.

Garvin, D. (2000). *Learning in action.* Boston: Harvard Business School Publishing.

Malloch, K, & Porter-O'Grady, T. (2005). *The quantum leader: Applications for the new world of work.* Sudbury, MA: Jones and Bartlett.

Porter-O'Grady, T., & Malloch, K. (2002). *Quantum leadership: A textbook of new leadership.* Sudbury, MA: Jones and Bartlett.

Porter-O'Grady, T., & Wilson, C. (1999). *Leading the revolution in healthcare: Igniting performance, changing systems.* Gaithersburg, MD: Aspen.

Suggested Readings

Albrecht, K. (2003). *The power of minds at work: Organizational intelligence in action.* New York: AMACOM.

Argyris, C. (1999). *On organizational teaming.* New York: Blackwell Publishers.

Coutu, D. (2002). Edgar Schein: The anxiety of learning. *Harvard Business Review, 80*(3), 100-106.

Fulmer, W. (2000). *Shaping the adaptive organization: Landscapes, learning and leading in volatile times.* Chicago: AMACOM.

Malloch, K., & Porter-O'Grady, T. (2005). *The quantum leader: Applications for the new world of work.* Sudbury, MA: Jones and Bartlett.

Oostendorp, H. V. (2003). *Cognition in a digital world.* Mahwah, NJ: Lawrence Erlbaum Associates.

Vaill, P. (2002). *Learning as a way of being.* San Francisco: Jossey-Bass.

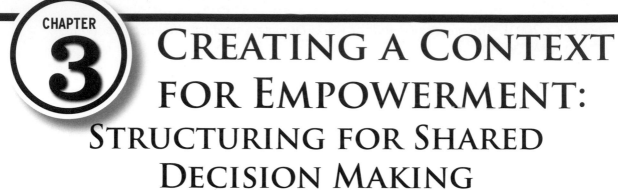

CHAPTER 3

CREATING A CONTEXT FOR EMPOWERMENT:
STRUCTURING FOR SHARED DECISION MAKING

Inclusion is not enough to ensure effective decisions and action. Building an infrastructure of engagement is essential to sustaining involvement and good decision making.

MAKING SHARED DECISION MAKING A STRATEGY

Developing a shared decision-making structure and shared decision-making approach to empowering the staff does not happen by accident. Development and application of a workable strategy require and advance major changes in how the organization operates and makes decisions. Strategy guides the change makers and provides a useful evaluation tool. An effective strategy for implementing shared decision making provides one plan for managers and another for clinical staff. Because implementation requires frequent adjustment for managers, they are the first focus of attention in the planning process. Problems and issues with a manager's understanding and role need attention at the outset so that a common basis for implementation is ensured. Planning and implementation usually take a minimum of 3 years. Anticipated time for full implementation is 3 to 5 years, although organizational and behavioral change will be evident before this time. The strategy uses rules already in place at the time implementation is initiated. This bridges the old and the new, allowing staff to see contrasts that move the vision out of the realm of theory and into practice (Porter-O'Grady, 1991b). Several things need to be in place:

1. A strong organizational commitment to engaging and investing staff in decisions that affect their practice and the goals of the organization
2. A clear understanding of the principles of shared decision making and clarification of accountability specific to management and the accountability of the staff
3. A willingness to undertake the necessary activities in changing both structure and behaviors, including confronting the vagaries and "noise" associated with this work
4. New leadership principles and practices that establish a partnership relationship of the staff, shifting the locus of control and building different interactions
5. A commitment to stay with it through the full processes of implementation, making shared decision making "our way of doing business"

Strategy Development

- Provide a roadmap and evaluation tool.
- Involve two parallel implementation patterns.
- Expect plan to take minimum of 3 years.
- Full implementation takes up to 5 years.
- Use an existing starting point for change.

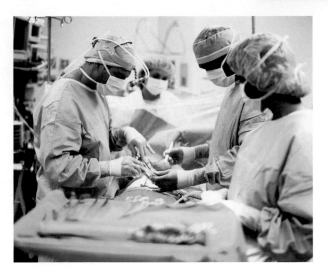

ESTABLISHING A COMMON PURPOSE

Staff accountability is the impetus for success and achievement of organizational purpose because it is tied to outcomes. Shared decision making depends on a new way of thinking, new roles, and different approaches to produce the outcomes. Outcomes are generated out of partnerships contingent upon role clarity, function, contribution, and a mutual understanding of purpose and mission. Shared purpose requires that every part of an organization have the right to access every other part in order to ensure each has what is needed to do the right thing the first time (Stack & Burlington, 2002). This concept is sometimes difficult to grasp because traditionally organizations have compartmentalized and isolated functions. Lack of accessibility to certain parts of the organization confounds the smooth operation and achievement of mission because the path of least resistance is to go around these obstacles rather than break them down. Given the right tools, commitment and ownership grow around shared purpose, which becomes more central with staff involvement.

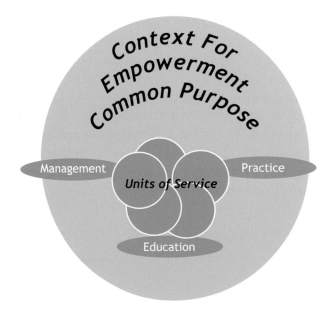

Achieving Shared Purpose

- Evolves from accountabilities sustaining it
- Enhanced by full accessibility to organization
- Grows along with commitment and ownership
- Becomes more central with staff involvement

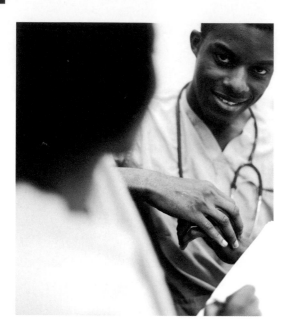

Structure Cultivates Ownership

- Empowerment increases accountability levels.
- Sharing decisions fosters staff involvement.
- Point-of-service focus facilitates relationships.
- Congruence contributes to stability and trust.
- Leadership vigilance removes barriers.

PARTNERSHIP AND OWNERSHIP

Partnerships require involvement, which is one of the requisites for ownership. Involvement and relationships are crucial at the point-of-service because control, leadership, function, activity, value, and determination of quality are mainly located there. The demand for increasing levels of accountability is met when staff are empowered with authority for practice. Shared decision making requires the application of ownership to the work of building new structures. The language, structures, processes, and outcomes must be congruent throughout the organization for true ownership to evolve. Congruence is reassuring and leads staff into trusting partnerships with management and coworkers. Ambiguity is the enemy of shared decision making. Leadership's awareness of unresolved issues, hidden agendas, personal biases, incomplete planning, and unexpressed concerns allows them to be addressed before sabotage of effective planning and implementation.

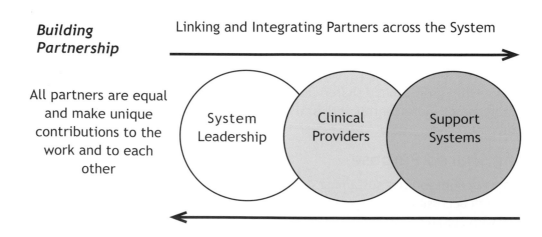

Building Partnership

Linking and Integrating Partners across the System

All partners are equal and make unique contributions to the work and to each other

System Leadership — Clinical Providers — Support Systems

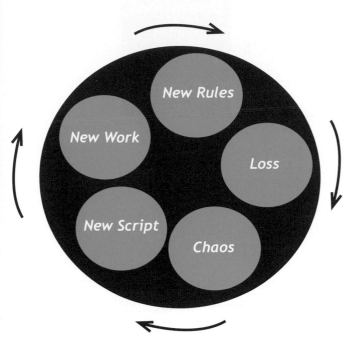

Work Changes

Work never stays the same. It must respond to the changing external and internal demand and to new and transformative technology that impacts how work gets done. Every person must recognize the fact that his or her work cannot remain the same. People must end addiction to ritual and routine, no longer allowing it to insulate them from necessary change and the learning of new ways.

New Principles

As work becomes different, the way work is determined, allocated, and delivered demands a different set of relationships between all the players. A new set of principles must now guide this relationship, inform it, and be demonstrated in the common work that results from it. Without commitment to these principles, the relationship necessary to sustain shared decision making is lost. Commitment to these principles must be pervasive (Porter-O'Grady & Wilson, 1997).

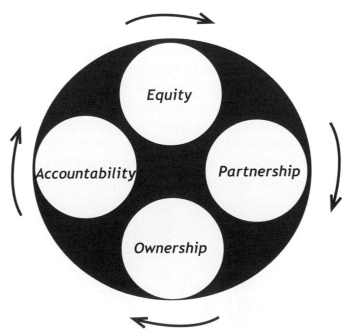

New Principles for a New Age

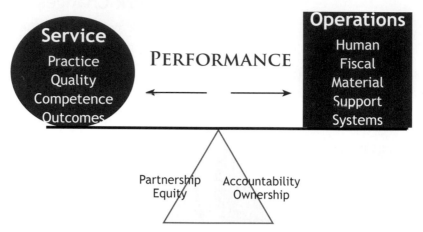

CLARITY REGARDING DISTRIBUTION OF ACCOUNTABILITY

Accountability requires a clarity around the locus of control for decision making. Accountability relates specifically to decisions and actions. Therefore, a specific understanding regarding the unique contributions to accountabilities that are played in the organization is a critical first step in ensuring the success in creating a shared decision-making approach. It should be understood that in all organized human systems there are management accountabilities related specifically to controlling resources. This is true regardless of what kind of management systems exist in the organization. Even in self-directed workplaces there are resource-driven management accountabilities that must be addressed in order to ensure that the context of work has been addressed (Porter-O'Grady, 1991a). These are human, fiscal, material, support, and systems functions that reflect specific management accountabilities. No matter what role is played, these resource or contextual accountabilities are always driven by the manager role. In a professional organization the profession also has distinct and unique accountabilities that relate specifically them. They are practice, quality, competence, and ensuring outcomes. In an effective shared decision-making environment these accountabilities are distinguished, separated, and clearly exercised within their locus of control at all times.

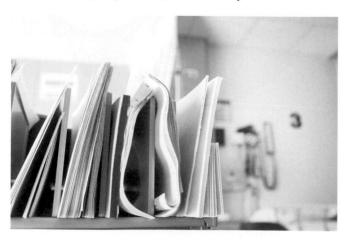

Note:

Because accountability abhors ambiguity it is important that clarity and role specificity in relationship to performance expectations and individual accountability be specifically enumerated.

MAKING ACCOUNTABLE DECISIONS

The continuous ritual of doing work often becomes seductive and steals the focus of attention away from the value of work, and focus is, instead, on the processes of work. All practitioners must be aware of the fact that, whereas the work is important, what is even more important is that it make a difference and has an effect on those to whom it is directed. The real workplace is rife with examples of individuals who are working diligently, undertaking a great many tasks, are very busy, yet actually produce few results. Work is valuable to the extent of its effect on purpose and out-come, not simply because someone is doing work. Work is not a value in and of itself. It becomes valuable when connected to its purposes and to the achievement of its results in a way that can be sustained (Hackman, 2002).

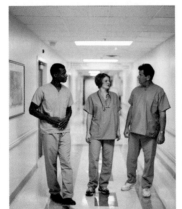

Responsibility of work relates to how individuals focus on their work, how well they do their work, and the amount and quality of that work. The focus is on action and activity, representing an orientation to process.

Accountability relates to the outcomes or the products of work. The focus of account-ability is on results, making a difference, having an impact, and producing meaningful and measurable results.

Responsibility (20th Century)	Accountability (21st Century)
Process	Product
Action	Result
Work	Outcome
Do	Accomplish
Task	Difference
Function	Fit
Job	Role
Incremental	Sustainable
Externally generated	Internally generated

BUILDING GOOD STRUCTURE

Achieving involvement in shared decision making requires creating a structure that ensures seamlessness between each component of the organization, covering decision making, operations, and service (McDonagh, 1991). This seamlessness provides the format for organizing decision making and paves the way for partnership development. Partnership demands dialog about the relationship between players and the way in which work gets structured and completed. In health care, provider relationships contribute greatly to the character and quality of care because they are inextricably linked. Shared decision making acknowledges this and frames work to promote this advantage. The effectiveness of shared decision making is a reminder that the organization needs the contributions of all its members because no one worker can know about or control all of the elements of the relationship necessary to consistently achieve desired outcomes. Partnerships enable the concerted effort required to effectively address the issues of change and their concurrent influence on outcomes (DePree, 1997).

Accountability Is Specifically Located within Its Locus-of-Control

*Clinical account-
ability is expressed
by the staff in their
role, and manage-
ment accountabil-
ity is expressed by
managers*

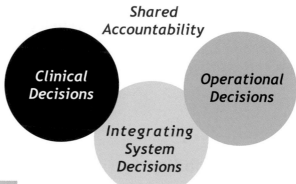

*Shared
Accountability*

*Clinical
Decisions*

*Operational
Decisions*

*Integrating
System
Decisions*

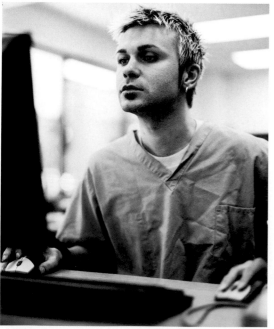

Revised Structure for Participation

- Seamless format for decision making
- Decision making, operations, and service linked
- Structure built from the inside out
- Begins with the provider-patient team
- Outcomes of work take precedence

Getting Ready for Staff Change

•Strong support from management team
•Committed relationship between leaders
•Nurse executive partnered with managers
•Individual understanding of role expression
•Transition from focus on self to groups
•Deserved trust and dependence on others

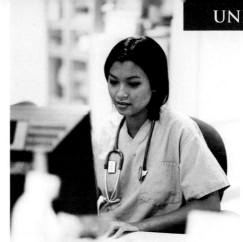

Shared decision making does not succeed without support of the management team. Support means the willingness to undergo personal and professional change and to lead that change in the staff (Nelson, 2000). The connection between the managers and the nurse executive signals to staff that the plan has unity. It is beneficial for managers to study their expression of the management role in order to understand how staff may perceive their influence. Managers are instrumental in providing a setting that emphasizes group or team values as focus shifts from self to group relationships and functions. Astute managers emphasize, early on that success is more a matter of relationship than function. The model of management striving for a mutually satisfying working relationship serves as a framework for the emerging relationship in the staff. Management's sincere trust and dependence on each other fuels staff commitment to change.

Unit (Point-of-Service) Leaders

● Change the decision-making accountability (locus-of-control).

● Develop new leadership competencies.

● Take back accountability for staff-driven decisions (greatest threat).

● Learn partnership leadership skills.

Unit Leader Skills

● New leadership skill-set development (facilitation, coordination, integration).

● Intentional surrender of past management practices.

● Develop staff accountability (practice driven).

● Model fails without leadership development and behavioral change.

PRINCIPLES OF SUSTAINABLE LEADERSHIP

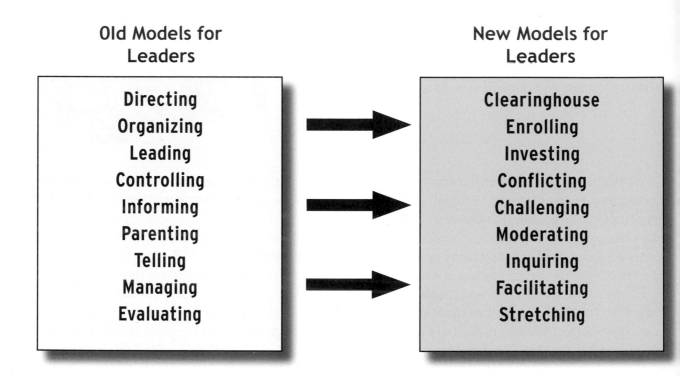

Old Models for Leaders	New Models for Leaders
Directing	Clearinghouse
Organizing	Enrolling
Leading	Investing
Controlling	Conflicting
Informing	Challenging
Parenting	Moderating
Telling	Inquiring
Managing	Facilitating
Evaluating	Stretching

NEW LEADERSHIP FOR SHARED DECISION MAKING

In a shared decision-making environment, leadership is critical to maintaining appropriate partnership and interacted behaviors and to sustaining the principles of shared decision making. Without clearly identifying the specific kinds of leadership behaviors necessary to succeed, it is difficult to adjust the leadership patterns so they fit a more horizontal, partnership-based approach to interaction than the traditional hierarchical, vertical orientation to the management-staff relationship.

It is important that leaders spend time in dialog with regard to the specific kinds of leadership changes that need to occur in order to support an empowered staff (Parker, 2003). As indicated in this chapter, specific accountabilities differentiate the role of manager from the professional. As these accountabilities are clarified and separated, as well as clearly enumerated with regard to performance expectations, it is important to develop the skills necessary to exercise the right accountabilities. The leader's role moves from directing, organizing, controlling, and disciplining to one of coordination, integration, and facilitation. Having played the hierarchical and controlling role as the major expression of the manager's role, the individual leader will need time to reflect, evaluate, and develop a plan of leadership and behavioral change that better fits a more partnership-based horizontal framework for leadership and managing relationships (Chrispeels, 2004).

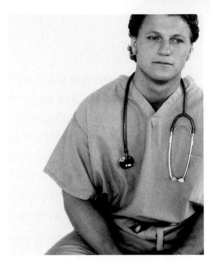

Relinquishing the Past

- Recognize losses felt by staff and leadership.
- Incorporate grieving time into change process.
- Understand steps creating a sense of ending.
- Develop formal process to begin change.
- Construct a realistic timeline for change.

Understanding the need for staff and leadership to deal with losses and incorporating this into the change process is essential for successful change (Lundin, 2001). Generally, three steps create a sense of endings. These steps are essential for a new reality to evolve, one that is so different from the old that this new reality eventually replaces the old way of doing things.

Disengagement is a period when issues of concern must be adequately addressed. This involves a significant shift that promises major adjustments in expectation and performance.

Misidentification is the point at which leadership and staff consciously deny the value of the tradition they are moving out of and are ready to apply a new set of values and principles as tests for their thinking and acting.

Disenchantment is the final step in initiating personal transition and allows for final separation. New behaviors that exemplify the values of the shared decision-making system begin to emerge and staff reject those of the past. Failure to move successfully through disenchantment can result in bitterness and rejection of the necessity to change.

Growing Leadership Importance

- Conduct continual ongoing surveillance of decision-making growth and development
- Determine needs for support and development and provide timely response
- Provide ego support and self-awareness
- Articulate clear expectations for performance
- Push developmental stages and evaluate effectiveness
- Create opportunities for small successes
- Measure and acknowledge progress and effectiveness
- Adjust and change elements and experimentation processes that are not working effectively
- Help staff develop new skills for effective decision making

> ### Note:
> Empowering staff means making sure that they have the right, power, and competence to exercise their accountability and achieve meaningful outcomes. Without all of these elements of accountability the ability to express it is compromised.

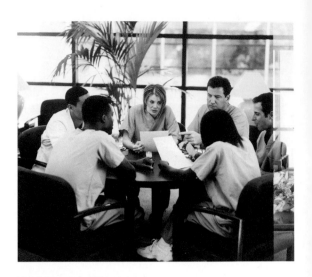

Empowered Staff Behaviors

Openness to new realities	Willingness to change
Sound practice standards	Clear sense of ethics
Engagement of their issues	Fundamental honesty
Emerging curiosity	Consensus seeking
Ability to express concerns	Structured risk taking
Committed to competency	Abide by consensus
Growing involvement	Increasing self-esteem
Exhibiting creativity	Initiating partnerships

INDIVIDUAL EMPOWERMENT CHANGES

Along with structural, organizational, and cultural changes, individual change must take place within point-of-service workers who drive the new processes. Structures and efforts that lead to empowered behaviors in the professional worker must be applied to successfully achieve changed behaviors. There are many signs that point to progress toward transformation. The characteristics and behaviors listed above are some that exemplify staff transition to empowerment. The most challenging part of implementing shared decision making is in the activities related to involving the staff and changing their perceptions about decision making and their role in it. Perceptions change as the organization's commitment to equity is demonstrated. Examples include the composition of group membership and the role of staff in decisions that affect their future. Demonstration of equity conveys that all outcome is sustained through the activities of the whole work team.

A Forum for Shared Decision Making

Staff transition may be impaired in the presence of personal feelings, insights, fears, and perceptions that might be responsible for preventing implementation from happening in the organization. Time in working out these issues is essential, if a strong premise and foundation for shared decision making are to be in place. Knowledge is only one of the conditions necessary to successful implementation. A safe forum should be ensured for dealing with the hard issues of practice and operating relationships. These issues are best dealt with in a nonthreatening place where frank and open discussions affecting the organization and the implementation of shared decision making get addressed (Surowiecki, 2004). Documented support from the nurse executive is a major consideration for success because shared decision making never works if senior management is not in support of it. Managers must be able to seek and get support during transition because their effectiveness is contingent on the support and encouragement of peers, as well as executive support.

Magnet Excellence and Shared Decision Making

The American Nurses Credentialing Center's Magnet Recognition Program has strongly identified shared decision making as a central component of the structures necessary to ensure professional action related to excellence in practice. For example, Force 2 and Force 13 (see the Magnet Recognition Program Manual) specifically identify shared decision-making as an element essential to the recognition of excellence. In fact, the program recognizes that without a structure of empowered shared decision making, the professional practice expectations for excellence cannot be sustained over time. Creating staff empowerment processes and building a shared decision-making infrastructure that supports it is essential to both obtaining and sustaining levels of excellence in nursing practice. Furthermore, an empowered professional staff is a strong indicator of the commitment, investment, and full participation necessary to assure engagement of decisions and practices that advance the interests of the profession and improve the quality of its services (Coffman & Gonzales-Molina, 2002).

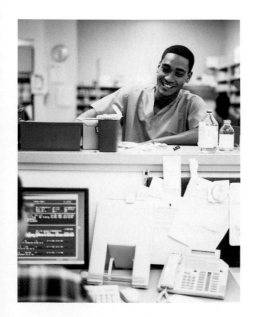

Conditions for Success

- Personal and professional issues addressed
- Time provided to build strong foundation
- Safe forum for frank and open discussions
- A learning and leader skills process for staff
- Staff involvement in creating a staff structure
- Shared decision making as a "way of doing business"
- Continual and active mentoring and support from management

SHARED DECISION-MAKING REQUISITES

- It is point-of-service driven.

- Stakeholders are involved in their own decisions.

- Decisions are made where the work gets done.

- Staff are focused on population/patient care.

- Managers are focused on empowering staff and creating a supportive work environment for staff decisions and practice accountability.

- The goal is to make the right decision as close to the point-of-service as possible.

- The structure of the organization is built to support point-of-service decision making and empower staff to decide and to act in a way that advances the exercise of their practice accountabilities.

21ST CENTURY PRACTICE-BASED ACCOUNTABILITY OF THE CLINICAL STAFF

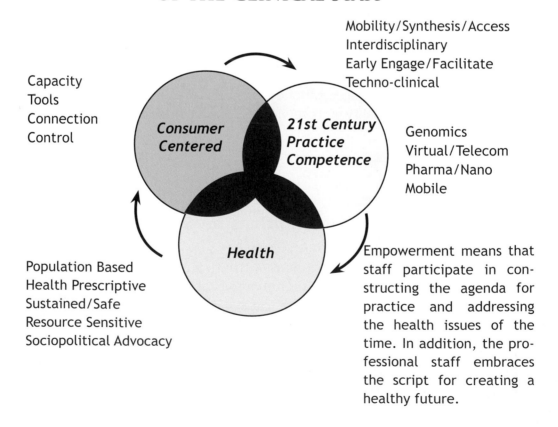

Capacity
Tools
Connection
Control

Mobility/Synthesis/Access
Interdisciplinary
Early Engage/Facilitate
Techno-clinical

Consumer Centered

21st Century Practice Competence

Genomics
Virtual/Telecom
Pharma/Nano
Mobile

Health

Population Based
Health Prescriptive
Sustained/Safe
Resource Sensitive
Sociopolitical Advocacy

Empowerment means that staff participate in constructing the agenda for practice and addressing the health issues of the time. In addition, the professional staff embraces the script for creating a healthy future.

A New Stye of Management

- Managers move from parent to partner, reflecting equity and value of all actions, differentiating value through role rather than position.
- Staff do not need permission to make decisions they own.
- Developmental approach for decision making and learning new skills, ensuring the staff is successful.
- Shift of control of practice and quality issues move from manager to staff.
- Managers move from the control and direction to facilitating, integrating, and coordinating good decision making and clinical action.
- Managers create a safe context for risk taking, confronting conflict, experimentation, and engagement of new processes.
- Managers recognize their own journey of learning in shared decision-making and concentrating on self-development, mentoring, and helping staff learn.
- Managers participate in determining accountability and role; expecting full participation and performance from staff, helping them evaluate and address progress.
- Managers develop strong peer processes regarding defining accountability, performance expectations, work processes, outcome achievement, quality assessment, and performance evaluation.

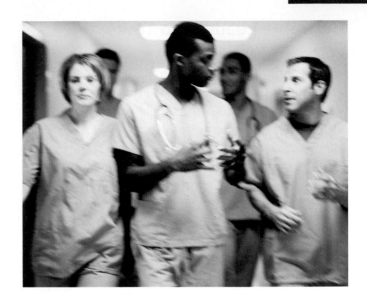

New Behavior

Managers move form the directing role to a facilitating role in shared decision making. This means more asking, less telling; more supporting, less doing; more group work, and less individual task assignment. Staff need accountability and skill to make managers understand that good decisions take time. Some control issues move to staff that, in the past, belonged to management. These issues are related to practice, quality of care, competence, and evaluation demonstrating a greater staff role in an empowered workplace. Managers must be comfortable with this transition of accountabilities. Managers select some of the issues to some of the issues to move to the staff based on preparedness, staff personal comfort, and the degree of risk in the decision. It is difficult for managers to avoid taking the more controlling and easy way of doing things. Extreme patience is demanded on the part of managers to allow staff to make decisions when it would be more convenient for the manager to do it for them.

Desirable Leadership Traits

- Willing to be vulnerable
- Eager to try new ways of doing things
- Not afraid to challenge the status quo
- Aspires to advance professional work
- Motivated to advocate for others
- Knows how to facilitate others' work/relationships
- Values the pursuit of knowledge/innovation
- Dedicated to keeping others fully informed
- Accessible, approachable, and trustworthy

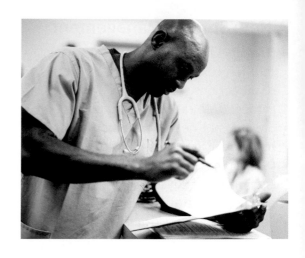

CHANGE LEADERS AND EMPOWERMENT CHAMPIONS

Change agents enable transition to shared decision making and take on the following roles to facilitate change. **Consciousness raisers** focus on issues by challenging authority and identifying dissatisfiers to give form to what everyone already knows. **Implementers** construct processes that undertake change and move them along a continuum. They generate ideas and identify ways of responding. **Outcome seekers** accept that change is going to occur and seek results of the change efforts. They are often characterized as having a bottom-line orientation because they look at what will be produced as the result of change. **Linkage creators** acknowledge that change makers alone do not achieve transition. They establish relationships, coalitions, and partnerships and link resources to ensure success. The role of **balancer** serves to normalize and stabilize a work environment experiencing change. This leader defines boundaries, establishes new values, and builds solidarity.

The wise manager always determines who are the informal change leaders and opinion makers. Managers recognize that informal relationships in any organization are as important as formal interactions. Often because of role or position, a manager cannot be as effective in communicating and relating with staff as can peers. Therefore, the manager uses the informal relationship structure to find catalysts and change agents that can be first engagers and can help address difficult issues and facilitate significant change.

Catalyst for Change

- Essential role for transitional process
- Catalyst and moderator of change
- Not exclusively a management role
- Aware of organization's unique culture
- Use various approaches to change

Note:

Leaders represent in their own behavior, openness, willingness, and engagement.

Values in Shared Decision Making

- Free-flowing information
- Mutual respect
- Diversity-infused collaboration
- Accountability for outcomes
- Empowered actions reflecting ownership
- Professional nursing model
- Shared decision making

Values are expressed through behavior and can often be elicited from observation. It is important to see values congruent with shared decision making, in the conduct of eveyone, if it is to work. Strong leadershio plays a key part in nurturing desired behaviors. Committed leaders work objectively on the road to change, model empowered behaviors, and encourage and praise mature behavior that correspond to a professional practice environment. The norms, rules, and rituals of the past are scrutinized in order to filter out behaviors that do not match the envisioned environment. Initiating forums for discussion or an educational process may be needed to bring a level of awareness to the forefront about negative behavior ingrained in past practice and historic relationships.

The implementation of shared decision making changes organizational culture, which is defined by values. The organizational systems and structures assist in supporting the values and behaviors. Concurrently, values and behaviors shape development of empowerment. As the organization moves toward changing values, the structure and support systems are redesigned to meet the values.

Transformation of the culture involves diligence, careful planning, and time. Requisites for change inlude a firm, consistent set of values, long-term commitment, constant evaluation and reevaluation of each element in the system, and education of all the parties to keep the vision alive. Role expectations impact behavior, as do skill and knowledge. Increasing knowledge and skill to affect changing values and behavior is helpful. Effective leadership guides behavioral changes that change culture.

The change leader recognizes that empowerment is a journey for both manager and staff. Clearly building change on a well-defined set of values with established parameters for behavior creates a firm foundation upon which to unfold new empowerment processes and actions.

Empowerment Values

1. Confirm and commit to new values.
2. Create a vision and enlist others.
3. Role model management changes first.
4. Promote and set expectations.
5. Build skills along the way.
6. Change sructure and systems to support the new values.
7. Define specifically the value of roles and link them to outcomes.

Historic Culture

- Unclear or uncertain about quality
- Inhibits creative behaviors; values rituals and routines
- Diminishes the loftiest goals
- Challenges what is formally communicated in an organization
- Can create a powerful Influence
- Requires laborious effort to alter

Changing Culture

- It is possible with a plan and creative and committed leadership.
- It requires planned time for change to take hold; staff need to mourn losses, embrace the new.
- Leaders create conditions for desired environment.
- Immediate and continual feedback combats immature behaviors.
- It includes key moments, celebration, and evaluation of incremental changes.

INFLUENCE OF CULTURE

It is important to acknowledge the influence of environmental culture on employees and work because of the powerful force it exerts. Staff are not typically familiar with management skills and practices. Historically, managers have taken accountability for all the areas of the practice system, including many of the decisions regarding patient care. Structure and education are necessary in order to achieve the smooth transfer of account- ability. In addition to the unfamiliarity with managing groups and systems, the staff has a level of fear related to change as an added element with which to cope. Many employees are afraid to ask questions and take positions. There often is an underlying culture that reinforces staff fear to initiate or act. It is obvious that this fear in a professional system severely hampers the organization's efforts to innovate and change.

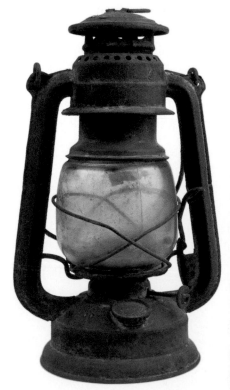

Culture magnifies or ameliorates the trepidation of caregivers encountering new expectations for accountability. For example, an individual, hearing encouragement to participate, summons courage to speak in a meeting and is rebuffed. A discrepancy exists between the system's message of openness and the "old" culture of suppression. Culture sends a contradictory message that communicates that "this is not the way things work around here." Culture begins to change when peer pressure is brought to bear to extinguish unwanted behaviors. Trust, or lack of it, has enormous consequences for organizations. Consolidated and integrated actions are needed to counteract the effect of old culture until it is changed to reflect more professional behaviors. Leaders, who develop strategies to address changing culture, are more likely to obtain support because of their willingness to

Leadership and Empowerment

- Everyone is learning.
- There is a plan for change all can engage.
- New culture invalidates the old.
- Manager adopts new facilitating behaviors.
- Managers/staff work on clarifying and applying new accountabilities.
- Reorient on principles of empowerment and ownership.
- Maintain focus on behavioral change, new

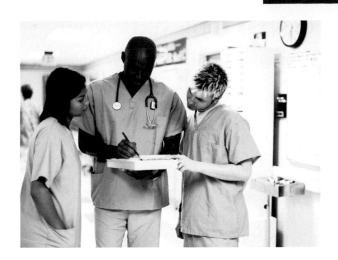

Leaders are products of the same work history as staff and face the same challenges; therefore, leaders may lack skills to lead an empowered, self-directed work team. Mangers plan personal and role changes because they learn along with staff. Empowerment exists when there is an expectation on the part of managers that those doing the work own the decisions affecting their work. Managers can let go of control of the decisions for which they have been accountable, and move on to facilitating, implementing, and coordinating accountabilities.

Focusing on the stated values and principles of shared decision making, in addition to achieving agree-upon outcomes, provides reference points amid the vagaries of change. The leader is always evaluating staff understanding and progress. Leaders must not short-circuit the timing and planning of the stages of movement from the hierarchical environment to an empowered workplace. It is a journey, and each stage has value and meaning. The leader works to assist both organization and people in making a meaningful transition that piece by piece builds the bridge to increased accountability, ownership, and investment on the part of leader and staff. This transformational work improves practice, outcomes, and accelerates provider and patient satisfaction.

In shared decision making, a manager's focus is different from those directly providing services to patients. Processes that advance patient care, such as development of the shared decision-making process, are shared with the staff as their means of participation. Managers create an environment that enables staff to be self-directed in dealing with clinical and service issues. They monitor the empowerment of teams to guide/advance their relationships and control. Managers are also concerned with the competence of staff in managing work and arrange for education, training, or contact with an expert within the organization when indicated. Overall, a manager effectively leads by giving staff the resources and support to address issues, resolve inherent conflicts, and achieve desired outcomes.

Leadership Support

- Resolves developmental issues
- Enhances the learning context
- Provides tools to problem solve
- Ensures access to expert resources
- Creates a self-directed environment
- Supports innovation and creativity in the staff

CONTEXT FOR STAFF WORK

- Authority and responsibility for professional practice invested at the clinical point-of-service
- Individual accountabilities and expectations clearly delineated in role description
- Shared decision making embedded in relationships/structures that intersect role descriptions
- Knowledge worker's decisions and participation at point-of-service of prime importance to an organization's success

One of the roles of the manager is to conceive ways to help staff recognize how their work integrates into the whole and perpetuates the mission of the organization. Placing competence, authority, and responsibility for practice at the point-of-service is the purpose of shared decision making. The manager explains how it fits with the work of others in the organization. Authority and responsibility for professional practice are invested with the staff in shared decision making. The knowledge and skills staff bring to their roles are applied to the goals of the organization. Knowledge, possessed by these workers is one of the major mediums of value and exchange in the workplace. Goals rarely get acted upon or fulfilled at the highest reaches of the organization. It is where the work is done, action is applied, and outcomes are achieved with the purposes and values of the organization that value is clearly exemplified. Managers recognize this context and work to build the infrastructure that supports it and create congruent leadership behaviors that advance and sustain it.

Empowered Practice

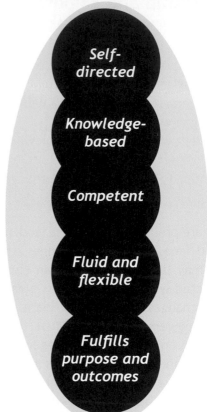

Self-directed

Knowledge-based

Competent

Fluid and flexible

Fulfills purpose and outcomes

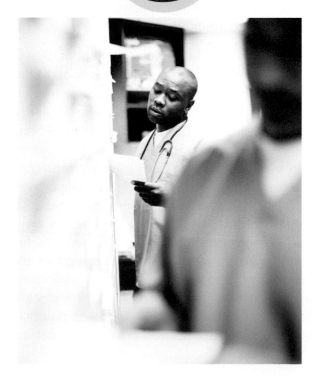

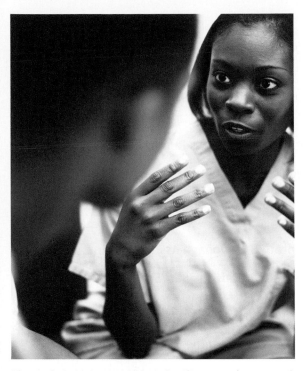

The Power of Empowerment

- System strengthened through integration
- Role of every player recognized
- System design ensures effective functioning
- Structure instills and sustains empowerment
- Flexibility key to cost-effective efficacy
- Order due to freedom to self-organize
- Delivery system supports all disciplines
- Optimum levels of performance/outcome
- Ownership cultivates desire for excellence
- Depends on staff competence and judgement

Shared decision making facilitates the creation of an effective organization based on a new professional practice paradigm. When empowerment takes hold, the relationship between work and the result of work is better defined. This reduces the waste of human energy and other resources because a streamlined system focuses on integration, ownership, and outcomes. Structural characteristics that sustain the empowered processes of shared decision making and leadership also provide a frame for work/worker flexibility. This flexibility is key to the viability of an organization confronting change. Responsiveness to change comes from the successful integration and goodness-of-fit between environment and the willingness of staff to alter and adjust their work. Integration, and interactions that are relationship based, strengthen the clinical system and promote continual improvement. Successful adaptation in the organization is accomplished because of the competency-based framework supporting the shared decision-making process.

The structure and culture of an empowered environment enable individuals to combine autonomy and teamwork to fulfill expectations and roles and achieve clinical outcomes. Shared decision making represents the valuation of the profession and the professional, while creating a real partnership between the professional and the organization. Good shared decision making creates and maintains a structural format for facilitating staff participation in decision making and dialog regarding decisions, requirements, and actions related to clinical practice. Additionally, interactions are relationship based, facilitating information flow and communication, a fundamental indicator of success. Shared decision making asserts the staffs right to control their practice and make decisions that influence practice, thus advancing the mission and work of the organization. The result is a more satisfying work environment, fulfilled professionals, and a more successful organization.

References

Chrispeels, J. H. (2004). *Learning to lead together: The promise and challenge of sharing leadership*. Thousand Oaks, CA Sage.

Coffman, C., Gonzales-Molina, G. (2002). *Follow this path: How the world's greatest organizations unleash human potential*. New York: Warner Books.

De Pree, M. (1997). *Leading without power*. San Francisco: Jossey-Bass Publishers.

Hackman, R. (2002). *Leading teams: Setting the stage for great performances*. Boston: Harvard Business School Press.

Lundin, S. (2001). *Fish*. New York: Hyperion.

McDonagh, K. (1991). *Nursing shared governance*. Atlanta: KJ McDonagh Associates, Inc.

Nelson, G. M. (2000). *Self-governance in communities and families*. San Francisco: Berrett-Koehler.

Parker, G. M. (2003). *Cross-functional teams: Working with allies, enemies, and other strangers* (2nd ed.). San Francisco: Jossey-Bass.

Porter-O'Grady. (1991a). Shared governance for nursing: Part 2: Putting the organization into action. *AORN Journal*, 53(3), 694-703.

Porter-O'Grady, T. (1991b). Shared governance for nursing: Part 1; creating the new organization. *AORN Journal*, 53(2), 458-466.

Porter-O'Grady, T., Wlson, C. (1997). *Whole systems shared governance: Architecture for integration*. Gaithersburg, MD: Aspen.

Stack, J., Burlington, B. (2002). *A stake in the outcome*. New York: Currency Doubleday.

Surowiecki, J. (2004). *The wisdom of crowds*. New York: Doubleday.

Suggested Readings

ANCC. (2005). *Magnet recognition program application manual*. Silver Spring, MD: American Nurses Credentialing Center.

Brown, J., Duguid, P. (2002). *The social life of information*. Boston: Harvard Business School Press.

Dotlich, D. L., Cairo, P. C. (2002). *Unnatural leadership: Going against intuition and experience to develop ten new leadership instincts*. San Francisco: Jossey-Bass.

Katzenbach, J., Smith, D. (1993). *The wisdom of teams*. Boston: McKinsey & Company.

Malloch, K., Porter-O'Grady, T. (2005). *The quantum leader: Applications for the new world of work*. Sudbury, MA: Jones and Bartlett.

Porter-O'Grady, T., Malloch, K. (2002). *Quantum leadership: A textbook of new leadership*. Sudbury, MA: Jones and Bartlett.

Porter-O'Grady, T., Wilson, C. (1997). *Whole systems shared governance: Architecture for integration*. Gaithersburg, MD: Aspen.

Porter-O'Grady, T., Wilson, C. (1999). *Leading the revolution in healthcare: Igniting performance, changing systems*. Gaithersburg, MD: Aspen.

Surowiecki, J. (2004). *The wisdom of crowds*. New York: Doubleday.

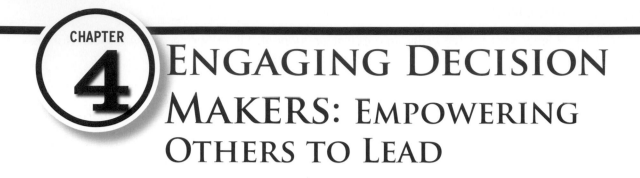

CHAPTER 4

ENGAGING DECISION MAKERS: EMPOWERING OTHERS TO LEAD

Embracing the power every person brings with him or her creates a strong community of decision makers and brings value to the contribution of every person.

EMPOWERMENT—THE BUZZWORD

The term *empowerment* has been used by leaders and managers for several decades. The assumption upon which it is based suggests that empowerment is something that one person can give another. The truth is that empowerment is recognition of the power that already exists in a role and allowing that power to be appropriately expressed within the role. Historically, workplaces have been operated in a hierarchical frame of reference, thus always putting the position of power in the hands

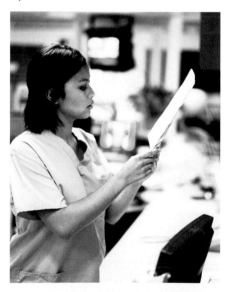

of those who were owners or managers of an enterprise. However, for work to be successfully advanced and sustainable outcomes to be obtained, the power in a role isn't absolute and is broadly spread and located in a number of places. The wise leader understands this and seeks to organize the workplace and the relationships in such a way that maximizes the power inherent in each role (Hackman, 2002).

Because of the history of power and control and perceptions related to it, real empowerment is much easier said than done. Because power is so strongly aligned with the role of owners and managers, it is difficult, even today, to define it in much broader terms. As a result, managers and workers behave as though the only legitimate locus of of control for power is in the hands of management leadership. This belief creates a range of untenable and unacceptable behaviors that, when applied, do not create effective and sustainable outcomes. Making sure that power is located in the right place and expressed appropriately is a fundamental task of good leaders (Stewart, 1997).

Expressing Power

Power is the ability to make decisions and to act on them. Good decision making is always:
- Right decision
- Right person
- Right place
- Right time
- Right purpose

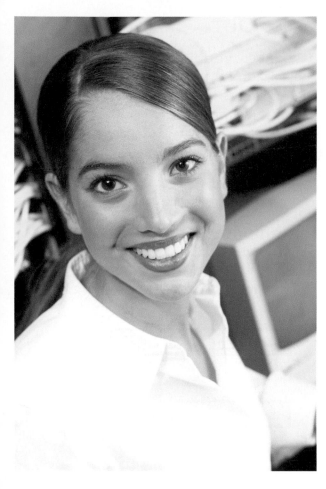

EMPOWERED ROLE

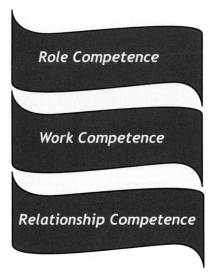

Role Competence

Work Competence

Relationship Competence

A Few Sources of Empowerment

- Organizations
- Actions
- Relationships
- Individuals
- Professions
- Special skills
- Competence
- Roles

Basic Requisites of Empowered Decisions

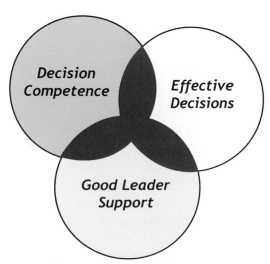

Decision Competence

Effective Decisions

Good Leader Support

Note:

Empowerment is not something that is granted. Instead, it is the power that exists inside the role and is legitimately and appropriately expressed there.

FROM THE CENTER OUT

Horizontal organizations (such as professional organizations) require a different leadership approach than traditional vertical organizations. The vertical organization of the past required superior and subordinate relationships. In empowered systems, the processes associated with communication and decision making require a different format for effective decision making. In these models the obligation for the success of the organization as well as the opportunity for individuals to grow and advance requires a different conception of the relationships necessary for organizations to succeed (Sveiby, 1997). Newer models of partnership need a much stronger orientation to shared decision making, shared risk, mutual goal setting, and collaborative relationship building.

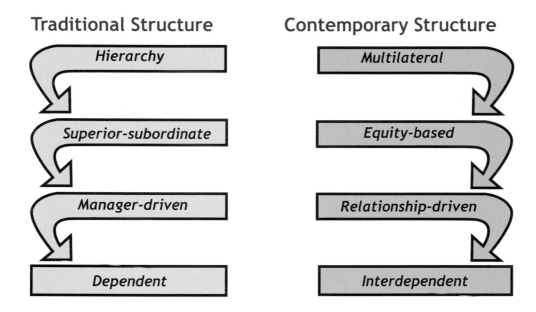

Traditional Structure

- Hierarchy
- Superior-subordinate
- Manager-driven
- Dependent

Contemporary Structure

- Multilateral
- Equity-based
- Relationship-driven
- Interdependent

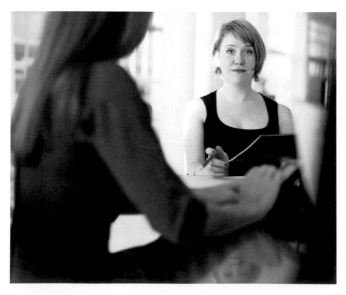

Note:

Empowerment requires a uniform valuing of the contribution of each member of the work community. Every role is considered important if it contributes to the advancement of the community and the achievement of work outcomes.

ELEMENTS OF PERSONAL EMPOWERMENT

Empowerment requires individual commitment and a willingness to fully invest in the activities of the work community recognizing that, as an empowered member, full participation is required.

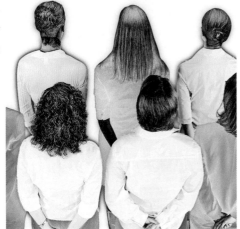

Commitment

Engagement

Willingness

Ownership

Communication

Interaction

Relationships

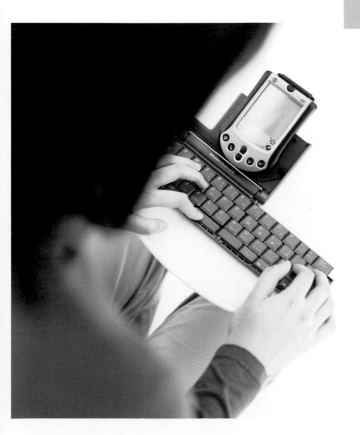

Note:

The empowerment-supporting leader ensures that full engagement has occurred on the part of all members of the work community.

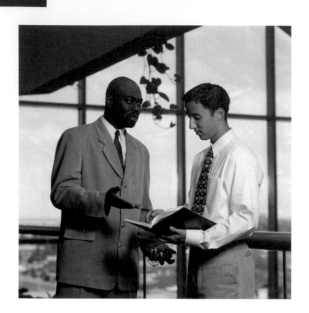

Note:

The structure of the workplace must be designed in such a way that the organization supports empowered work processes. If structure does not support process, empowerment becomes more fiction than reality. A structural frame is always important to ensure that the context for empowerment supports the expression of empowerment.

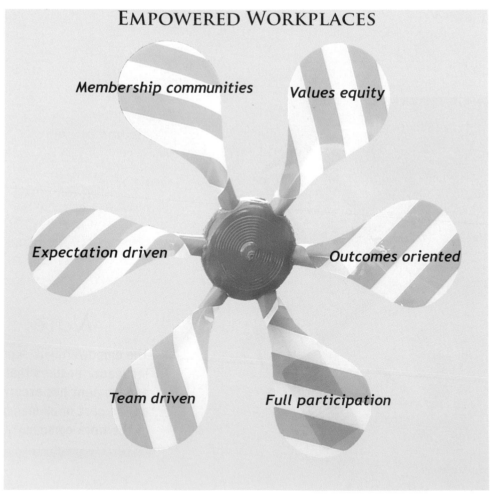

EMPOWERED WORKPLACES

Membership communities

Values equity

Expectation driven

Outcomes oriented

Team driven

Full participation

EMPOWERED BEHAVIORS

The concept of partnership is the driving force for empowerment in the workplace (Coffman & Gonzales-Molina, 2002). This means that risk sharing and undertaking process and work arrangements will be influenced by issues of balance roles and equity in the workplace. This notion of partnership allows the work system to establish relationships that reflect necessary interactions between workers, payers, and consumers. Decision-making partnership reflects the understanding in the workplace of the essential collaboration between all members of the work team. It is expected that all work roles converge to create the conditions that produce positive work relationships and achieve desirable work outcomes. These empowered behaviors are essential to developing a strong and effective work environment. The leader must reflect in his or her own behaviors a commitment to empowerment and engagement:

- Words and behaviors of a leader always reflect the importance of individuals as the greatest assets of the organization.

- Leaders recognize the value of individualism and meet individual workers where they are, looking to address the unique skills and talents that must integrate with those of the work team.

- The leader can listen effectively to a wide variety of people and is open to consistently learning new insights and gathering new resources to better integrate and coordinate the work of the team.

- The leader can identify the specific unique characteristics and strengths of each individual, aggregate them, and coordinate and integrate them into a mosaic of contributions facilitating the achievement of work outcomes.

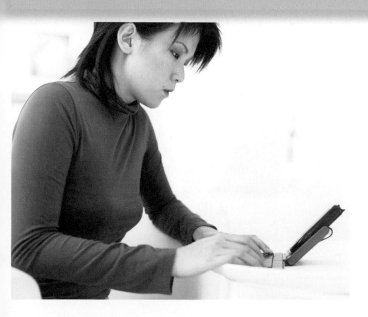

Note:

The leader who values empowerment sees the workplace as a **community of individuals** gathering together for common purpose, each committed to making his or her contribution toward an agreed-upon outcome.

EMPOWERED LEADER EXPECTATIONS

1. Team members will be committed to advancing the collective work effort.
2. All members of the work community will be equally valued by the leader in the organization.
3. Mechanisms will exist to help people find agreement and avoid conflict.
4. Critical thinking skills will be developed as a vehicle for problem solving and solution seeking.
5. People's individual needs and concerns will be considered in work expectations and building relationships.
6. Each individual will be assigned and assessed in relationship to the agreed upon work expectations they bring to their membership in the organization.
7. The inevitable problems and issues that come from working together will be addressed frequently in a nonpunitive, responsive environment.
8. The leader will encourage growth and work relationships, problem solving, and goal seeking between and among all members of the work team.
9. Trust emerges in the work relationship when people are valued and included in decisions and actions.
10. The continual focus on outcome will be facilitated by leadership, and evaluation mechanisms will be incorporated to determine effectiveness and progress toward such goals.

These expectations don't operate independently. The leader links all the behavioral elements together to create a mosaic of responses resulting in an effective, successful workplace.

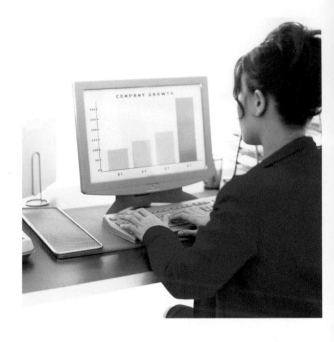

Driven by Purpose

- Everyone is clear on purpose.
- Staff Participate in defining and interpreting purpose.
- Accountabilities related to fulfilling purpose are clearly defined with staff and in each individual's role.
- Leaders help staff make a connection between the meaning of their own work and the purposes of the workplace.
- The purposes of work are clear enough that they give direction and indicate the specific values related to doing the work.

The Clarity of Empowered Decision Making

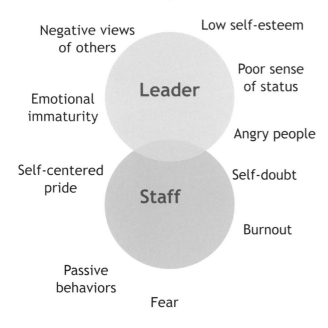

Negative Forces:
Ensure No Empowerment

Negative views of others

Low self-esteem

Leader

Poor sense of status

Emotional immaturity

Angry people

Self-centered pride

Self-doubt

Staff

Burnout

Passive behaviors

Fear

Empowered Decisions

- Are made by those who own them
- Are clear and specific
- Are related to achieving a pre-determined outcome
- Reflect the competence of the decision maker
- Result in a defined action or behavior
- Achieve specific results as defined and expected

Empowered Decisions

- Direct people to action
- Are evaluated regularly
- Form the basis for performance evaluation
- Indicate the level of commitment to the goals of the organization
- Relate to the process of rethinking and reconfiguring action when necessary
- Guide individuals with regard to the priorities related to establishing direction and undertaking the work

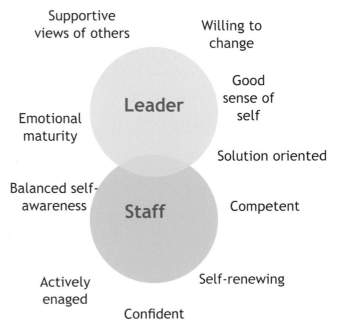

Positive Forces:
Ensure Empowerment

Supportive views of others

Willing to change

Good sense of self

Leader

Emotional maturity

Solution oriented

Balanced self-awareness

Staff

Competent

Actively enaged

Self-renewing

Confident

EMPOWERED DECISION MAKING REQUIRES PERSONAL OWNERSHIP

Victim Mentality Characteristics

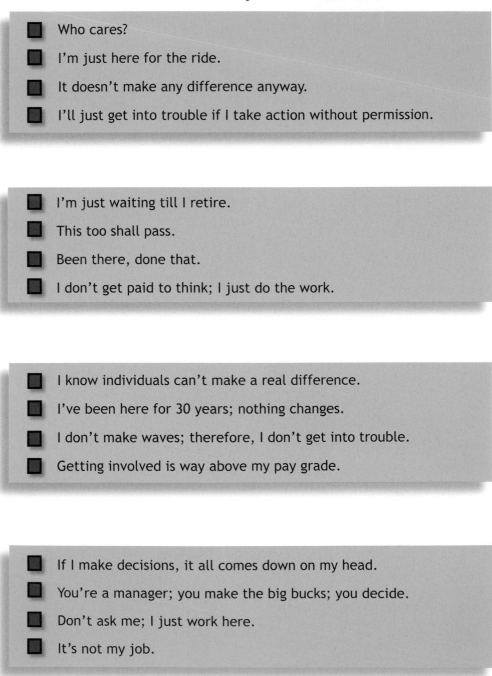

- ☐ Who cares?
- ☐ I'm just here for the ride.
- ☐ It doesn't make any difference anyway.
- ☐ I'll just get into trouble if I take action without permission.

- ☐ I'm just waiting till I retire.
- ☐ This too shall pass.
- ☐ Been there, done that.
- ☐ I don't get paid to think; I just do the work.

- ☐ I know individuals can't make a real difference.
- ☐ I've been here for 30 years; nothing changes.
- ☐ I don't make waves; therefore, I don't get into trouble.
- ☐ Getting involved is way above my pay grade.

- ☐ If I make decisions, it all comes down on my head.
- ☐ You're a manager; you make the big bucks; you decide.
- ☐ Don't ask me; I just work here.
- ☐ It's not my job.

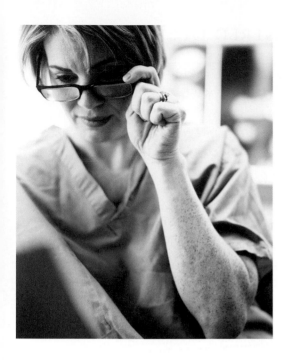

Empowered Decisions Require:

- Accurate information about process
- Good direction regarding outcome
- Effective tools for decision making
- Consensus decision methods
- Contribution from all participants
- Each participant knows own role
- Enumerated elements of evaluation
- Mechanisms for corrective action
- Opportunity for presenting new insights
- Openness to experimentation
- Nonpunitive error correction

TEAM DECISIONS AND INTERACTIONS LEAD TO OUTCOMES

There's no point in making decisions in the workplace if they are not ultimately going to lead to some action. It is action that moves individuals and teams to achieve outcomes. Discourse and dialog, negotiation and consensus seeking are all precursors to action. The team dynamics is established to create a framework for the application of collective wisdom in making appropriate decisions from which subsequent action will take form (Surowiecki, 2004). Each element of the relationship contributes to the decisions that will be made upon which subsequent direction and applied action will unfold (Lansdale & Papas, 2000).

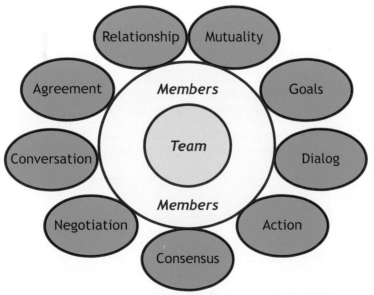

12 Factors Affecting Good Empowered Decision Making

1. The right information, in the right hands, at the right time is the support motto of the leader in advancing the action and success of the team.
2. Power is not the exclusive right of the individual but, instead, is the means of whoever is necessary to good decision making.
3. The leader does not control information flow; he or she facilitates its generation to those who need it.
4. Each member of the team grows and works in different ways—the leader incorporates this in assignment, roles, and expectations.
5. Individuals need different kinds of support in undertaking their work—application of decisions reflects the individuality of the worker.
6. The leader is always coaching others to more effectively manage their own decision making and coordinating their actions with others.
7. The leader always assumes the teaching-learning relationship, generating to others the information, tools, skills necessary for work.
8. Leaders help staff sort fiction from truth, real from perceived, actual from mythical, in order to accurately apply data to decisions.
9. The leader does not assume unilateral exercise of power over the collective wisdom of group participation in effective decision making.
10. The leader sees her- or himself as a servant to the team, supporting it with all of the information and tools necessary to act well.
11. If the team succeeds, everyone succeeds. Individual acknowledgement occurs from within the team, in the action of peers.
12. The leader encourages constant team evaluation of decisions, actions, and outcomes, always advancing skills and abilities of the team.

DECISION-MAKING CHALLENGES

Unclear Frame for Decisions

- Unclear information
- Uncertain goal
- Unidentified roles
- Duplicating accountability
- Undefined expectations
- Undefined process

Unclear Role in Decision Making

- Unclear role
- Uncertain performance
- Unidentified behaviors
- Undefined accountability
- Unclear tasks
- Undefined relationship(s)

Making decisions requires a context for the decisions be in place in a way that ensures that they will be effective and have an effect on work outcomes. Perhaps one of the most difficult issues affecting the exercise of work is ambiguity and a fundamental lack of clarity with regard to expectations and role (Lundin, 2001). It is critical for the leader to make sure that all participants in the work process have a good understanding of individual and collective role responsibilities and relationship in light of the outcomes to which the work is directed. Without a sense of clarity and understanding, work performance is negatively affected.

Unclear Direction in Decision Making

- Ambiguous language
- Lack of specificity
- Inadequate skills
- Lack of role clarity
- No measure of progress
- Undefined results

Unacceptable Expectations

- Beyond role capacity
- No adequate skills
- Unaddressed learning curve
- Inadequate role development
- Insufficient resources
- Inadequate time

SETTING STAFF UP FOR FAILURE

Frequently, on the path to empowerment, staff are inadvertently or intentionally set up to fail in their decision making. If there is a power shift that is untenable or unacceptable to the leader, processes can be undertaken that ensure staff-based decision-making is unsuccessful. Sometimes this is unintended and accidental; other times it is a determined process whose outcome is directed to ensure staff cannot succeed in their own decision making. Regardless, the outcome is the same. In an empowered system in which full engagement of staff in their own decision making is fundamental to success, the leader must guard against preexisting performance roles and expectations in which the leader is always the locus of control for making decisions and directing action (Morgan et al, 2005). This requires a level of self-assessment, an examination that includes the following elements:

Effective Transfer of Decision Making

- How do I as a leader express my need to participate fully in decisions in a way that has an impact and can be valued by all members of the team?

- Have I thought carefully about skill and role transfer to the staff, and do I plan a structured developmental process that ensures them the skills they need to succeed in decision making?

- Am I clear about which accountabilities belong to staff roles in decision making and which decision-making roles remain my accountability, and have I had dialog and communication regarding this locus of control with staff?

- Am I clear about where the staff is individually and collectively with regard to their own maturity in decision making and have I constructed developmental processes that operate at their level of skill and ability?

- Can my ego needs be satisfied through the reflected decisions and work of the staff when they are acclaimed and rewarded for their outcomes in place of my own individual acknowledgment?

Helping Staff Succeed in Decision Making

Collective Understanding about Role

- ■ Every staff member is a decision maker.
- ■ All staff will have the skills necessary to fully participate.
- ■ Participation in decision making is an expectation, not an invitation.
- ■ Staff will be clear about their specific accountability regarding decisions.
- ■ The team will play the chief role in defining models and processes of decision making.
- ■ Staff participation in decisions is always directed toward organizational and team goals.
- ■ Ambiguity of accountability avoided; each member is clear about role and expectations.
- ■ The leader is coach and mentor, modeling decision making and helping staff develop skills.

Developing Decision Skills

EXPECTATION

ABILITY

ACCOUNTABILITY

ROLE

RELATIONSHIP

TEAM ROLE

EVALUATION

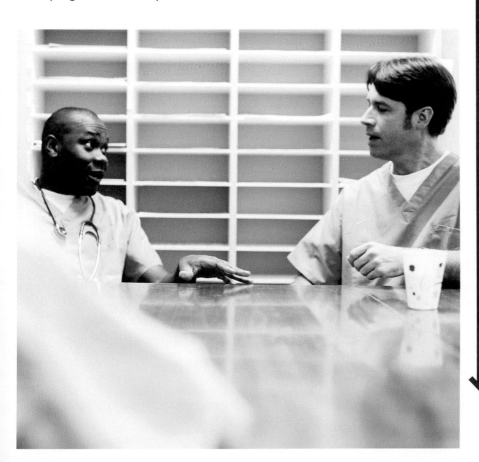

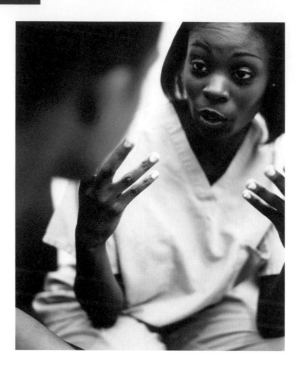

Note:

Mentorship and good role development are essential to effective, empowered decision making. A good mentor can help staff move through the rough or developmental stages of team decision making and build a high level of team success in decision effectiveness.

ACCOUNTABILITY AND DECISION MAKING

Three Stages of Accountability

Stage 1 Clarity: Each team member must know clearly how her or his work relates to the goals to which the work is directed.

Stage 2 Specificity: No generalizations with regard to expectations are acceptable; each rule must be specifically enumerated in relationship to its team contribution.

Stage 3 Outcomes: All team members must know their specific and unique role contribution to obtain results.

Avoiding Unilateral Agendas

- Personal goals conflicting with organizational goals
- Conflict-based methods of communication
- Unresolved disagreements with regard to appropriate process
- Variable commitment to achieving outcomes
- Interpersonal conflicts and competition
- Special personal relationships impeding team effectiveness

COLLABORATION IN DECISION MAKING

Requisites for Collaboration

Collaboration is a skill, not a gift (Porter-O'Grady & Wilson, 1997). It can be learned, but not without a process of inclusion, engaging all team members. Good process is always necessary for effective teambuilding and establishment of the kinds of relationships necessary to collective decision making. The requisites for good collaboration are:

- Learning processes built on a specific set of principles

- Situations requiring collaboration clearly enumerated

- Barriers to collaboration outlined and understood by all members

- Individual performance expectations with regard to group process clearly understood

- Action learning and developmental processes well defined and applied in the team

- Problem areas are focused upon and dealt with directly by team members

- Organized and systematic methods are used for confronting and resolving conflicts

- Regular time is set aside for evaluating team learning and progress

Collaboration Barriers

- Inability to address real issues
- Personal dishonesty of team members
- No methodology for problem solving
- Unsafe space for dialog
- Poor team relationships
- Individually ego-driven member(s)
- Variable commitment to teamwork
- Poorly developed relationships skills
- Problems with personal accountability
- No clear team development program
- Poorly developed decisional skills
- Inadequate mechanism for evaluation

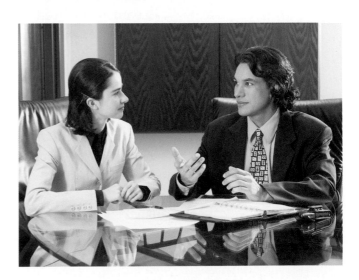

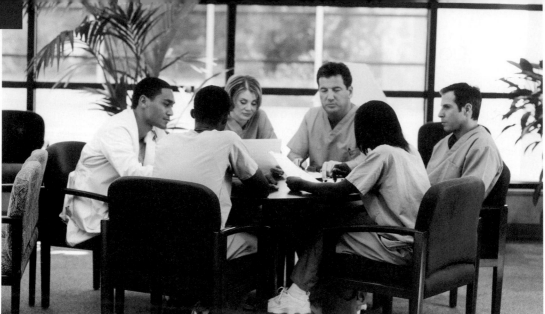

Decision Success

- Members agree regarding the decision
- Group conflict resolved
- Specific problem resolved
- Customers satisfied
- Team meeting is a success
- Cost saving achieved
- New approach has worked well
- New procedures mastered
- Team-staff survey indicates satisfaction
- Learning occurred
- Challenges were successfully met

COMMITTING TO EMPOWERED DECISION MAKING

Individual to Group

- Individual talents and skills
- Learning needs
- Specific contribution to group goals
- Individual needs from the group
- Individual commitment to good group process
- Willingness to solve group problems

Group to Individual

- Support individual contribution
- Make use of individual skills
- Facilitate the individual's learning process
- Set clear group expectations
- Evaluate performance within group norms
- Fully invest individual as team member

MEASURING DECISION-MAKING EFFECTIVENESS

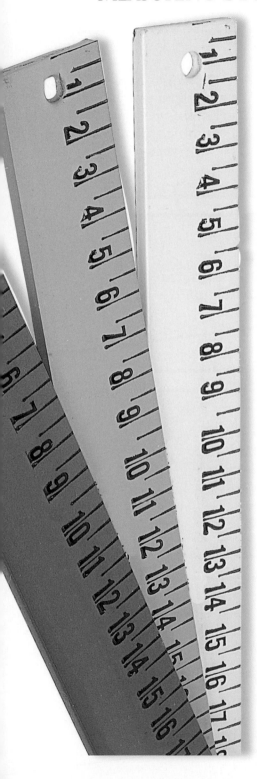

Determine the standard of measure for making decisions that can be used consistently over time.

Define specific measurement criteria that can be applied to particular decisions and evaluated.

Clarify the team's understanding of the performance expectations and the measurement elements.

Incorporate the performance consequences for noncompliance and achievement of anticipated goals.

Define process expectations and time frame for measuring team's achievement of goals.

Dialog evaluation/data results, plan corrective action and undertake revised processes.

MAKING EFFECTIVE EMPOWERED DECISIONS

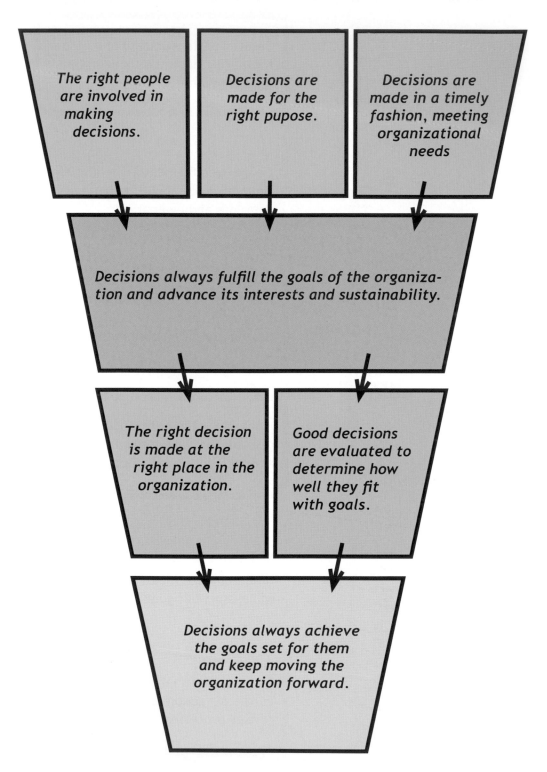

The right people are involved in making decisions.

Decisions are made for the right pupose.

Decisions are made in a timely fashion, meeting organizational needs

Decisions always fulfill the goals of the organization and advance its interests and sustainability.

The right decision is made at the right place in the organization.

Good decisions are evaluated to determine how well they fit with goals.

Decisions always achieve the goals set for them and keep moving the organization forward.

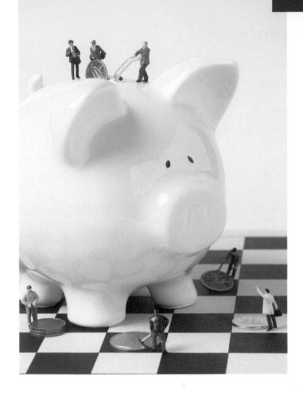

> ## Note:
>
> Good decisions reflect the interdependence of all decision makers and their effective commitment to the goals of the organization.

Principles of Effective Team Decisions

- Partnership
- Equity
- Accountability
- Ownership

EMPOWERED TEAM DECISIONS

Team decisions are effective insofar as they advance the work of the team and achieve the goals of the organization. The collective decision making of the team reflects the individual contribution of each decision maker. Each empowered team member advances the concerted and integrated effort of the team as a whole and contributes to the work outcomes of the team (Plas, 1996). Empowered decision making reflects valuing and placing decisions in the hands of the team for those issues that affect the work of the team and represent its accountability in advancing the interests of the organization. Continuing good team-based decision making requires constant commitment to the following principles:

1. Applying the principles of partnership, equity, accountability, and ownership, governs the effectiveness of all teams.
2. Good decision making in teams is driven from their relationship to the goals and the customer satisfaction.
3. Good team decision making focuses on the work, which is always guided by the standards of the team and the values each member brings to it.
4. Effective decision making requires continual learning and development.
5. Good decision making is a "weak" process. Team members seek to contribute unique talents to advance the decision-making effectiveness of the team.

References

Coffman, C., & Gonzales-Molina, G. (2002). *Follow this path: How the world's greatest organizations unleash human potential*. New York: Warner Books.

Hackman, R. (2002). *Leading teams: Setting the stage for great performances*. Boston: Harvard Business School Press.

Lansdale, B. M., & Papas, W. (2000). *Cultivating inspired leaders: Making participatory management work*. West Hartford, CT: Kumarian Press.

Lundin, S. (2001). *Fish*. New York: Hyperion.

Morgan, H. J., Harkins, P. J., Goldsmith, M. (2005). *The art and practice of leadership coaching: 50 top executive coaches reveal their secrets*. Hoboken, NJ: John Wiley.

Plas, J. M. (1996). *Person-centered leadership: An American approach to participatory management*. Thousand Oaks, CA: Sage Publications.

Porter-O'Grady, T., & Wilson, C. (1997). *Whole systems shared governance: Architecture for integration*. Gaithersburg, MD: Aspen.

Stewart, T. (1997). The new power game. *Fortune*, 135(1), 66-75.

Surowiecki, J. (2004). *The wisdom of crowds*. New York: Doubleday.

Sveiby, K. (1997). *The new organizational wealth*. San Francisco: Berrett Koehler.

Suggested Readings

Chrispeels, J. H. (2004). *Learning to lead together: The promise and challenge of sharing leadership*. Thousand Oaks, CA: Sage.

Ciampa, D., & Watkins, M. (1999). *Right from the start: Taking charge in a new leadership role*. Boston: Harvard Business School Press.

Cloke, K., & Goldsmith, J. (2002). *End of management and the rise of organizational democracy*. San Francisco: Jossey-Bass.

Donaldson, G. A. (2001). *Cultivating leadership in schools: Connecting people, purpose, and practice*. New York: Teachers College Press.

Dotlich, D. L., & Cairo, P. C. (2002). *Unnatural leadership: Going against intuition and experience to develop ten new leadership instincts*. San Francisco: Jossey-Bass.

Keller, E. B., & Berry, J. L. (2003). *The influentials*. New York: Free Press.

Meredith, G. E., Schewe, C. D., Hiam, A., & Karlovich, J. (2002). *Managing by defining moments*. New York: Hungry Minds.

Parker, C. (2002). *The open corporation: Effective self-regulation and democracy*. Cambridge, MA: Cambridge University Press.

CHAPTER 5

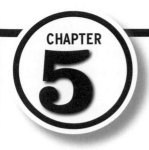

THE PERSON OF THE LEADER: HOW DO I LEAD

Self-knowledge provides the leader with a clarity regarding the skills and abilities necessary to express competence and commit to the journey of leadership growth.

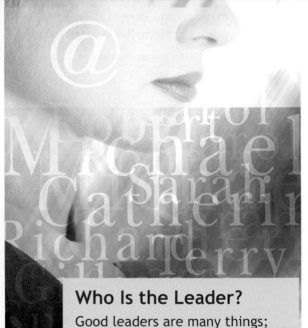

CREATING CONTEXT

The leader is the frame for the organization, the individual who most represents the values, purposes, and direction of the organization. Leaders do little other than create the context that gives a foundation for the organization and provides a mirror to the staff regarding who the organization is, what its work is, and where it is going (Lussier & Achua, 2003). Leadership is its own work and should not be cluttered with the activities and tasks that belong to the team and the staff. The greatest deficit with regard to most leaders is how easily leaders are co-opted by the work of the day in such a way that the work overwhelms their leadership and impedes their performance of the role.

Who Is the Leader?

Good leaders are many things; they also play many roles. In the 21st century the leader must be:

- A transformer
- A visionary
- A translator of direction
- Communication central
- A pursuer of truth
- A generator of creativity and innovation
- A seeker of the very next thing
- A team expert and role model
- A model of the journey to excellence

Note:

The leader creates a context that frames the behavior of the organization in a way that helps the organization achieve its objectives.

The Person of the Leader   197

WHO ARE YOU?

The most important level of self-knowledge is reflected in how leaders represent themselves to others. The world reflects great change, and that is where the work of leadership begins. But the real work is for leaders to change fundamentally who they are, the work that they do, and, even more important, how they lead. Contemporary challenges are exciting and intimidating. In order to lead people within the context of contemporary change, leaders need to achieve the behavioral shifts necessary to develop and build new organizational formats and create a new environment for meeting the challenges of change (Fitzgerald & Kirby, 1997).

This new organizational form demands that leaders understand the process of transformation and the need to change current management paradigms and behaviors as well as to accommodate the awareness through which these changes are made. Sustainable behavioral change happens within the context of continuing relationships, something that does not always go well in contemporary organizations.

For leaders to understand the world in which they live they must understand the relationships with each other and with those they are linked. Relationships are the oil that enables organizations and people to work effectively. Leaders who understand the relational dynamics of the contemporary age know that relationships operate at the center of all organizational life. As relationships are managed, the health of the organization is ensured. Leadership is really about building and sustaining long-term relationships that effectively converge around common goals directed to meeting the mission and purposes of organizations.

Note:

It is time for leaders to change who they are, how they do their work, indeed, transform the very work itself.

Who Am I as a Leader?

Good leaders constantly ask themselves questions that relate to their value and relevance to the goodness-of-fit between their leadership practices and the changing demands of the organization:

1. Are my leadership practices consistent with the changing goals of the organization?
2. Do I focus my leadership practices on building strong relationships and creating a good fit between people and the work they do?
3. Am I aware of my own continuing developmental needs, always exposing myself to the challenges of changing developments and new learning?

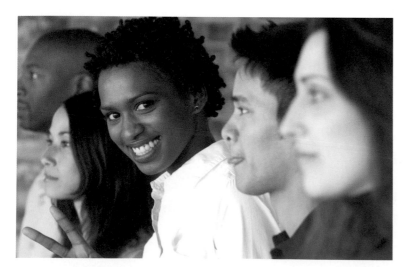

THE LEADERSHIP MIRROR

Leaders have to reflect to the people in their organizations the new realities of society, culture, and business. The increasingly technologically driven arena of work calls organizations and systems to move away from outdated systems and structures that limit the ability to be relevant in a viable and fast-paced technologically driven work environment. This new paradigm for work has a number of elements and characteristics that must be reflected through the role of the leader:

1 A continuous and constant acknowledgment of the value of collective wisdom.

2 The application of collective wisdom to the shifting world of work. Leaders now recognize the systems foundation of everything and the inter-connections that drive all decisions and actions in a system.

3 The industrial age is passing; the world is, instead of a great machine, a great set of continual intersecting relationships.

4 The leader is servant to the system and all that makes the system work—coordinating, integrating, facilitating all the elements of a system to ensure sustainability.

5 Meaning is informed by purpose and a leader is always reminding those who do the work to search for meaning in it and to reflect what the purpose of work is and how each contribution to work moves the organization to sustainable success.

6 Leaders understand all the elements of the change process from reaction to engagement and help those they lead move seamlessly through each stage in a way that ensures their success as well as the viability of the organization.

7 Leaders must make sure that enough time is devoted to transforming individuals as they make the transition to new roles and accountabilities, recognizing it is a personal voyage contributing to the broader transformation that ensures the organization's relevance.

8 Leaders must recognize that they are exemplars of personal transformation, constantly being observed by those they lead and assessed with regard to the their level of engagement, commitment, and consonance with the demand for new behaviors and skills.

Note:

If leaders want to know what kind of leaders they are, they need only look into the mirror of their staff; reflected back will be the quality of their leadership.

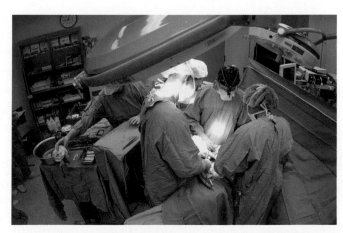

The Person of the Leader   199

21ST CENTURY LEADERSHIP CHARACTERISTICS

Interpersonal competencies

> RECEPTIVITY AND SIMILARITY

> IMMEDIATELY AND EQUALLY

> INTEGRATION

> FACILITATION

> COORDINATION

> COACHING

> FRAMING NEW LEADERSHIP LANGUAGE

Conceptual Competencies

> SYSTEMS THINKING

> ACCLIMATION TO CHAOS

> PATTERN RECOGNITION

> CONTINUOUS LEARNING

Participation Competencies

> PARTNERSHIP

> EQUITY

> ACCOUNTABILITY

> OWNERSHIP

> INVESTMENT

> INVOLVEMENT

> EMPOWERMENT

Leadership Competencies

> VULNERABILITY AND OPENNESS

> SYSTEMS SKILLS

> EMOTIONAL MATURITY

> SELF-MANAGEMENT

> TRANSFORMATION SKILLS

> GROUP PROCESS SKILLS

> CHANGE MANAGEMENT

> FLUIDITY AND MOBILITY

New Leadership Skills

Leaders must recognize that the 21st century has created a new frame for management and movement of people and organizations. These new realities in a sociotechnical age call for leaders to be more fluid and flexible in understanding the organization's dynamics and in moving people through all change. The contemporary "quantum" leader recognizes that movement and fluidity are the essential constituents 4 of continual and dynamic change; the central context of all life. Adaptation, transformation, and adjustment are constants that must be incorporated into everyone's lives. Leaders reflect this within the context of their own lives and leadership, making it normative so that movement simply is a matter of pace or rate of change rather than the "reality" of the change itself. Reflecting transformative and mobility-based dynamics within the context of the leader's own role becomes a frame of reference and an exemplar.

OLD VS. NEW LEADERSHIP SKILLS

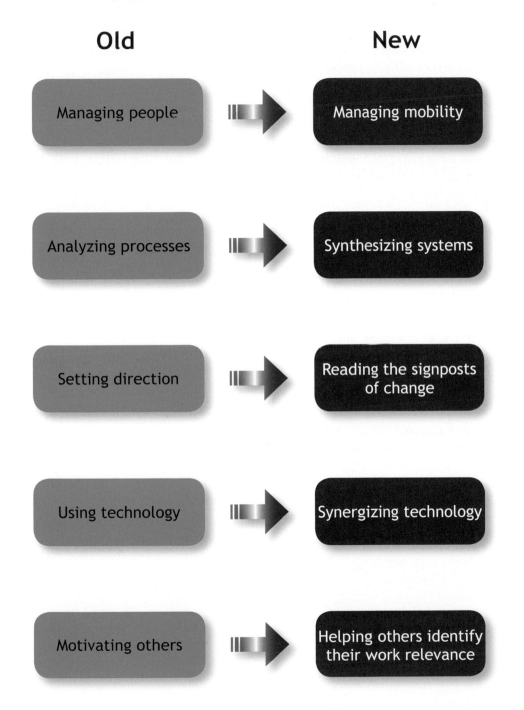

Old

New

Old	New
Managing people	Managing mobility
Analyzing processes	Synthesizing systems
Setting direction	Reading the signposts of change
Using technology	Synergizing technology
Motivating others	Helping others identify their work relevance

CHECKING OFF BASIC LEADER ATTRIBUTES

☐ Do I like people? I will be leading many people, sometimes in directions they may prefer not to go. I must be willing to relate with many types of people and will need a positive sensitivity to the needs of others. I must like this work.

☐ Can I live with a high degree of ambiguity and uncertainty? I will be dealing with a great amount of change. I will have to be an example of excitement and engagement of this change and demonstrate a will to implement it in my own life before I ask anyone else to implement it.

☐ Are my communication skills well developed? I will be communicating with others almost constantly and will need to be informed and articulate in my expressions. Others must understand me and must respect the validity of the information I communicate.

☐ Do I have the courage to handle the discipline issues that my leadership role will demand? Can I make tough decisions and follow through with action when required without fear and uncertainty.

☐ Can I stand alone on an issue when it appears that others are not embracing it? If the position is ethical and appropriate, can I defend it with clarity and firmness, incorporating others' concerns in my own development and position?

☐ Am I a good team player? I can make a contribution to the planning and implementing processes and then take leadership in translating decisions to others and helping them act in concert with the goals and direction others may have developed for them.

THE COURAGE TO LEAD

Leadership is hard work. The committed leader must see the work as a full-time job. In many organizations leadership is not always looked at as requiring the full attentions of the individual leader. However, nothing could be further from the truth. Any compromise in the leader's role is an assurance that the effectiveness of the role is diminished.

> ## Note:
>
> **Leadership is a full-time obligation requiring the full skills of the leader. Playing other roles at the same time as holding the leader role creates role confusion and ambiguity of accountability.**
>
> **Any suggestion that the leader role has no discernible content that creates a full-time demand compromises both the role and the effectiveness of it. In this case, the staff lose sight of its value and develop expectations for performance that further compromises its exercise.**

Many leaders are promoted into the role from staff jobs. Often, their promotion was a reflection of what good work this individual did as a staff person. In the staff role, this individual became an expert at their work. This expertise and effectiveness ultimately led this individual into the role of "new leader." The greatest problem with this process relates to the conflict between really great preparation in the work process and the demands of a good leader—often they are not aligned. Leadership skills are unique to the role. Staff expertise may be an indicator of potential competence, but it is no guarantee of transferability into the leader role. The emerging leader must understand this differentiation from the outset. Not doing so skews the new leader's understanding of the role and affects the quality of how the role is applied.

A common occurrence in many organizations is the frequent transferability of the leader from the staff role to the leader role and back to the staff role depending on staffing and scheduling or issues of workload. This role "schizophrenia" creates discordance between the leader and the role and between the leader and the staff. Although this situation can occur, it should happen rarely. Such a routine compromise of the role can create severe challenges in its successful application (Kottler & Brew, 2003). Additionally, it institutionalizes this functional ambiguity and never really addresses the concerns related to inadequate staffing. The leader fulfilling staff roles becomes a surrogate for the real issues and ensures that they never get expectations addressed. In addition the leader never really fully expresses the leader role, and its full expression thereby becomes compromised.

LEADERS ENGAGE STAKEHOLDERS

Good leaders know that they are not the answer to all the questions that staff raise. The leader must recognize that accountability for answers always rests with the questioner. The minute the leader answers the question, a transfer of the locus of control for the answer moves to the leader, essentially absolving the questioner of any ownership of the solution to his or her own question. This transfer occurs thousands of time every day in the life and role of the leader.

The wise leader recognizes that the accountable answer to any question is the next question. The leader recognizes that ownership of the issue should remain with the person who brings it and that person must be encouraged and enabled to respond and seek the solution that can most be sustained (Fisher, 2000).

The Leader Seeks to Have the Questioner:

- Retain ownership and control over the issue
- Identify the resources necessary to pursue a solution
- Name the barriers impeding a solution
- Identify the best deliverables related to a sustainable solution
- Enumerate a mechanism for selecting the best alternative
- Outline the process steps necessary to address the issue
- Indicate the impact of the selected approach
- Evaluate the results of the approach(es) selected
- Undertake corrective action related to an effective solution
- Validate the action of the staff
- Celebrate the success for the staff in resolving their own issues

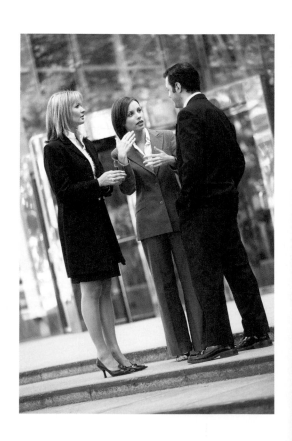

Note:

Leadership requires a strong sense of self. It is next to impossible for a tentative leader to influence the life and choices of others. A context of competence and confidence can sometimes be the only difference between encouragement and failure.

Affirming Leader Competence

> Has a solid self preception

> Is strongly self-directed

> Relates to others well

> Possesses effective verbal skills

> Willing to interact

> Is able to clarify issues

> Is unafraid of ambiguity

> Is willing to face conflict head-on and early

> Embraces the noise of creativity

> Allows others to be innovative and break the rules

> Lands running

> Is not good at avoiding anything

> Can live in the reflected glory of other's accomplishments

> Doesn't mind a little chaos

> Demonstrates empathy

> Loves to celebrate other's successes

PAYING ATTENTION TO LEADER SELF-DEVELOPMENT

Every leader, no matter how experienced, must be aware of the need to continually develop and grow in the role. Competence in the role is neither static nor ensured. Each leader must recognize how dynamic change is, constantly shifting the work landscape and calling all who work to continually reflect on the value of their contribution and the currency of their skills (Murphy & Riggio, 2003). This means participating in an endless assessment of competence and the need to adjust and grow in the role as it responds to new demands:

- Am I able to see the whole picture, not just the part that applies to me?
- Do I work in systems models and not merely reflect a process orientation?
- Am I able to look past the current issues and see where I am?
- Can I "envision" the journey and reflect on where I am in it?
- Am I good at translating reality and change so that others understand?
- Am I willing to face issues first before others must contend with them?

- Do I anticipate the needs of the system and of others in it?
- Do I explore different ways of seeing things and expand my thinking?
- Will I experiment with and evaluate options to current routines?
- Is there place in my life for the uncertain and the chaotic?
- Can I find the energy in stress and use it to good advantage?
- Am I disciplined in my work and my life without being limited by it?
- Can I see the pain and noise in others and respond with empathy?
- Do I push others into their own challenges and support them in it?

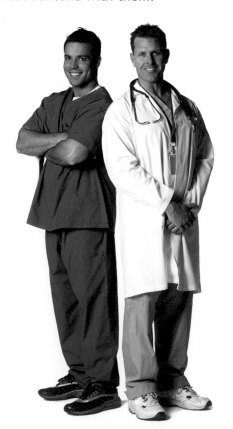

Note:

Self-awareness ensures that a leader is able to confront the challenges that lie within and adjust for the conflicts and challenges that move the individual to grow and develop in a way that takes the person beyond limitation and into the arena of true innovation and creativity. Today, most organizations are hungry for just such people.

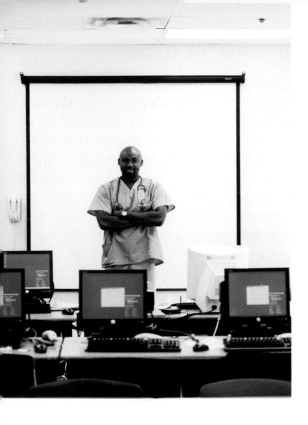

THE LEADER AS CREATOR

Leaders are inventors. They must be mentors and encouragers of the innovative and creative in every person. Sustainability depends on a leader's ability to get out of others the unexpected. This means that the leader values the unusual and "out of the box" processes and ideas that do not always fit in the current model of doing business. The challenge for the leader is in creating a context for the innovative ideas and actions of others by making it safe and appropriate to be and do differently (Eitington, 1997).

Often people get caught up in their own rituals and routines and become inured of emerging trends or changes in their own circumstances. It is the role of the leader to "pull staff out" of their rituals and routines. The leader exposes them to the demand for change and encourages in them a response to the call to confront the new and emergent in their lives and work. Making it safe for innovaton and modeling acceptance of what is different and emerging make it possible for people to risk stretching toward new ways and work with all the excitement and joy that come with it.

Honoring the Creative

- Establish a "new idea of the day."
- Make old practices "unsafe" to continue by creating gentle barriers.
- Reward ideas with as much energy as rewarding work processes.
- Have an innovation learning session at least once a week.
- Expose the group to another person's (and profession's) way of thinking.
- Set priorities for changing internal events to make them work better.
- Celebrate error and take advantage of it; learn what it is trying to teach.

New Age Content for the Leader

- *Outcomes driven*
- *Systems Oriented*
- *Chaos context*
- *Value based*
- *"User" driven*
- *Work portability*
- *Flexible*

CONFRONTING ORGANIZATIONAL REALITIES

For the leader, it is sometimes not the staff who are a problem in confronting the challenges of change and creativity. At times, the barrier to engaging in real change is imbedded in the behavior of the leadership of the organization. There is great uncertainty and fear in the "bowels" of any change event. Innovation and change always call for a shift in the order of things and the rituals associated with maintaining them. The leader must be willing to confront the vagaries of the change itself—inadequate attention has often been paid to the processes associated with legitimizing the change in the organization through the action of the leadership at every level of the organization (Clark, 2003). Staff are often blamed for not embracing a change soon enough when the real issue is the leader's ability to visualize the needed change and create the conditions that allow the change to have life in the organization.

Leaders must always remember that their primary role is to create a supportive context for the action of change in the organization. This means that the leader recognizes the forces influencing the leader's own expression of encouragement and facilitation of the change process. Understanding the issues of "fit" between the leader's practices and the conditions that affect them is critical to the good selection of approaches that make change successful. The leader is always aware of this need for good choices and best represents those good choices in her or his own behaviors and practices so that they become a model for the staff and the signpost of how best to respond to the inevitability and engagement of continual change.

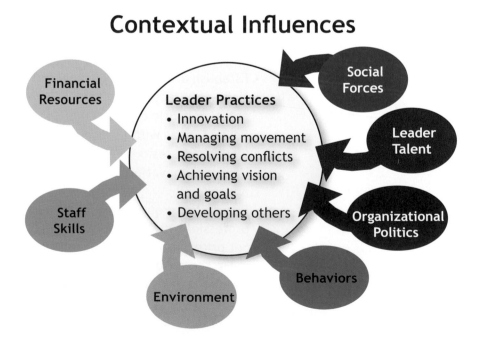

Contextual Influences

MORE LEADER CORE BEHAVIORS

- Leaders reflect flexibility in their approach to all problem solving and in confronting all issues.

- Leaders describe the changes that will affect the staff well in advance of the staff actually experiencing them.

- Leaders translate the goals of the system in a language that others can understand and apply to their own work.

- Leaders represent in their own behavior the patterns and practices they expect to see in others.

- Leaders anticipate the changes that staff will have to make in their work and carefully design approaches to guide staff in accepting and implementing changes.

- Leaders recognize the chaos imbedded in all change and are not afraid of it, demonstrating engagement of it to others, mentoring acceptance and use of its energy.

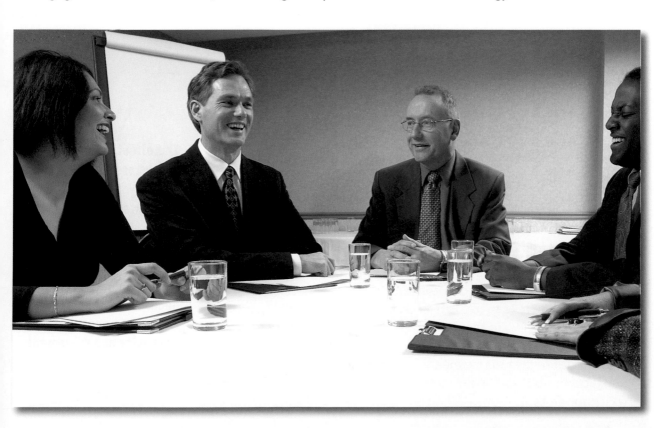

LEADERSHIP AND THE DYNAMICS OF A GOOD PROCESS

How many times do we hear, "If we could just get to the end of this and know it was over and done with"? Whereas there is certainly some truth to the incrementalism of this statement, there is no truth to its substance. Nothing is ever really "done." Everything is always and forever in movement. If the movement of the universe should stop, so would everything in it. We may achieve specific objectives, but if we're seeing them correctly, they are really a small component of a much larger journey—one that never ends. The good leader puts all movement within the context of this larger reality and helps others understand the essential movement (very much as in a symphony). This leader gathers all the stakeholders around the "story" of the journey and helps them make it a part of their own movement (very much like a concert where each instrument interacts to create the collective symphony.)

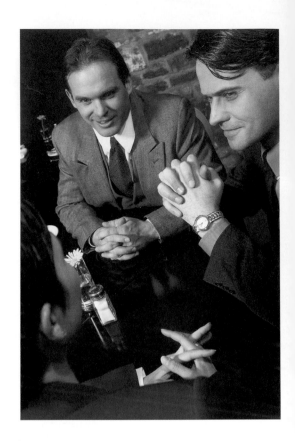

The Leader as Storyteller

People get easily inculcated into their own rituals and routines. The problem with this is the risk they undertake by getting lost in their work and losing sight of its purpose. The leader's role is to create sufficient context for the work in which people can create a broader image of the meaning and value of the work they do. Work needs a context with which to define meaning. Work is not an end in itself.

Every leader must understand his or her role in describing for others the larger context and the greater journey of which every person is a part. Without this conception of the greater context, it is easy for people to get lost in their work and forget to ask the question "why" in the midst of the work effort. It is tragic to see so many folks working hard and doing much with little insight with regard to this meaning and value. It is the leader's obligation to tell the larger story and enumerate the individual's contribution to it.

Note:

The effective leader always prefers chaos over stability. Stability is a momentary respite in the endless movement and creativity of essential change. Although occasional stability is necessary, stability over time is the enemy of creativity and movement.

WHAT STAFF WANT FROM THEIR LEADER

Honesty
Clarity of Role
Open Communications
Personal Caring
Respect
Trust
Opportunity
Good Problem Solving Skills
Engagement
Meaning in their Work

THE OPENNESS OF THE LEADER

Perhaps there is nothing more important than the ability of the leader to be humanly present. The notion that the leader is somehow imbued with supernatural or special characteristics is untrue. Leaders are people who hold an important role in relationship to others. Often the role is formal and structured within an organizational frame of reference. Although the expression of the role of leader is consistent regardless of the position, its formal expression will be differentiated by context and culture. Still the leader must not forget that humanity essentially defines the role and is the primary context for its expression. Leaders must be able to communicate to others their common humanity in a way that allows others to more fully identify with it and be encouraged in their own personal and work journey.

It is important that the leader represent and express a level of openness and availability to others in a way that helps them identify with the person of the leader. Rather than traditionally presumed, the leader should not be identified as separate and unique from those he or she leads. Instead, the leader should be most identified with the led and exemplify for them the best of human characteristics in a way that affirms their common roles and combined purpose. This openness and availability of the leader represent to others their connection to the leader, their common identity, and their collective commitment.

Note:

The wise leader identifies with those led so intensely that he or she is the visualization of what is best in those led and what is most vital and filled with potential in them.

Leader Vulnerability

Leaders must acknowledge and articulate their common humanity with those they lead. A part of the reason for this is to expel and extinguish any notion that the leader has characteristics or capacities beyond those of others. The leader expresses vulnerability through frank disclosure and sharing of common humanity. As well, the leader seeks identity with the staff and finds strength in the collective relationship and common wisdom of the group. This vulnerability dispels expectations and projections that are mythological or beyond the capacity of the leader. Wise leaders guard against being placed on a pedestal or being emulated beyond normative behaviors and expectations.

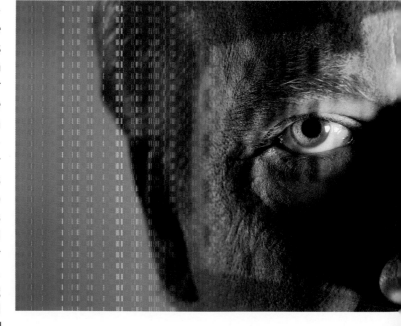

LEADERS MOVING PAST THE AGE OF CONTROL

It has been said that control was the cornerstone of organizational leadership in the 20th century. As organizations seek to function in the 21st century, much of the characteristics of change are driven by a different set of principles. Recognizing the impact of complexity thinking and quantum theory, organizations are looking at an emerging significant set of relationships and intersections that require coordination and synthesis. This means that control is no longer the central issue of stability and organization in systems. The good leader recognizes that issues of fit, linkage, interaction, and relationship are the critical elements of all human dynamics.

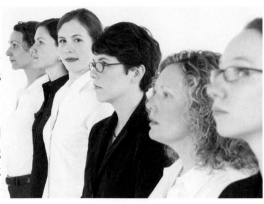

Note:

The leader who must control others is expressing a basic insecurity that ultimately results in negative forces and behavior impeding achievements of the organizations's goals.

Leaders recognize that building complex relationships requires constant attention and continual reflection on interaction of all elements in an organization including that of the people who comprise it. Building an infrastructure for relationships calls for leaders to understand linkage and intersections and to provide staff with clarity of meaning and purpose. The leader ensures those who are led that there is value in the work and relationships necessary to advance the purposes and values of the organization. In this, the leader fully engages the participants in an interaction that invests them in the commitment of their work with the purposes of the organization, advancing the meaning and value of their contribution, and to growing and improving their own personal skills and participation. This can only be done through invitation, gathering, inclusion, and encouraging the best and the most vital in all who participate.

Eliminating the Focus on Control

- Help people understand what is happening to them
- Engage others in defining the content of their own work
- Reduce hierarchy to its lowest necessary levels
- Involve stakeholders in setting their own goals
- Eliminate secrets—disclose whatever is necessary to help others do their work

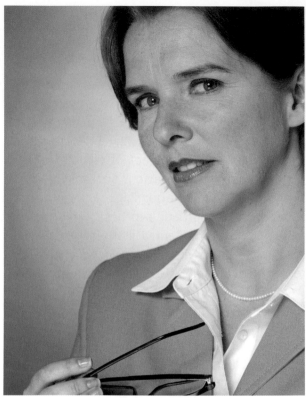

> **A Personal Plan for Learning**
>
> An endless commitment to learning is fundamental to the role of the leader. Three things are critical:
> 1. A good assessment of leadership skills and needs
> 2. A good plan with strategies for action and implementation
> 3. A 360-degree evaluation of the effectiveness of the application of leadership skills

THE LEADER'S COMMITMENT TO LEARNING

The leader cannot expect in others what he or she is not willing to find within. It is important to the consideration of the role of leader to recognize the value of continuing growth and development. The person of the leader represents to others the general commitment to a continuing development that is fundamental to competence and effectiveness. Like all roles, the leader cannot be competent and static at the same time. The leader must expect the willingness and ability to expand the skill-set necessary to exercise the role and role model to others.

It is important for leaders to develop a formal and structured approach to their own development. The individual leaders should assess skill level and competencies as a foundation for determining abilities and deficits in support of establishing a learning program. This self-assessment provides an opportunity for the leaders to enumerate clearly the elements of leadership upon which development will be based. In this way the leader can design a developmental process specific to his or her own needs around which particular skills can be refined. Furthermore, individual leaders can depend on one another for supplementing learning and development through use of other leaders' skills and talents. In this way, the community of leaders can provide a supporting infrastructure and process through the creation of a dynamic and continual process of collaborative leadership development.

Of course, the leader should evaluate progress against initial goals for skill development. Learning leadership only has value if it ultimately affects the role of the leader. Without specific change and effectively applied and improved skills, development alone has little value. Leadership must always be translated into behaviors and have an effect on those who are positively led.

LEADERS ARE ALWAYS RESPONSIVE TO CHANGE

> **Reading the signs of change**

> **Translating the language of change for others**

> **Guiding others in adapting to change**

> **Applying change in the process of work**

> **Entering into dialog regarding change impact**

> **Evaluating the results of change**

> **Renewing energy for the very next change**

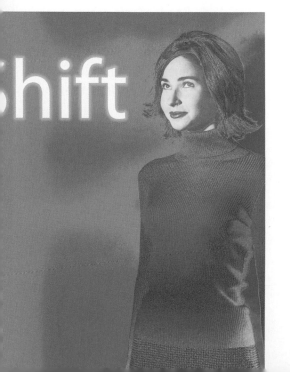

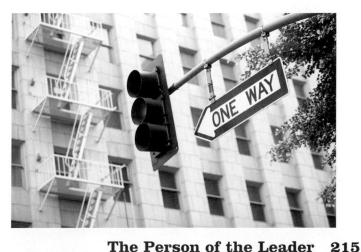

A Leader Is Inspired and Is Inspiring

The ability to encourage others and to continue supporting their effort through modeling, motivating, and the leader's own personal commitment is critical to good leadership. The inspiring leader always recognizes that who one is, is as important as what one does.

This Leader Always Remembers That:

- Individuals need to know that their work has meaning and value.
- Individuals hope that their work makes a difference and has a positive effect on the lives of others.
- Everyone wants to know that they are personally valued and have a place as well as play a key role in the world.
- Everyone seeks, at some level, to make a difference and to hear that difference in the words and language of others.
- People want to know that they matter; that their lives have personal value, and that they have an opportunity to express that value in their work and actions.
- The leader always seeks what is good in others, identifies it, and makes other team members aware of the value that an individual brings to their efforts.
- The value of collective wisdom is shared between and among all team members so that their collective impact is recognized by all.
- Nothing is sustained without concerted effort of all stakeholders committed to a common purpose.
- The leader creates the context within which others live and work in a way that encourages engagement, stimulates creativity, and builds commitment.

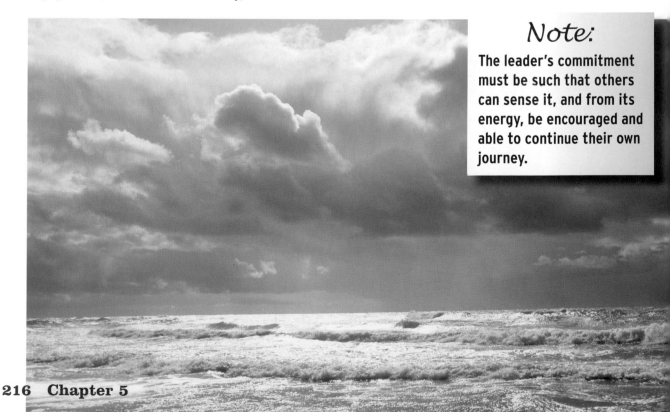

Note:

The leader's commitment must be such that others can sense it, and from its energy, be encouraged and able to continue their own journey.

References

Clark, C. C. (2003). *Group leadership skills* (4th ed.). New York: Springer.

Eitington, J. E. (1997). *The winning manager: Leadership skills for greater innovation, quality, and employee commitment*. Houston: Gulf.

Fisher, K. (2000). *Leading self-directed work teams: A guide to developing new team leadership skills* (rev. and expand ed.). New York: McGraw-Hill.

Fitzgerald, C., & Kirby, L. K. (1997). *Developing leaders: Research and applications in psychological type and leadership development: Integrating reality and vision, mind and heart*. Palo Alto, CA: Davies-Black.

Kottler, J. A., & Brew, L. (2003). *One life at a time: Helping skills and interventions*. New York: Brunner-Routledge.

Lussier, R. N., & Achua, C. F. (2001). *Management effectiveness: Developing leadership skills*. Cincinnati: Thomson Learning/South-Western College Publishing.

Murphy, S. E., & Riggio, R. E. (2003). *The future of leadership development*. Mahwah, NJ: Lawrence Erlbaum Associates.

Suggested Readings

Bell, C. (1996). *Managers as mentors: Building partnerships for learning*. San Francisco: Berrett-Koehler.

Buckingham, M., & Coffman, C. (2000). *First break all the rules*. New York: Simon & Schuster.

Goleman, D., Boyatzis, R., & McKee, A. (2002). *Primal leadership*. Boston: Harvard Business School Press.

Kotter, J. (1996). *Leading change*. Boston: Harvard Business School Press.

Porter-O'Grady, T., & Malloch, K. (2002). *Quantum leadership: A textbook of new leadership*. Sudbury, MA: Jones and Bartlett.

UNIT 3: ACCOUNTABILITY

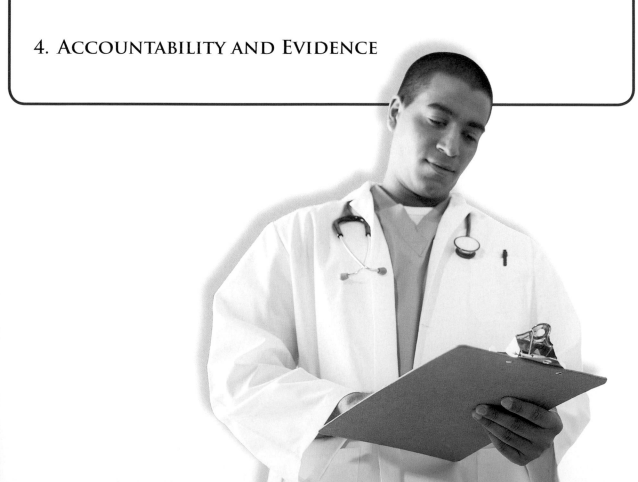

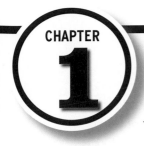

PERFORMANCE ACCOUNTABILITY: COMPETENCE FOR THE WORK

Accountability calls for commitment to achieving outcomes. There is no accountability if it is not informed by purpose and disciplined by results.

Accountability and Clarity

Perhaps one of the most challenging elements of accountability is the lack of clarity with regard to what it means in the context of work. Furthermore, there are many challenges with regard to how it is evidenced in the work of the team and how it influences the outcomes of work. There is no other concept in work that is used as much as accountability, yet is so little understood.

Accountability most simply reflects the achievement of sustainable outcomes. Responsibility, on the other hand, is the effective performance of actions in the exercise of doing work. One (accountability) is about the achievement of results and the other (responsibility) is about the quality of the work effort. One can be responsible without being accountable. In fact, responsibility without accountability is one of the work crises of the current age. Many people do good work and work very hard on processes or activities that have a questionable relationship to the achievement of sustainable outcomes.

Because of the traditional business fixation on process and action, short-term and interactive products are evaluated as signs of performance effectiveness and progress. However, sustainable results can be achieved only over much longer periods of time. To achieve them means to better tie the actions of work to their products. Good research relates to creating a very tight goodness-of-fit between the effort of work and its results. Effectiveness is best indicated by the directness of the work effort to the expectations for results and the actual results. The better the relationship, the more sustainable the outcome and the more valuable the relationship between the two. It is this set of circumstances that creates the ideal work relationship in that it directly connects responsibility and accountability.

To achieve this direct connection between responsibility and accountability requires a clear understanding of the elements of accountability and the expectations for performance of each of the parties. Without it, there exists no foundation for defining or delivering accountability.

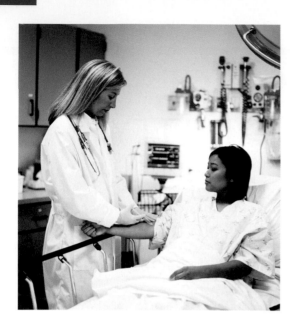

Note:

Expectations are the foundation for performance. Every worker has the right to know what is expected and the skills necessary to meet expectations or he or she shouldn't be in the role.

CLARIFYING EXPECTATIONS

Every person should know the elements of their work and the criteria for performance.

Each worker should be fully aware of the competence requirements of the role before taking or filling the role.

Those performance factors that advance the system's viability and success must be identified and emphasized.

If expectations shift or change, time must be taken to reorient or train for new behaviors or competencies.

Team expectations are the sum of the individual performance factors and can be advanced only by individual accountability.

SOURCES OF EXPECTATION

Role Descriptions

1. Performance criteria
2. Work elements
3. Job Factors
4. Time considerations
5. Hygenic factors
6. Functions
7. Competence
8. Reporting relationship
9. Role characteristics
10. Evaluation premises

Team Expectations

1. Team criteria
2. Member elements
3. Role Factors
4. Relationships
5. Team role fit
6. Member functions
7. Team competence
8. Communication
9. Conflict process
10. Team outcomes

Expectation Definers

■ The criteria for performance are identified in advance.

■ Stakeholders share in the process of defining role expectations.

■ Team members determine the degree of necessary fit between roles.

■ Expectations are defined in a language individuals can understand.

■ Each expectation relates well to the set of expectations for a role.

■ Each team member's role intersects with all team members' roles.

■ No team member is expected to perform beyond expected level of skill.

CLARITY ELEMENTS

■ Make it simple.

■ Use short statements instead of complex ones.

■ Use precise language specific to the role.

■ Use clear statements of competence.

■ Array critical elements in order of priority.

■ Create well-defined team relationship expectations.

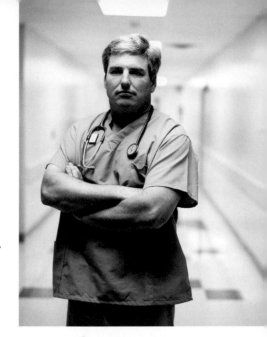

Issues of Clarity

Ambiguity is the enemy of accountability. It is essential that performance expectations be clear and understandable at the outset or performance will always be negatively affected. Some basic elements for role clarity are:

- Precise language that states role in terms that are clear.

- Performance factors that relate well to role tasks and functions.

- Terms of reference that are precise and expressed as single items.

- Competence factors that are clearly enumerated as role foundation.

- Clearly stated factors that will comprise evaluation of the role.

- Individual performance that is tied together with team performance.

Problems of Clarity

Clarity is both a gift and a challenge. The gift of clarity is the directness of understanding and application of the role. It provides simple terms that can be readily applied to an individual role. The challenge relates to problems with subtleties and elements within the role that are not amenable to simple notions and basic functional processes. Every role has in it those things that are intangible, yet if missed can readily affect the value and viability of the role and its effect on team members' ability to work together.

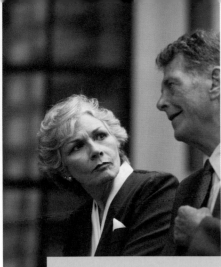

Expectation Dialog

- Is bidirectional between manager and staff
- Is free of punitive content
- Is directed toward raising performance
- Is open and free
- Is practical and applicable
- Is directed at performance, not person
- Results in a change in behavior
- Is evidenced in better outcomes

Voicing Expectations

Expectations must be made explicit. People should not have to read the minds of managers and/or the organization to gain some understanding of what is expected of them. It is surprising how often so much of what is expected of others is assumed. As a result leaders are often surprised that people did not know what was required and often fail to meet expectations (Clegg, 2000). Assumptions are a dangerous commodity in leadership circles because they so often lead to misunderstanding and to failure.

The good leader always (Smither, 1998):

1. Gives a voice to the roles and expectations that unfold in a way that can be both heard and understood by those who must perform.
2. Assumes nothing. If any assumptions are made, they err on the side of not knowing and facilitate the leader to raise questions regarding what is known and what is expected.
3. Knows simplicity is the best approach to understanding regardless of how "smart" the person in a role may be. It is critical that the foundations be laid upon which a further level of complexity and a deeper understanding can be built.
4. Identifies personal and organizational priorities for the work and the work environment, in order to make sure team members know what the givens and the nonnegotiable items are with regard to work expectations.
5. Communicates expectations, making sure that they are understood and can be acted on. Getting agreement with regard to performance is a central condition of accountability and essential to obtaining outcomes.
6. Acknowledges deficits that are identified in relationship to work expectations, making sure they are clarified up front as to whether they are foundational expectations or can be developed in the course of the work. If they are to be developed, the organization must have both the means and the time available to make sure that they can be acted on.

ACCOUNTABILITY-BASED PERFORMANCE FACTORS

Roles are defined in such a way that job expectations are clear and performance outcomes are well outlined.

Recruitment policy ensures that there is a good fit between the role expectations and the person who will ultimately fill the role.

Performance factors clearly outline the performance specifics in a way that can ensure that they can be acted on.

Configuring any one role reflects the relations of that role to other roles both influenced by and influencing the individual role.

Functional expectations flow easily from the role definitions and tie the role functions to the results to which they are directed.

The team values each role that makes up the composite of roles and can relate all roles with the purpose of the work of the team.

Note:

Effective accountability implies that all team members understand each role as a reflection of the team and must contribute to reflecting the purposes of the team and advancing the achievement of its outcomes.

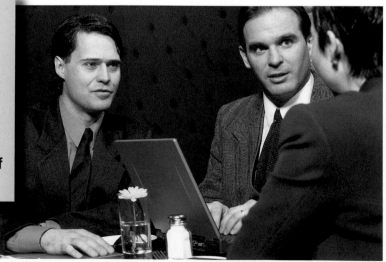

REVISITING INVITATION AND EXPECTATION

In a performance-driven organization, it should be clear to all participants that contribution, commitment, performance, and participation are expected (O'Reilly & Pfeffer, 2000). Team members should feel that they must be invited into ownership and participation in decisions and actions that represent the obligations of the team. Invitation indicates that accountability is optional. In effective team configurations, this is simply untrue. Membership implies ownership and accountability and each team member must represent that in his or her role.

Invitation

- External orientation
- Passive engagement
- Other directed
- Functionally driven
- Process oriented
- "Job" mental model
- Task fixed
- Event based
- No ownership
- Past active

Expectation

- Internal orientation
- Active engagement
- Self-directed
- Purpose driven
- Outcome oriented
- "Role" mental model
- Relationship based
- "Journey based"
- Full ownership
- Proactive

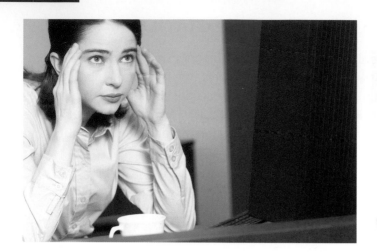

Note:

Staff often lose sight of the meaning imbedded in their work and become focused on the work itself. Effective leaders are always helping staff refocus and center their activities on the purposes and values that drive the work.

WORK AND MEANING

Work must reflect purpose if it is to have any meaning (Runco, 2003). Slavish attachment to ritual and routine is the best evidence that meaning is missing or that the workers are not aware of what meaning might be present. In the absence of meaning, people create their own structure and form that often acts as a poor replacement for consistent team meaning and value. It is important for leaders to help people stay in touch with this issue of meaning and value in relationship to work, if only to keep them reality oriented regarding the nature of the work and its inevitable changeability. By so doing, the leader keeps the question of meaning and value ever before the staff and makes it an important part of the dialog. Steps in keeping an orientation to the meaning of work in the staff are:

■ Make work purpose visible to the staff through storyboards or displays that publicly demonstrate the meaning and values driving the work.

■ All job descriptions and performance expectations should evidence the values and meaning driving performance.

■ Team members should actively participate in forming and implementing meaning and values in order to actualize ownership for them.

■ Expectations for outcomes cannot be sustained if there isn't a value or purpose driving the work. Each team member must be able to articulate that value within the context of individual and team expectations for performance.

■ Evaluation of performance and productivity should include how individuals and teams have advanced the purposes and values of the organization and how that is demonstrated in the process and products of work.

■ Leaders adjust the processes and activities of work as the demand, technology, and conditions change. At the same time they work to reconfirm the purpose and reconfigure it within the context of new activities.

PERFORMANCE COMPETENCE

Clearly, performance expectation includes the competence necessary to do the work. Although this goes without restating, leaders need to set up work expectations and performance accountability at the outset through making competence requirements clear to potential team members before they become members of the team and the organization (Harris, 2003). The ability to perform compatibly and equitably at the level of other members of the team is a reasonable expectation of all team members. Whereas development and growth are an expectation of orienting to work expectations, there must be reasonable hope that the individual can and will grow into the role in an appropriate period. Many organizations orient and train and re-train to death those workers who frequently have demonstrated that they cannot meet expectations for performance and likely never will. By the time this reality hits home, it is too late, the employee is often with you to stay. Remember:

1. Competence is not static or permanent; it is constantly changing with the work and technology. It is the expectation of leaders and workers that changing work expectations will include adequate time to learn the new reality and processes related to the work.

2. Leaders are reading the signposts of change, prepared in advance to alert team members of the potential for change and the role and functional shifts that might require. Determine what the demands will likely be and prepare the staff as far in advance as possible of expected behavioral changes.

3. Competence isn't what people bring to their work; it is instead, evidenced in the work reflected in its value, quality, and appreciation by those who are the direct beneficiaries of the products of the work.

4. Competence assumes adequate preparation for the role. Leaders should not compromise preparation by personality. Often a dynamic, exciting individual will appear on a team's doorstep with all the requisite charm and with effective communication skills but is shy on talent. Outcomes cannot be achieved or sustained through force of will alone, a basic and underlying competence that grows with the demand is necessary to sustain work and necessary change.

5. Competence is as competence does. The best exemplar of competence is not excellent work but great results. Staff and leaders should not be captured by the concept of "doing a great job." Manual dexterity and technical proficiency are not competence; they are simply means. The competent worker always sees the work as an element of the goals it produces or the results it obtains.

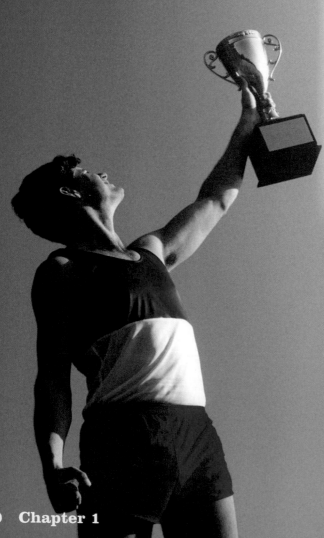

ELEMENTS OF PERFORMANCE COMPETENCE

■ Basic skill and performance expectations are clarified for the role in advance of expecting role competence.

■ Competency expectations are written in language that is clear yet relates to the level of technology the role demands.

■ As the work changes, so do performance expectations. These adjustments must be noted in advance as workers change practices to accommodate newer realities.

■ The organization addresses developmental needs of team and individuals as a change in expectations ushers in a change in performance.

■ Opportunities are available to advance skills and improve contribution to the team and to the work. Advancement programs provide incentives for staff to keep growing.

■ The team changes and adjusts demand to shift the focus on team expectations for performance and changes team competency expectations to match new demand.

BARRIERS TO COMPETENCE

■ A lack of openness from the management team toward sharing information with the staff

■ A punitive environment that constrains freedom of expression and individual contribution

■ A controlling manager who must maintain his or her own authority and needs to take credit for everything

■ A staff attitude of nonparticipation and job orientation, seeing the role simply as a conduit for functions and tasks

■ A formal and rigid hierarchical structure that is strictly "top-down" and does not locate decisions at the point-of-service

■ Ambiguity regarding role and performance expectations and nonspecific evaluations and no consequences for nonparticipation

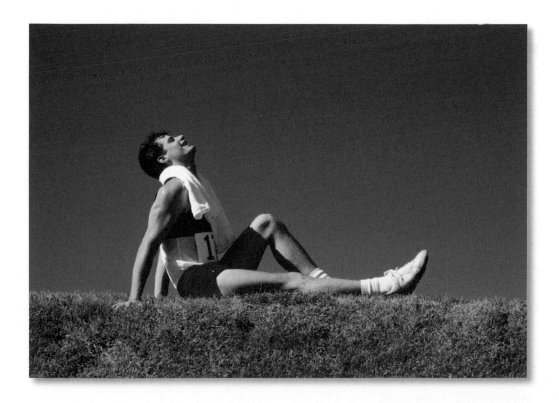

SCENARIO

Competence Management

Nancy, the nurse manager, has been approached by a staff member for the fifth time regarding Patrick, a nurse new to the unit. They expressed real concerns about Patrick's competence and understanding regarding his role and related performance expectations. Sharon had talked with Patrick before and he seemed responsive and willing to adjust his practices. Each of the new staff complaints, however, focused on differing areas of competence.

In addition to the concerns regarding Patrick's clinical competence was a real concern for the staffing shortage on the unit. Having Patrick aboard had filled a position that had been vacant for a long time. Nancy really needed Patrick to "work out" because she didn't want to have to fill the position again with someone else she would have to orient and train.

Place yourself in Nancy's position and using the information already shared in this chapter, address the following questions:

1. What should Nancy have done to prepare for Patrick's arrival on the unit?

2. How could the other staff have been involved in the initial interview and assessment of Patrick before his coming to the unit?

3. What are the important management questions Nancy needed to ask of Patrick before his coming to the unit?

4. What are the critical questions the staff needed to have answered about Patrick before his coming to the unit?

5. What possible barriers could exist on the unit influencing Patrick's ability to be successful there?

6. What about Patrick's preparation and previous experience do the staff need to know in deciding whether there is a goodness-of-fit between Patrick and the unit staff?

7. What questions should Patrick have asked about the unit, staff and work before his agreeing to join the staff there?

8. What is the purpose of orientation and precepting programs and how would this affect Patrick's experience as a new member of the unit?

9. Now that Patrick is a member of the unit, how do the manager and staff address their concerns regarding his performance?

10. How can trust between Patrick and the staff be reestablished?

11. What are the key elements of Nancys plan of approach to addressing this concern and where should she begin?

12. How will Nancy and the staff evaluate progress or change in their relationship with Patrick and in his performance and what do they do if no change occurs?

The "Buck" Stops at Competence

Competence is perhaps the single greatest factor in determining the effectiveness of individual work and its integration with the collective work of the team (London, 2001). Leaders have a great deal of difficulty with the whole issue of competence when applied to roles and articulated through performance expectation. All kinds of social pressures and relational factors strongly influence how leaders and team members deal with each other's personal performance and in evidencing defined competence and role outcomes.

Performance means just that—performance. Specific expectations for individual performance are usually identified at the outset of a work role. The good leader provides short increments of information and feedback at defined periods in both the individual and the team's performance against specific goals (Malloch & Porter-O'Grady, 2005). These short-term interventions around the expression of performance create an opportunity for identification of issues, dialog with regard to any shift in performance, and an opportunity to discuss the development of new skills. Aso, smaller increments of time spent in performance evaluation activities help reduce the intensity and drama related to performance changes that might otherwise occur over longer periods. Perhaps the best example of the least effective approach to performance is the annual performance evaluation. After having waited a long time for definitive evaluation of performance and progress, the person being evaluated finds that the volume and the intensity of information related to performance becomes overwhelming. Too much volume of material is covered over too long a period of time and in a way that cannot adequately address personal issues, incremental elements of function and action, and issues and factors related to measuring real-time performance.

Incremental Performance Evaluation	*Annual Performance Evaluation*
• Fequent review of progress	• Long-term review of progress
• Identification of specific issues	• Identification of larger issues
• Addressing of problems as they arise	• Dealing with aggregate problems
• More personalization of response	• More generalized in valuation
• Opportunity for immediate change	• Long-term change plan
• Timely addressing of concerns	• Addressing of problem patterns
• More relevant to the work at hand	• Relevant to broad issues of progress

Performance competence is one of the most serious factors related to individual and team action. It should never be left unaddressed over long periods. The least effective way of addressing performance evaluation is waiting until the annual performance review.

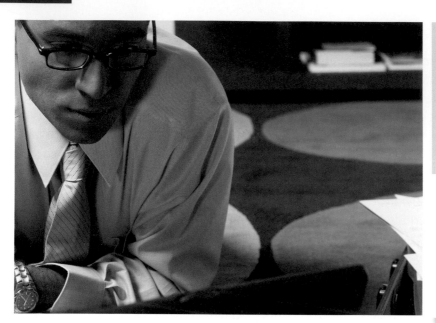

Competency Sources

- Learning
- Experience
- Reflecting
- Relationships
- Practice
- Serendipity

Note:

Competence is not a capacity; it is a journey of growth, development, and continual improvement to whic every individual is committed.

INTERSECTION OF COMPETENCE FACTORS

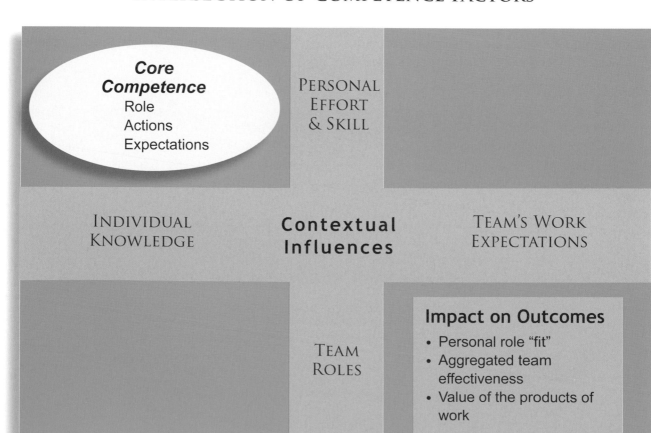

Core Competence
Role
Actions
Expectations

PERSONAL EFFORT & SKILL

INDIVIDUAL KNOWLEDGE

Contextual Influences

TEAM'S WORK EXPECTATIONS

TEAM ROLES

Impact on Outcomes

- Personal role "fit"
- Aggregated team effectiveness
- Value of the products of work

RESPONSIBILITY VS. ACCOUNTABILITY

Responsibility (20th Century)	*Accountability (20th Century)*
Process	Product
Action	Result
Work	Outcome
Do	Accomplish
Task	Difference
Function	Fit
Job	Role
Incremental	Sustainable
Externally generated	Internally generated
Quality effort	Quality impact

Differentiating Accountability from Responsibility

The terms *accountability* and *responsibility* are frequently used interchangeably. However, these terms and the dynamics to which they relate mean entirely different things. Perhaps the most important distinction between responsibility and accountability relates to their orientation. Responsibility focuses on the work, the competence of the worker, the effectiveness of the processes, the quality of the effort, and the excellence of its application (Porter-O'Grady, 2003).

Accountability, on the other hand, focuses on the products of work rather than the processes of work. Accountability relates to issues regarding the impact of the work, the products or results of work, a difference the work makes, and whether the work mattered in relationship to performance and expectations. Quite simply, accountability focuses on issues of outcome and calls attention to the effects of the work rather than the processes related to the work itself. Today, questions of accountability have become increasingly important as the relationship between work effectiveness, outcome, and work process becomes more important.

PROCESS VS. OUTCOME

Elements of Process

- Action oriented
- Task related
- Functional proficiency
- Manual dexterity
- Time bound
- Progressive
- Incremental
- Fixed effort
- Applied

Elements of Outcome

- Results oriented
- Value driven
- Satisfaction based
- Impact
- Expectation
- Satisfaction
- Product of work
- Fluid
- Making a difference

Focusing on Process

So much effort is built on creating effective process, reducing error, identifying and saving costs, and ensuring good work productivity that questions of real value almost get lost (White, 2001). Whereas there certainly is recognition of the issue of value, it is almost secondary to the efforts of creating a good process. Accountability asks questions related to the value of the outcome, the impact of the difference that's made, and the conditions and circumstances that are advanced by having undertaken the work or produced the product. Work is not inherently valuable simply because there is a desire to do it. The value of work is driven by purpose, meaning, and the enhancement of the value and quality of human life and experience. Accountability suggests that these questions have been raised in all places of the organization, from strategy through tactics to application. Good leaders recognize that the issue of accountability is always the question of the time and that defining the relationship between the work and its impact at various levels of measure is a critical element of good leadership.

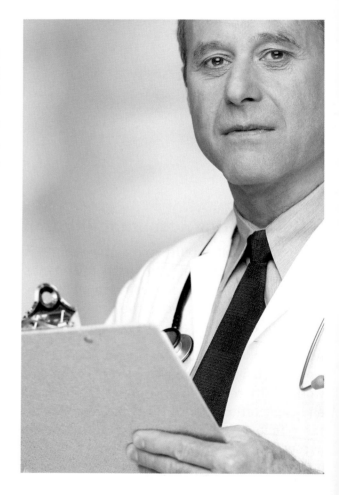

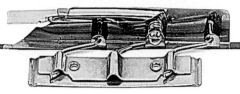

ACCOUNTABILITY AND IMPACT

■ Accountability always asks, what difference does the work effort make?

■ Accountability focuses the effort of the worker on the products of work rather than the processes of work.

■ In accountability, the discipline is focused on creating a goodness-of-fit-between work effort and results.

■ Accountability suggests that evaluation and comparison occur between work and the products of work.

■ Accountability implies that quality improvement focuses on work as a reflection of the value of its products/result.

■ Accountability seeks to identify what specific elements of work make the key difference in its results.

■ Accountability requires an internal generation or motive for excellence, not merely an external demand.

A Brief Note about Work Effort

Much has been written on the value of work. Clearly, work is important to the people that do it. Most people want their work to be meaningful and valuable and to be an expression of their personal commitment. The reality, however, is that work itself can never be a source of meaning and value. When work becomes a source of meaning and value it begins to create serious problems for the worker. The truth about work is that it is constantly shifting and adjusting to the ever-changing landscape of life and the external forces that provide the context for work. Work is always changing; becoming something different, new, improved, ever adjusting to the changing social, economic, and technological characteristics that influence it (Goad, 2002).

Instead of providing meaning, work should be the expression of the meaning the individual brings to it. That set of principles, values, and other sources of meaning that inform individuals actions and pursuits should be the foundation upon which individual personal meaning is developed. As one's own meaning and work becomes clear, the individual can better evaluate how much the action of work reflects the expression of meaning. When meaning fails to drive work, before long, work ceases to be meaningful.

It is important for workers and for teams to stop occasionally to raise questions of meaning and value, exploring the reasons and insights behind the individual and team efforts in undertaking work. In working, one is often overwhelmed with the actions, functions, and processes associated with it, such that these can sometimes cause individuals and teams to lose sight of the direction and purpose of those efforts. The wise leader stops individual and team action periodically to spend some time in reexamining the relationship between the work effort and the meaning and purposes that drive it.

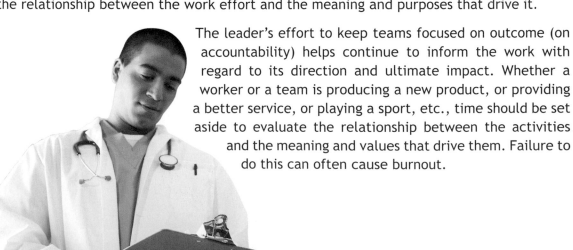

The leader's effort to keep teams focused on outcome (on accountability) helps continue to inform the work with regard to its direction and ultimate impact. Whether a worker or a team is producing a new product, or providing a better service, or playing a sport, etc., time should be set aside to evaluate the relationship between the activities and the meaning and values that drive them. Failure to do this can often cause burnout.

ROLE CLARITY AND ACCOUNTABILITY MODEL

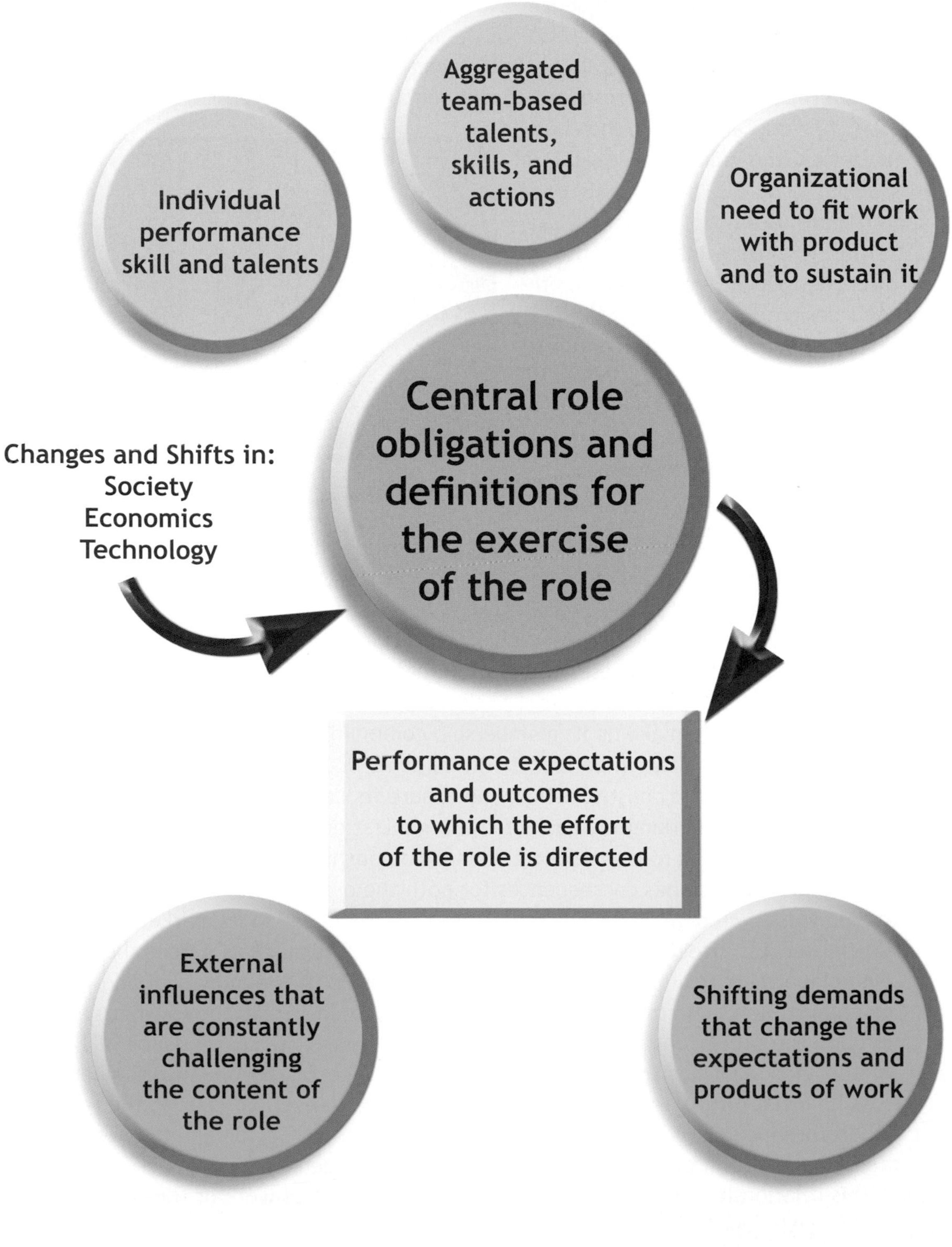

Aggregated team-based talents, skills, and actions

Individual performance skill and talents

Organizational need to fit work with product and to sustain it

Changes and Shifts in:
Society
Economics
Technology

Central role obligations and definitions for the exercise of the role

Performance expectations and outcomes to which the effort of the role is directed

External influences that are constantly challenging the content of the role

Shifting demands that change the expectations and products of work

COMPETENCE AND CONSEQUENCE

There is no accountability without consequence. Everyone must understand that the performance of work is not directed merely to the satisfaction of the individual, but instead is more specifically directed to fulfilling the purposes and goals of the organization. People work in organizations and groups in order to create a collective response to the demands of an enterprise. In this way, the

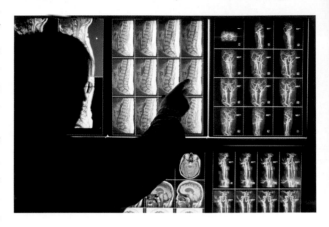

aggregated efforts of work can advance the viability of the organization, the individual's quality of life, and the social good. In a free and open economy, the relationship among these three factors is vital to ensure their sustainability. Although there are many challenges with regard to the ethics, efficacy, and design of organizations, work, economics, and social impact, the intersection of all these dynamics is continually operating, influencing and affecting the action of work. Every individual must know that performance effectiveness and advancing outcome is the cornerstone upon which effective work is built.

Every worker must produce. There must be a relationship between the work effort, the expectations for it, and outcomes. Every worker must incorporate this understanding into his or her set of behaviors with regard to the personal exercise of work. Whereas organizations and workplaces do have a clear and ethical responsibility to create a quality of work life, to reward equitably, and to assist in the improvement of the quality of life of those who make up its membership community; to do this requires that the organization be successful, meet its financial and economic goals, satisfy its constituencies, and ensure its continuing ability to thrive. Each working member of the organizational community has a clear and specific role and obligation in accomplishing these objectives. Failure to do so has consequences for both the orga-

> *Note:*
>
> **Neither the organization nor the individual lives in isolation from the other. Each has an obligation to advance its best efforts in creating the conditions for mutual thriving.**

nization and the individual. An organization unable to thrive, to succeed in its marketplace, and to advance its financial success affects the individual's quality of life as much as it does the organization's. In the workplace there is an intertwining of the relationship of the individual and the work community. The organization that combines them, entwining them in a relationship where each has a direct impact upon the other contributes to its sustaining success. The consequence of the non-performance of the individual has an impact on the performance of the organization, and ultimately affects its financial future and the ability to thrive at every level. Of course, the reverse is also true. It is therefore incumbent upon the relationship between the person and the organization to recognize their inherent relationship and to acknowledge the consequences that occur when they fail to consider this relationship in either the individual commitment to work or the organization's commitment to those who do its work and advance its ends.

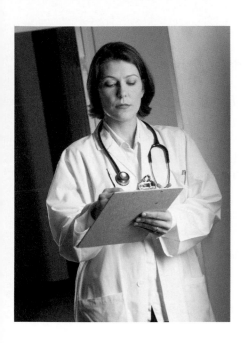

A Message about Ownership

Owners are different from renters. When one owns something, one is considerate of it, caring for it and protecting it from harm. When one owns the effort of work, the same care and concern are required to advance it and value it as well as create the conditions for sustaining it.

Advancing Personal Ownership

Every individual owns his or her own work. Wise leaders never impede this sense of ownership by acting as though the organization owns the work.

The leader is always a consultant regarding the individual's expression of work, guiding and articulating work effort with organizational goals.

Ownership of work suggests full engagement and participation in decisions that affect the exercise of that work and its effect on the organization.

Individual ownership calls for a movement away from "job orientation" and task focus. Ownership calls for a focus on work value and outcomes.

References

Clegg, B. (2000). *Creativity and innovation for managers*. Philadelphia: Butterworth-Heinemann.

Goad, T. W. (2002). *Information literacy and workplace performance*. Westport, CT: Quorum Books.

Harris, C. (2003). *Building innovative teams: Strategies and tools for developing and integrating high performance innovative groups*. New York: Palgrave Macmillan.

London, M. (2001). *How people evaluate others in organizations*. Mahwah, NJ; London: L. Erlbaum.

Malloch, K., & Porter-O'Grady, T. (2005). *The quantum leader: Applications for the new world of work*. Sudbury, MA: Jones and Bartlett.

O'Reilly, C., & Pfeffer, J. (2000). *Hidden value*. Boston: Harvard Business School Publishing.

Pfeffer, J., & Sutton, R. (1999). *The knowing-doing gap: Turning knowledge into action*. Boston: Harvard Business School Publishing.

Porter-O'Grady, T. (2003). A different age for leadership, part 2: New rules, new roles. *Journal of Nursing Administration*, 33(3), 173-178.

Runco, M. A. (2003). *Critical creative processes*. Cresskill, NJ: Hampton Press.

Smither, J. (1998). *Performance appraisal*. San Francisco: Jossey-Bass.

White, S. (2001). *New ideas about new ideas*. New York: Perseus Publishing.

Suggested Readings

Hickman, C., Smith, T., & Conners, R. (2004). *The Oz principle: Getting results through individual and organizational accountability*. New York: Portfolio Hardcover.

Malloch, K., & Porter-O'Grady, T. (2005). *The quantum leader: Applications for the new world of work*. Sudbury, MA: Jones and Bartlett.

Miller, J. (2004). *Qbq! The question behind the question: Practicing personal accountability in work and in life*. New York: Penguin.

Riggio, R. E., & Orr, S. S. (2004). *Improving leadership in nonprofit organizations*. San Francisco: Jossey-Bass.

CHAPTER 2

ROLE ACCOUNTABILITY: THE OWNERSHIP OF WORK

Every worker has a stake in success. Failing to create stakeholders commited to the purpose, value, and outcomes of work ultimately endangers the enterprise and the energy people bring to sustain it.

Each individual brings to the team a specific set of characteristics, skills, and contributions to the work and the team's relationships. Vital to undertaking this work is a clear understanding of both the contribution and its relationship to the range of contributions that each member brings to the action and work of the team. It is important to understand this contribution and to know what skills and talents one brings to the workplace. What is more important, however, is a clear understanding of the contribution those skills will make when aggregated with the individual contributions of all members (Porter-O'Grady & Krueger Wilson, 1998).

Teams should reflect the total range of skills, talents, abilities, and interactions necessary to collectively fulfill the work obligations they have. It is important that each team reflect in its members the necessary facility in addressing the demands of performance and productivity. Furthermore, each member of the work team must know that the entire team depends on each member's specific gifts and talents. Individual member contributions complete the array of requisites necessary to fulfill the work obligations of the full team. In fact, each member must "own" his or her contribution to the team to the extent that the individual affirms, extends, and develops personal contribution to the processes and work of the team.

Ownership implies investment, creativity, and a commitment to personal growth. Each member of the team must bring this understanding into the role and recognize the expectations of one's own work and its relationship to other members of the team. This calls each member to have a commitment to personal growth.

Note:

Ownership implies full engagement and contribution to the work and the life of the team. Ownership suggests that the individual will take good care of the talent, relationship, and contributions he or she brings to the team effort.

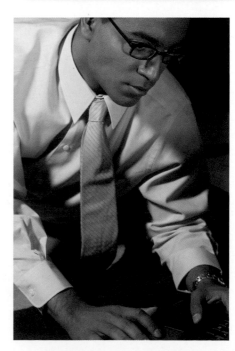

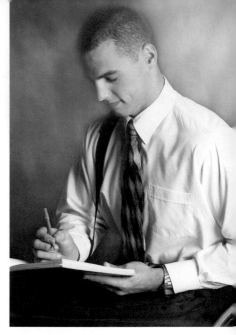

Ownership Is Commitment

- To fully applying one's own skills.
- To growing and learning to enhance talents.
- To development of others.
- To evaluating effectiveness of contribution.
- To continual lifelong learning.

THE CRITICAL ELEMENTS OF OWNERSHIP

Individuals value their specific talents and skills and commit to the full application of them in the workplace.

Individual team members recognize that learning is a lifelong experience and needs to be incorporated into the work experience.

Skill enhancement depends on a collective commitment to sharing, developing, and learning from each other in the team.

Ownership implies a commitment to help others learn and develop, thereby increasing the value of the team.

Problems or issues with role or relationship are identified early with each team member committing to resolving these challenges.

INDIVIDUAL ROLE ACCOUNTABILITY AND TEAM PERFORMANCE

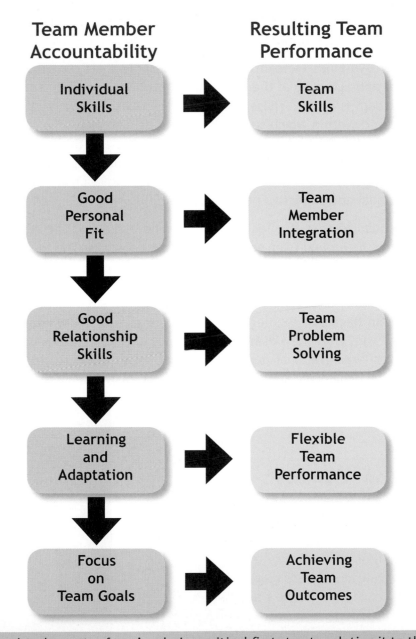

Team Member Accountability	Resulting Team Performance
Individual Skills	Team Skills
Good Personal Fit	Team Member Integration
Good Relationship Skills	Team Problem Solving
Learning and Adaptation	Flexible Team Performance
Focus on Team Goals	Achieving Team Outcomes

Defining the elements of one's role is a critical first step to relating it to the work of the team. Knowing the contribution that one can make to the team before joining it is an important foundation for team effectiveness. The lack of a goodness-of-fit between individual and team is one of the greatest causes of team problems. Clearly enumerating what an individual brings to the team facilitates team effectiveness.

INDIVIDUAL ACCOUNTABILITY FOR TEAM GOALS

Every team member has a specific accountability for achieving the team's goals (Gottlieb, 2003). All team members must work in concert with others in order to ensure that individual and collective effort is contributing to the achievement of team goals.

There are basically two kinds of team goals to which individuals contribute. First are those that relate to the needs and activities of the team and fulfill the purposes and direction of the organization of which the team is a part. These goals and objectives are the work priorities of teams and provide the framework within which team action unfolds. Secondly, the team has its own specific service or functional goals that relate to the work that it does and the manner in which that work is completed. Here the team focuses on the application of standards, protocols, processes, pathways, and plans. These goals sets identify the frame for individual and team action and provide the context within which individual and collective performance unfolds.

Team members recognize that if effectiveness is to be achieved, the effort of individual team members must converge around team goals. All activities related to the function of the team should coalesce in a way that advances performance against the anticipated goal achievement. It is in failing to recognize this fundamental reality for all teams that infrastructure and relationship begin to break down. When any one member's performance operates out of concert with the team, the integrity of the team begins to disintegrate. It is important for team members to recognize that although individual work is unique and important, it must ultimately advance the team's work effort as well as fulfill the organizational purposes for that work. Good teams assess the relationship between the work of individuals and the collective work of the team and its effect on achieving outcomes.

Focusing on Team Goals

- Incorporating team goals and individual work
- Defining the fit between individual and team
- Clarifying organizational work expectations
- Identifying team performance factors
- Specifying individual needs related to work
- Supporting each other in the collective work
- Removing impediments to team effectiveness
- Ending incongruent individual performance
- Evaluating progress regularly and often

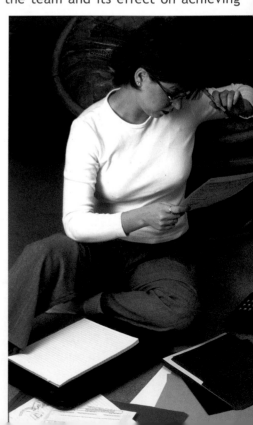

FITTING INDIVIDUAL AND TEAM GOALS TOGETHER

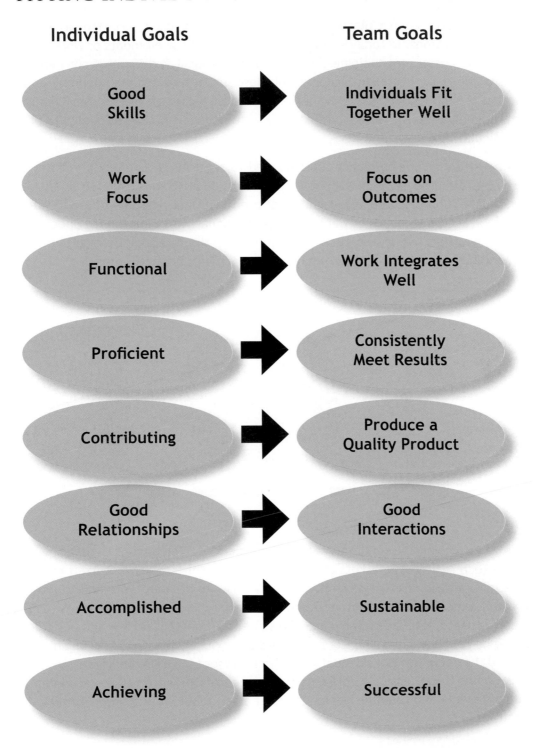

Individual Goals

- Good Skills → Individuals Fit Together Well
- Work Focus → Focus on Outcomes
- Functional → Work Integrates Well
- Proficient → Consistently Meet Results
- Contributing → Produce a Quality Product
- Good Relationships → Good Interactions
- Accomplished → Sustainable
- Achieving → Successful

Team Goals

ACCOUNTABILITY VS. JOB DESCRIPTIONS

Most organizations and leaders place a great deal of stock in job descriptions as a framework for performance expectations. In today's work world, so many of the elements of work are being transformed by new processes, technologies, and approaches that it is difficult if not impossible to permanently affix job descriptors. In fact, the job description as a tool for defining and identifying specific work is probably no longer relevant. Leaders must recognize that in an accountability based workplace, defining long lists of responsibilities and functions is no longer adequate or appropriate to clearly articulating roles.

In order to be effective, performance must be tied to the role as a reflection of the outcomes to which the role is directed (Thompson et al., 2002). This focus on outcomes calls for an entirely different orientation to role. Job-oriented approaches that are functional, incremental, and event based are not adequate or accurate means of delineating professional work. Identifying specific components of work is not as effective an approach as is identifying the direction or results of the work and clarifying, within current technologies, what work activities will obtain them.

Job
- Fixed
- Finite
- Functional
- Activity
- Incremental

Transition
- Unbundling
- Adapting
- Moving
- Refocusing
- Sustaining

Role
- Fluid
- Flexible
- Focused
- Mobile

This change to new roles and functions reflects the speed at which work is adapting and adjusting to a new high-tech reality. As markets change and demand shifts, the work itself must also be fluid and flexible (Tilley & Watson, 2004). The ability of the worker to be adaptable and to move seamlessly from one set of expectations to another is now a cornerstone of the future of work. Role expectations and performance descriptions now must be subject to constant review and periodic adjustment if they are to be relevant. Permanently prescribed and defined job descriptions do not meet these conditions and therefore are not adequate tools to represent both the character and the content of work. Transitioning to professional role versus job orientation will require considerable rethinking on the part of leaders and redefine approaches to better adapt work to transforming demands and shifting realities.

FROM PROCESS TO OUTCOME

The primary focus of accountability is on the achievement of results and the effect of those results over the long term. Sustainable organizations do not simply look at the next increment of time with regard to sustainability. Instead, they establish a long-term vision and tie their work processes to all of the efforts necessary to achieve it. Ultimately, individuals and teams must define their accountabilities as a reflection of this long-term viability. This focus on accountability instead of process responsibility calls for rethinking of a unilateral focus on job elements and process.

Focus on Accountability

■ Accountable organizations clearly identify who they are and their relationship to those they serve. They are continually committed to redefining their processes to fit their identity.

■ Individuals who understand accountability continually redefine their work effort as a reflection of their work goals. They also redefine goals as their work landscape and customers change.

■ Organizations understand accountability in light of fulfilling the real needs of those they serve, not just their wants. The ability to sort through and distinguish need from want is key to success.

■ Processes always lead to defined outcomes. As the outcomes adjust or advance (or are enhanced), work processes are adaptable and redesigned to create a better fit.

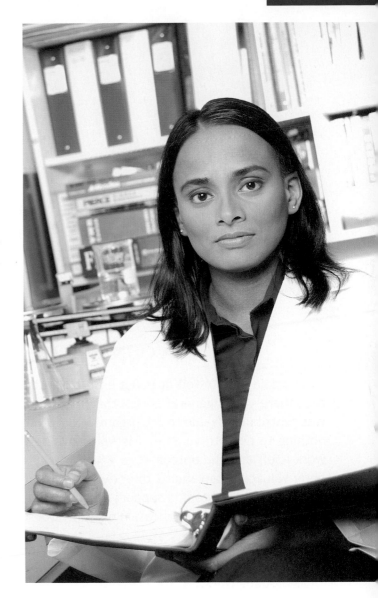

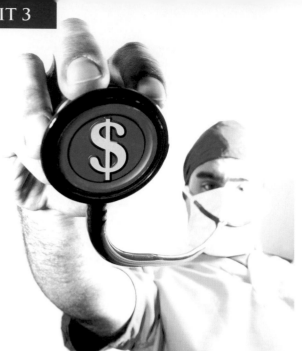

Note:

Value is more than controlling costs and achieving specific goals. Value reflects meaning and purpose and not only relates to the outcomes achieved but also reflects the relationships and processes necessary to sustain success over time. Value is as much about people as it is about the products of work effort.

ACCOUNTABILITY AND ADDING VALUE

Simply doing a job well does not ensure that the work was valuable or made a difference. In times past there was a general notion that if an individual did good work and worked hard, that person was contributing value to the organization. What is increasingly apparent, however, is that value has nothing to do with volume. The value of one's work depends on the goodness-of-fit between the work itself and the outcomes to which it is directed (Malloch & Porter-O'Grady, 2006). Work is not inherently valuable. Its value is directly related to how it contributes to the purposes and ends of the organization or system in support of its sustainability. This notion of adding value is critical to both the meaning and the application of work. Questions related specifically to value that every worker must ask are:

- Does the work I do relate well to the purposes of the team?
- Do my work efforts integrate well with the efforts of others on the team?
- Am I clear on the essential value of each of the elements of mywork?
- Do the efforts of all team members link and integrate well around expectation?
- Do I reassess my functions and activities regularly to determine their relevance?
- Do I join with the team in evaluating effectiveness of work effort?
- Is there clear evidence that my work and the outcomes directly relate well?
- Am I willing to adjust my work activity when a change is clearly indicated?
- Do I actively problem solve with team members to resolve critical issues?
- Am I flexible in adjusting my work activities when the team needs to change?
- Do I join actively with team members in identifying specific work changes?
- Do I initiate discussions and dialog when problems in work processes emerge?
- Is there willingness on the part of all team members to confront each other?
- Do I join with the team in celebrating successes and accomplishments?

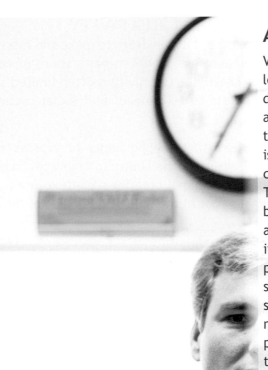

Accountability and Value

Value is a critical element of measure that looks at a number of variables and makes a decision about the integrity of the relationship among them. From purpose, meaning, expectation, and outcomes, the expression of value is the reflection of how these factors work in concert to produce success and sustainability. This notion of the application of value works both for the individual who is applying skills and talents in the accomplishment of an activity and the organization that is looking to provide a service or produce a product that, in some way, advances the interests of those it serves and improves the viability of the organization. This "dance" between individual and personal applications of value and the collective and organizational expression of value is a vital element of all human endeavor.

Accountability and Time

We've all heard the saying "Time is money." Although true, the commitment to one's work should include the valuing of time. Time is valuable because it is an element of the measure of work and therefore calls each person to be reflective of how well time is being used to meet the purposes of work. One can be either efficient and effective or slow and wasting time in the course of doing the same work. Time must be considered as an element of value in the accomplishment of work. One is as accountable for the use of time as for any other measure of effectiveness. There should always be a balance between work effort and time; exceeding or underappreciating either one creates the opportunity of losing balance and ultimately increasing work effort and cost and depreciating the value of time.

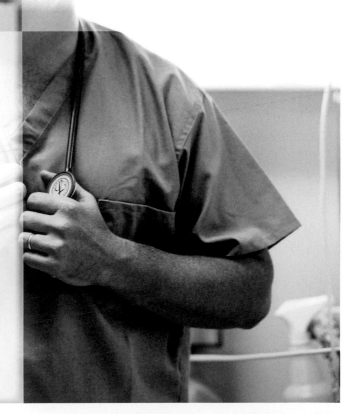

ACCOUNTABILITY AND INDIVIDUAL CREATIVITY

Accountable individuals use the greatest resources they have in order to make the most sustainable difference. All people are born creative. The course of life, however, has a series of variable kinds of impact on the ability of individuals to express creativity. Creativity is often limited by childhood experiences, challenges to personal growth, threats to self-image, and social occurrences that limit its expression.

Creativity and innovation demands openness, freedom, the opportunity to express and to move beyond habits, rote, ritual, and routine. Creativity reflects the ability to embrace, to challenge, to think in new ways. The greatest deficit of leadership is in not creating a context or an environment where the most creative and innovative can emerge out of the minds and hearts of those who work and relate together (Pearce & Longer, 2003).

Accountability assumes the openness and availability to the creative urge and the impulse to create in each individual. Individuals must expect creativity as a part of their own role, and leaders must expect it as a part of creating an environment that will support creativity. This calls for the leader to embrace self-creativity and to recognize the innovative within. Unable to do so, the leader fails to recognize the value of doing it with others and becomes unable to identify the most creative in the action of others.

It is often difficult to live creatively at work. There's always some regulatory or procedural requisite that impedes the ability to be expressive and spontaneous. The need to be socialized and well integrated in the organization often values sameness at the expense of innovation. The uncertainty and disattachment to ritual that is necessary to stimulate the urge of innovation is simply absent. Also, the time necessary to explore and discern "outside the box" related to one's own work is often missing and not valued sufficiently to allow time to reflect and simply explore thinking differently. Yet, creativity is absolutely essential to the life and sustainability of the organization. The wise leader knows there is no option but to create the conditions and circumstance that generate the opportunity and accountability for creativity.

Generating the Creative Urge

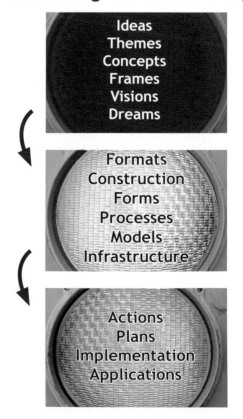

Ideas
Themes
Concepts
Frames
Visions
Dreams

Formats
Construction
Forms
Processes
Models
Infrastructure

Actions
Plans
Implementation
Applications

ISSUES OF OWNERSHIP

Accountability relates to decisions and their actions. It is important to clearly align decisions with those who are accountable for them (Malloch & Porter-O'Grady, 2005). Empowered work environments reflect a distribution of decisions based on their most appropriate locus of control. Central to this notion is the understanding that decisions are not reflective of position power but, instead, represent role power. Position power reflects that power is distributed to a role in the organization and vertically aligned to other positions over which it has authority. Accountability suggests that power is located where the decision has the best chance of being effectively carried out. Accountability has no dependence on position power because such power does not reflect a focus on effective location and exercise of a decision based on its characteristics rather than the positioning of a person. In an accountable organization, decisions are always located where they can be best exercised. If decisional competence is missing there or inadequately or inappropriately exercised or there is a preference for moving the decision away from its legitimate locus-of-control, the potential for negative outcomes is dangerously accelerated.

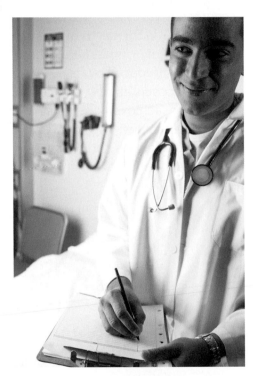

Note:

Decisions are located close to the places where they are exercised by those who own the accountability for action and sustaining the products of work. This locus-of-control reflects the fact that decisions are best made by those who most directly affect or achieve their outcomes.

Accountability and Outcomes

Accountability:
-Right decision
-Right person
-Right place
-Right time
-Right purpose

Decisions are located closest to where they will be acted on.

Outcome:
-Evidence based
-Applicable
-Acted on
-Defined results
-Effective

ACCOUNTABILITY AND LOCUS-OF-CONTROL

Accountability reflects the individual ownership of the decisions that attend to a particular role. A role holds decisional authority not so much because that authority is "assigned" to it but more because it is legitimate to the role because of the role's opportunity and obligation to directly affect outcome. The necessity to act in a certain way necessary to effect a related, defined outcome is the authority basis for determining location and making decisions related to a particular work effort. A role is empowered to make specific decisions because of its direct relationship to the specific decisions and actions that result in the fulfillment of the purpose or products of the work. An accountability-driven organization has an infrastructure that supports and recognizes this approach to accountability and performance.

Accountability reflects the location of power in the hands of those who ultimately undertake the actions that produce results. Ownership of accountability is necessary to the achievement of sustainable outcomes. Without this dynamic interaction, all work is, at best, incremental and short term.

Accountable Decisions and Action

Accountable decisions flow from individual role through the actions necessary to directly achieve outcomes and sustain an effective work-outcomes relationship.

Role:
-Location
-Accountability
-Performance
-Competence

Decisions:
-Authority
-Autonomy
-Competence
-Applicable

Actions:
-Applied
-Appropriate
-Implemented
-Good process

Outcomes:
-Evaluated
-Good fit
-Effective
-Sustainable

SHARED GOVERNANCE AND ACCOUNTABILITY

Much has been written about shared governance and its principles and implementation. Because this is not a text on shared governance, it is not discussed here. Readers are encouraged to review the literature and apply it to the culture of their own setting.

What IS important to say about shared governance here relates to the importance of creating a structure for accountability. Leaders cannot change behavior by addressing the behavior alone. The leader must create an infrastructure that emulates and expects particular kinds of behavior. Structure demonstrates the values, relationships, roles, and priorities of an organization and tells others how these variables are expressed and how they affect work and outcomes. In organizations that employ professionals, there must be a stronger partnership orientation and equity-based structure between the organization and the professional. This balance is necessary to maintain the integrity of the profession and the purposes of the organization. Structure creates the frame for this relationship and encases the mechanisms and processes that demonstrate the alignment of this partnership between profession and system.

Shared governance focuses on this demand for equitable structure and creates an infrastructure for professional practice that reflects the accountability of the profession and the obligation of the organization. This model frames the principles, decisions, roles, and processes associated with the professional work and the requisites of professional practice. Shared governance provides a context for defining the profession's work and relationships and the elements necessary to advance them. It requires the involvement and full participation of the members in the governance and decisions of their profession and the implementation of its work in relation to that of other disciplines and of the organization.

The relationship between structure and accountability is direct and dependent. Accountability is the expectation of the performance of the professional. Structure is the frame that is created to obtain and advance that accountability in performing the work of the system and in fulfilling its purposes. The professional "owns" the work of the profession and operates in a structure (shared governance) that supports the action of this ownership and the products of its work. Shared governance fully engages the professional and provides the means for the profession to act in concert and to apply the value of its collective wisdom to the work and purpose of the system in meeting the needs of those it serves. The context of shared governance provides means through which genuine professional relationships, performance, and outcomes emerge, and the individual and collective value of practice converges to make a difference that is consistent, integrated, measurable, and valued. In it, both professional and system can partner around a clearly articulated and concerted agenda that aggregates the efforts of the stakeholders and creates a relationship that supports them and coordinates all efforts around the common purposes of service, quality, value, and outcome.

SCENARIO

Accountability

Stephen was the newly elected chair of his unit-based practice council. He was not familiar with the demands of the role but wanted to respond with his best effort. He looked at the rules of engagement for the council and reviewed the terms of reference for its actions on the unit. Stephen was a little concerned when he saw the statement "The practice council has the accountability for the practice decisions on the unit; since the council represents the clinical staff and reflects its accountability for practice decisions, its deliberations and decisional processes always lead to action and therefore require staff compliance." He was unaware of this level of authority and sought to clarify it with his manager.

Upon clarification, it was clear that his role was seen as a clinical leader who fully participated in decisions that affected the work of others. His manager explained that her role was to support the council's decisions and to help him in the processes associated with dialog, discussion, negotiation, and making and implementing decisions. She also encouraged him with her personal commitment to help him develop leadership skills and facilitation processes.

Stephen was encouraged by this support but a little intimidated that he would be responsible for the staff making decisions that could affect practice and patient care in a direct way. This was a powerful break from the past when the manager was the prime mover and controller of decisions. Now accountability means that clinical decisions are placed with the staff where they have the best chance of being implemented and evaluated. This clearly increases staff engagement and extends their role in having an effect on the work of the organization.

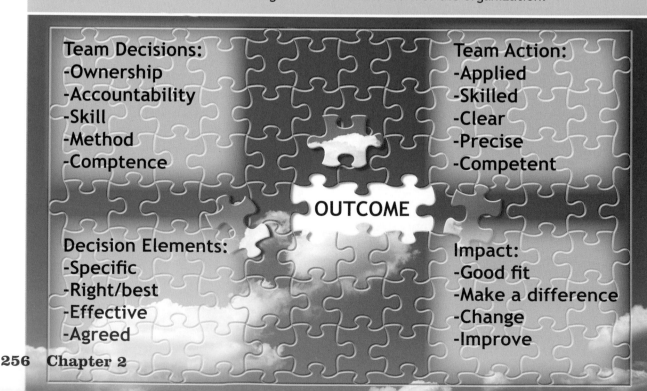

Team Decisions:
-Ownership
-Accountability
-Skill
-Method
-Comptence

Team Action:
-Applied
-Skilled
-Clear
-Precise
-Competent

OUTCOME

Decision Elements:
-Specific
-Right/best
-Effective
-Agreed

Impact:
-Good fit
-Make a difference
-Change
-Improve

OWNERSHIP—THE CENTER OF ACCOUNTABILITY

The central theme of accountability is the ownership of work. There is much controversy and disagreement about the locus of control for decisions and actions related to the work of organizations. In a private enterprise system, it is often assumed that the owner of the enterprise owns the means and processes associated with the organization.

In truth, however, this is an incomplete view of the work relationship. Although the organization owns the products of work and influences the processes of work, unless a real partnership exists between those who do the work and those who own the means and products of work, there is no sustainable, consistent, and accelerating outcome.

The challenge here is to incorporate the understanding that workers also have an ownership capacity. Because outcomes generate from the efforts of the worker as well as the resources of the owner, a fundamental partnership exists between them. When this partnership is well described and shared, the processes and products of work have the potential to be continually effective and sustainable (Pearce & Longer, 2003).

The wise leader understands this fundamental relationship and does everything to clarify its elements and to better describe the contribution that both people and resources make to the achievement and sustainability of the organization. This leader continually balances the needs of workers and demands of the organization in a mosaic or dance of effort that ensures the energies of the worker (human capital) and the resources (financial capital) of the organization continue to contribute to success.

Accountable Decision Making

Ownership of Work:
-Internally generated
-Skill based
-Continual improvement
-Conscious contribution
-Full engagement
-Good processes
-Effect on outcomes

Resources:
-Externally generated
-Adequate
-Relate to need
-Cost-benefit value
-Shared with workers
-Gain shared
-Return on investment

VOLUME VS. VALUE

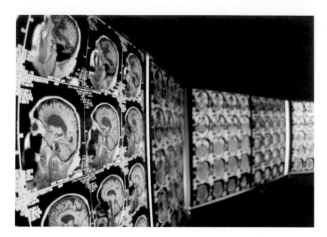

Note:

So often workers feel or sense value if they accomplish a job or do good work. The problem is that simply accomplishing work is not real value; making a difference with the work is a stronger indicator of real value.

So many times the professional worker will indicate that the amount of work done should be evidence of importance of work. Of course, nothing could be further from the truth. The amount of work one does has nothing to do with its meaning or value. Value is found in the effect of the work, or with its outcome (Malloch & Porter-O'Grady, 2005). The inputs of work relate directly to the outcome and should advance or increase the value of the outcome at a faster rate than the cost associated with the input. There is no positive value if this exchange of the relationship between input and outcome is negative. Increasing the work one does does not increase value. It is just increases the effort. Value is better represented when there is an expenditure of just the right amount of effort to maximize the products or outcome of the work and not an ounce more. In most effective workplaces, this relationship is important enough to be constantly defined and measured as a way of obtaining as much value as can be derived from the work effort.

Volume and Value Indicators

Volume of Work:
- Task focused
- Functional
- Process oriented
- Focus on the work
- Task completion
- Many processes
- Worker centered
- Immediate
- Short term

Value of Work:
- Results focused
- Action based
- Outcome oriented
- Effect of the work
- Achieving expectations
- Goodness-of-fit of effort
- Making a difference
- Sustainable
- Renewable

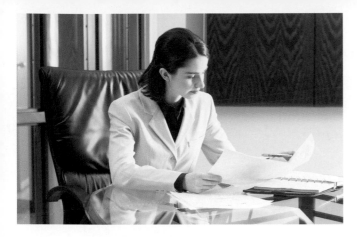

STAFF CANNOT GO WHERE THE LEADER HASN'T BEEN

Leaders create context; in fact, it is the only real work they have to do. Leaders create a safe space for staff to do their work and to risk the effort necessary to make the work a success. That means that the leader has to always be prepared to create the conditions and circumstances necessary to facilitate the work that will get the organization to where it is going. Leaders can't ask others to go to places they are not willing to go themselves.

The leader always lives in the potential. The leader demonstrates a willingness to go into unfamiliar territory and explore the possibilities that lie ahead of the work and experiences of the staff she or he leads. Creating context for the work of others is the primary work of the leader. This context should be the frame for the future action of the staff. It prepares the groundwork for the action of the staff as they move into new or enhanced experiences associated with the quality of the work they do. Changes, adjustments, shifts, and challenges to the current work of the staff are all anticipated by the leader, discerning their impact on the work or the worker. From this perspective the leader is able to prepare the staff in a way that is congruent with the changes that ultimately affect them or challenge the work they do or the way they do it.

Leader Risk Taking

The leader must demonstrate willingness to confront the vagaries of change. By so doing, she or he models behavior that can be replicated by the staff. The leader makes it safe for the staff to reach out and risk new approaches or patterns and confront change directly and harness the possibilities embedded there. If the leader cannot embrace and model risk behaviors, it is likely the staff will not be able to either.

Looking over the Horizon

Anticipating the inevitable
Redescribing the journey
Translating future events
Creating context for change
Expecting functional shifts
Noting economic shifts
Perceiving new technology
Identifying role enhancements
Reviewing data-driven change
Noting shifting markets/demand

CYCLE OF ENGAGING RISK AND ACTION

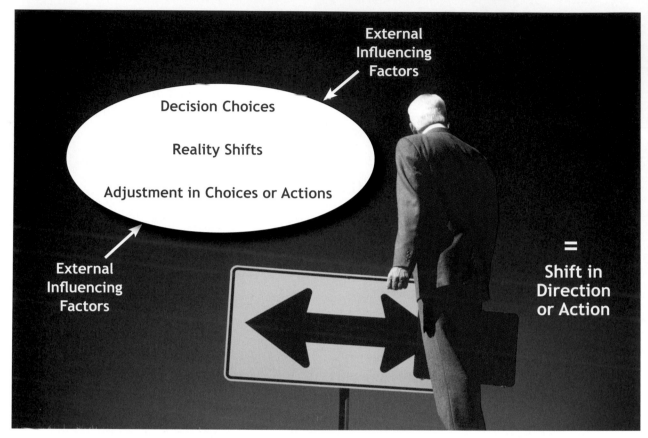

External
Influencing
Factors

Decision Choices

Reality Shifts

Adjustment in Choices or Actions

External
Influencing
Factors

=

Shift in
Direction
or Action

MAKING RISK NORMATIVE

There is risk embedded in all human action. It is not possible to eliminate risk. If there were no risk life would be flat, indeed, lifeless. Risk is a sign of reaching out in new ways or in new directions without a compass or ability to absolutely predict what will happen. Risk can only be accommodated and managed. The more the leader understands the nature and occurrence of risk, the better able he or she is in predicting it and designing responses that accommodate it or manage it well (see the model above). In fact, the good leader is able to anticipate the degree of risk inherent in a change and to predict it with a level of accuracy. In this way, the leader can help the staff grapple with the implications of risk and to maximize their own response to the changes in the work. The risk management mechanisms of the leader help the staff normalize risk and more easily engage it.

SOME RISK-DEALING RULES OF ENGAGEMENT

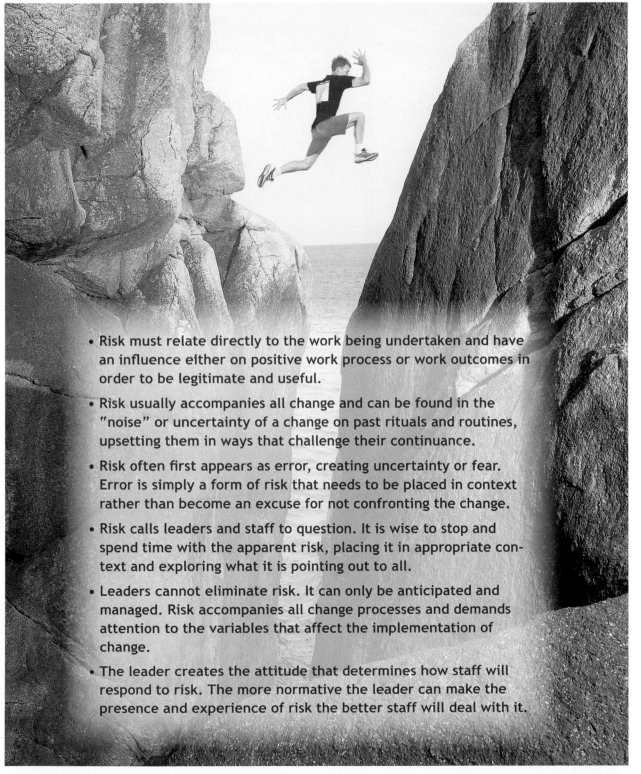

- Risk must relate directly to the work being undertaken and have an influence either on positive work process or work outcomes in order to be legitimate and useful.

- Risk usually accompanies all change and can be found in the "noise" or uncertainty of a change on past rituals and routines, upsetting them in ways that challenge their continuance.

- Risk often first appears as error, creating uncertainty or fear. Error is simply a form of risk that needs to be placed in context rather than become an excuse for not confronting the change.

- Risk calls leaders and staff to question. It is wise to stop and spend time with the apparent risk, placing it in appropriate context and exploring what it is pointing out to all.

- Leaders cannot eliminate risk. It can only be anticipated and managed. Risk accompanies all change processes and demands attention to the variables that affect the implementation of change.

- The leader creates the attitude that determines how staff will respond to risk. The more normative the leader can make the presence and experience of risk the better staff will deal with it.

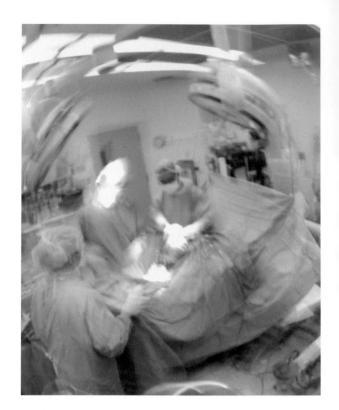

Note:

Accountability requires a discipline like any other aspect of leadership. The leader always disciplines the work of staff with questions about purpose and meaning in order to keep them oriented to the value of the work, not just its processes.

Clarifying Accountability

Accountability demands action, but not just any action. Action of work must reflect the need to have an effect or to make a difference. Accountability is always asking the worker to think of action in light of its value and effect on service or product of work. This fit between action and value is the best indicator of the presence of accountability. Good leaders frequently set time aside with staff to reconnect with the meaning and value of work as a way of keeping them focused on purpose and value. Failure to have this focus often results in a loss of meaning for workers. They can descend down the ladder of motivation and increase the risk of addiction to ritual. They can even burn out from the routine of doing the same thing without any relationship to meaning and value. This focus on value is the one thing that distinguishes accountability from other elements of work.

Ensuring Outcomes

Remember that work is not simply about doing work. The notion of getting work done makes the work an end rather than the means it really is supposed to be. Focus on the work alone is often the greatest contributor to the formation and support of ritual and routine as a major element of work. Forming repetitive habits is perhaps the most significant barrier challenging effective work and its achievement of potentially sustainable outcomes. It must be remembered that all work serves a purpose and if that purpose is forgotten, the work loses value and meaning. Leaders and staff must spend time reviewing the reasons for action in the work and tie them to the purposes and outcomes. That is how work keeps in touch with its value. Leaders continually ask: "What are we doing this work for and are we doing it?"

ACCOUNTABILITY AND ACTION

Accountability is not complicated, but it does demand a consistent understanding of what it means and of the performance that demonstrates its presence. Some summary principles are:

■ Accountability always reflects the individual commitment to performance and action. It is this individual ownership of work processes that is necessary for accountable action.

■ Personal accountability fits well with the collective team effort to do work and achieve desirable outcomes. Individual and team are one as they are reflected against their work products.

■ Accountability suggests congruence among ownership, action, and outcome. The individual must link all three in order to sustain impact or results.

■ Individual accountability cannot be expressed if it does not demonstrate the power to deliver the personal performance effort necessary to be effective.

■ The team has a right to expect that each member perform to the fullest extent of competence and that individual skills integrate well with group process and work.

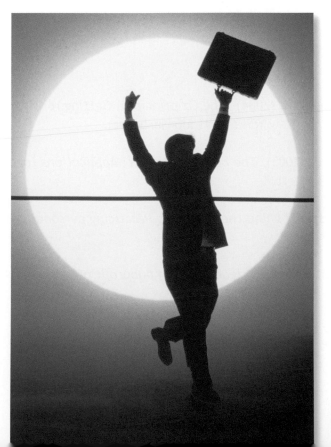

References

Gottlieb, M. R. (2003). *Managing group process*. Westport, CT: Praeger.

Koerner, J. (2001). Nightingale II: Nursing in the new millenium. In: *The nursing profession: Tomorrow and beyond.* Thousand Oaks, CA: Sage Publications.

Malloch, K, & Porter-O'Grady, T. (2006). *Introduction to evidence-based practice in nursing and health care*. Sudbury, MA: Jones and Bartlett.

Malloch, K., & Porter-O'Grady, T. (2005). *The quantum leader: Applications for the new world of work*. Sudbury, MA: Jones and Bartlett.

Pearce, C. L., & Conger, J. A. (2003). *Shared leadership: Reframing the hows and whys of leadership*. Thousand Oaks, CA: Sage.

Porter-O'Grady, T., & Krueger Wilson, C. (1998). *The healthcare teambook*. St. Louis: Mosby, Times Mirror.

Thompson, L., Aranda, E., & Robbins, S. (2002). *Tools for teams: Building effective teams in the workplace*. Boston: Pearson Custom Publishing.

Tilley, S., & Watson, R. (2004). *Accountability in nursing and midwifery* (2nd ed.). Oxford, UK: Blackwell Science.

Suggested Readings

Hickman, C., Smith, T., & Conners, R. (2004). *The Oz principle: Getting results through individual and organizational accountability*. New York: Portfolio Hardcover.

Malloch, K., & Porter-O'Grady, T. (2005). *The quantum leader: Applications for the new world of work*. Sudbury, MA: Jones and Bartlett.

Miller, J. (2004). *Qbq! The question behind the question: Practicing personal accountability in work and in life*. New York: Penguin.

Riggio, R. E., & Orr, S. S. (2004). *Improving leadership in nonprofit organizations*. San Francisco: Jossey-Bass.

CHAPTER 3

ACCOUNTABILITY AND EXCELLENCE

Doing good work is important. Doing work that makes a difference is even more valuable. If one doesn't know the "why" of the work, it is difficult to maintain the energy for the "how" of the work.

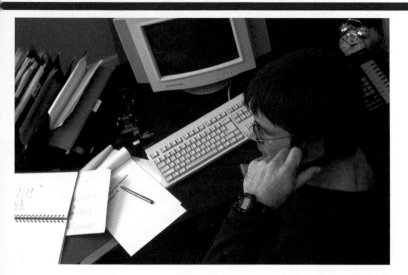

Note:

Excellence is as excellence does.

Accountability for excellence rests with those who do the work!

STRIVING FOR EXCELLENCE

In today's world, process is outcome. The desire for excellence is becoming the clarion call in most of the workplaces in America. One wonders whether there is any relationship between achieving excellence and the commitment of leadership to achieve and sustain it. There are requisites for excellence just as there are for any pursuit. After all, excellence is as excellence does.

To achieve levels of excellence requires the engagement of all stakeholders in an effort that challenges and changes the whole culture of work. It is not simply an effort to improve things such that by so doing excellence will have been obtained after which everyone can rest and celebrate. What is critical to know about excellence is that it is a way of life that must be maintained if it is to be sustained. Once recognized as excellent, the real work of excellence begins. The truth is that excellence really can't be obtained or achieved, it can only be demonstrated every day as a way of life, a pursuit that one lives everyday. It is a way of being and the work is simply the reflection of "the way." It reflects how an organization actually lives its work experience and addresses its challenge in a way that continues to write the script of improvement as a journey, not as an event.

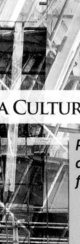

The Culture of Excellence

- It is safe to observe for irregularities.
- The group norm is the journey of excellence.
- Leaders exemplify commitment to excellence.
- Excellence is not more than the norm; it is the norm.
- The philosophy of the organization sets the stage.
- Every role has a definer for excellence within it.
- Competence is a special concern for the organization.
- Excellence is not considered a behavioral exception.
- Everyone understands the engagement of excellence.

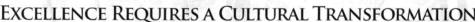

EXCELLENCE REQUIRES A CULTURAL TRANSFORMATION

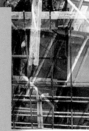

Cultural shifts are evidenced by a change in the following:
- *Vision*
- *Desire*
- *Framework*
- *Discipline*
- *Support*
- *Infrastructure*
- *Systems*
- *Methods*
- *Learning*
- *Resources*
- *Measurement*

Personal shifts are evidenced by a change in the following:
- *Willingness*
- *Insight*
- *Commitment*
- *Self-discipline*
- *Teamwork*
- *Participation*
- *Ownership*
- *Engagement*
- *Learning*
- *Dialog*
- *Self-evaluation*

EMBRACING ERROR

Error is a normal aspect of all lived experience. There is no life without error. Many people believe that error can be completely eliminated from life experience. Of course, it can't. Error is not an untenable and unacceptable part of life. It is, instead, a fundamental element of live experience that demands concerted attention on the part of everyone (Porter-O'Grady & Wilson, 1999).

Error is essentially a teaching moment. It attempts to point out to the observer that there is distance between the actual and the desired. The first experience of error is always a teachable moment. It is the second error and all subsequent error that is unacceptable since it demonstrates that nothing was learned from the first incidence of error or corrective action was essentially unaddressed (see the error flow below). The secret is in honoring error when it is first discovered. Indeed, it is wise to look for it so that upon discovering error, action can be taken and the bar can be raised to a new level of action. Failing to recognize the value of error ensures that it will be repeated with the negative impact that implies (see below).

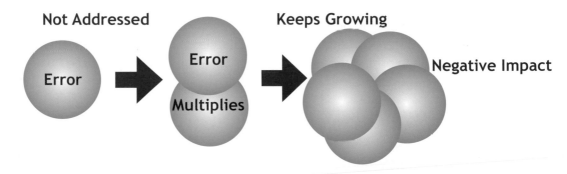

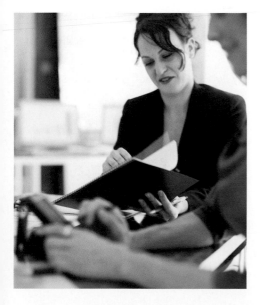

Note:

The only error that is unacceptable is the error unaddressed. Error is desperately trying to demonstrate a teachable moment. If error is unaddressed it is always destined to be repeated.

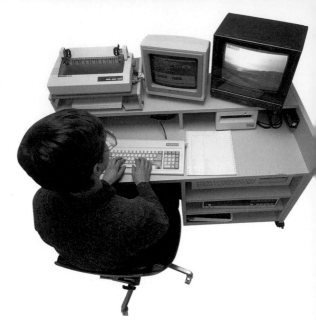

Error Leadership Tips

- Create error seekers, not avoiders.
- Create an "error finding quota."
- Help staff recognize error potentials.
- Have error celebration sessions.
- Acknowledge the best error solutions.
- Create storyboards of errors resolved.
- Tie error to quality improvement activities.
- Identify best practices in error management.

LEADERSHIP IN ROLE ERROR MANAGEMENT

The leader has to set the environment that makes the engagement of error safe and appropriate. If error results in punitive action, staff will avoid, even hide, error. One wonders how many error incidents are simply ignored in order to avoid the negative consequences of having "committed" an error. The reporting and recording, counseling and classes, time spent in enumerating incidents, etc. really make it simpler and easier to ignore or cover up error so that the "pain" of dealing with it can be avoided (Malloch & Porter-O'Grady, 2005).

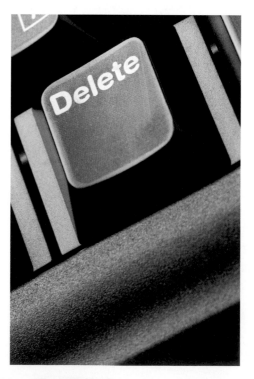

> Create a "zone of safety" around error, removing fear.

> Celebrate error, don't punish it.

> Build a culture of "error finding" in order to address it.

> Address error very early, when its impact is the lowest.

CREATING THE CULTURE OF ACCOUNTABILITY

■ Bring people on board with the clear understanding of their role and contributions as members of the team.

■ Make sure everyone knows that participation is not optional and that every member of the work community must contribute.

■ Include participation and ownership behaviors in the performance assessment process; review at least quarterly.

■ Identify skill levels and developmental needs and make sure they are addressed as a part of the individual's growth plan.

■ Advise all members that accountability is about the achievement of outcomes, not just good work performance.

■ Identify and resolve interpersonal conflicts early; the later they are engaged the less likely they can be resolved satisfactorily.

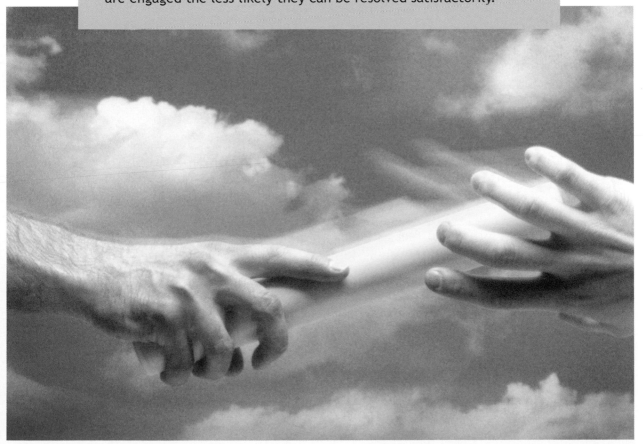

ADDRESSING THE HUMAN FACTORS IN ACHIEVING EXCELLENCE

1.	Self-awareness is central to the ability to safely engage issues of risk and change. Accountability cannot be achieved if individuals lack an awareness of their own levels of skill and performance.
2.	Self-deprecation is a critical barrier to individual engagement. Leaders cannot eliminate all personal fear, but they can address it early and make it untenable in the expression of work.
3.	Partnership is an essential element of team behavior. Leaders must emphasize the role of partnership behaviors in all team members.
4.	Addressing conflict in its earliest stages helps avoid the painful noise of conflict when it becomes war in the workplace.
5.	Communication skills in team members are not an optional skill. The leader must address communication talent in the team early in order to adjust team members to each other's styles and to the acceptable and unacceptable patterns of communication.
6.	Relationships are the lifeblood of the team. "Special" relationships, be they romantic or friendships are often an impediment to the team's ability to function and should be monitored closely for their negative impact on team solidarity.
7.	Drive all fear out of performance as soon as practical because it does nothing to promote honesty and openness with regard to error and corrective action.
8.	Commitment is a personal affirmation to the process of collective change and should be expected from all members of the team. Commitment is an expectation of accountability, not a invitation to participate.
9.	People need to feel safe at work. The leader has an obligation to create a "zone of safety" for work in order to offset normal uncertainty.
10.	The final value for all leadership and decision making is the choice to do the right thing. The leader must demonstrate this commitment through personal behavior and transfer the expectation and the skill necessary to ensure all team members are committed to the right decision and right action (Peters, 2003).

RISK TAKING AND ACCOUNTABLE BEHAVIOR

Good Risk Management

- Have access to the right information.

- Spread information around generously.

- Eliminate fear from the responses of staff.

- Embrace risk as a normative component of the work.

- Fight silence or secret keeping.

- Dig deeper into error to find a root cause.

- Make good use of time; respond quickly.

Create an Ethical Environment

- Establish a foundation for the rules of engagement in the team.

- Make sure people hear the real messages that are communicated.

- Make expectations clear and make sure they are understood.

- Develop principle-centered policies and practices.

- Consistently adhere to the rules; do not bend them for anyone.

- Talk out the areas of disagreement until common ground is found.

- Create an environment of trust and hold people to their bond.

- Respect each other's contribution and build on the team values.

- Work out new ethical situations quickly and establish new rules.

EXCELLENCE IS AS EXCELLENCE DOES

Excellence is not a point of arrival, it is a way of traveling. Many people believe that excellence is a place. Instead, it is a process that is lived and represented by who we are, rather than simply what we do. Excellence calls for a commitment to a particular way of doing and being that demonstrates a standard that operates at some difference from the acceptable; the norm. The challenge with regard to understanding excellence is helping people see it as a way of life instead of a condition or circumstance.

Excellence always operates at a level above the norm. It sets a template for the highest level of achievement and demonstrates what excellence looks like. It is an exemplar for all others as to what the foundations of "the best" look like. Although it is often an arbitrary determination, it does reflect the commitment to raise the standard and to engage it at a higher level of acceptable performance.

Excellence Is...

■ A level of performance that operates in a way that distinguishes the very best and separates it from all other standards of measure.

■ A target level of performance that others aspire to in a way that sets people apart at a level that is desirable but not easy to achieve.

■ An exemplar of the most desirable state that is achievable and sets the expectation as to what it will take to go there.

■ A way of practicing or working that incorporates best practices and uses them to raise the level of performance and establishes the baseline for the next level of achievement.

■ A journey that represents the road to the very best and reflects an agreement that performance will always be evidence of the very best in all a person seeks to do.

■ A definitive process that moves inexorably toward a definitive goal that reflects a commitment to sustaining the best possible outcome that can be achieved through human effort.

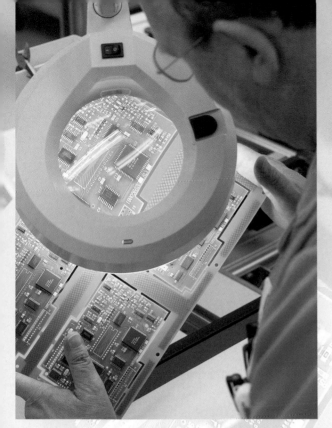

Elements of Excellence

- Evidences personal commitment
- Specific standards of performance
- An agreed-upon goal
- Change of behavior
- Method of process
- Great performance
- Units of measure
- Evidence of excellence
- A definable difference in the outcome
- Moments for celebration
- Continual renewal of new effort

ACCOUNTABLE EXCELLENCE

Excellence cannot be achieved without a defined level of expectation and accountability. It is a challenge to build performance on clear accountability because it requires a discipline that most do not seek to achieve. Yet there is no sustainable excellence without that discipline built into the organization's way of doing business and represented by every person in the system.

1. Accountability seeks to personalize the commitment to excellence by making it the agenda of every member of the team.

2. The team defines excellence as its central work and structures it so that it is the way of doing business in every activity.

3. Team members clearly define their personal contribution to the efforts necessary to maintain excellence.

4. The team evaluates and adjusts its priorities and activities when the evidence suggests a different course of action necessary to support excellent practices.

5. The team undertakes any necessary corrective action to reconfigure the path of excellence so that nothing impedes the movement that maintains their level of excellence.

6. The team has the authority to decide and act when excellent performance requires necessary changes in course.

Excellence Pitfalls

- Externally defined expectations
- Failure to agree on common goals
- Misunderstanding of performance objectives
- Lack of clarity about role expectations
- Highly variable levels of skill
- Inadequate direction around team objectives and strategies
- Lack of collaboration between the team and other stakeholders
- Unresolved conflict between team members
- No consistent measures of performance
- Missing elements of outcome measures

Failures in Accountability

- Unclear role definitions
- Expectations that have not been accepted
- Assumptions about what is agreed to
- Lack of clarity regarding performance expectations
- Lack of fulfillment of personal agreements
- Uncertain level of skill
- Undefined program of skill development
- Failure to perform as expected
- Lack of follow-up on performance challenges
- Poor fit of personal behavior with team action

Note:

There is no excellence without accountability. Personal accountability is necessary to give excellence form and to translate it into a set of behaviors that best represent the actions necessary to provide the visual evidence of the presence of excellence.

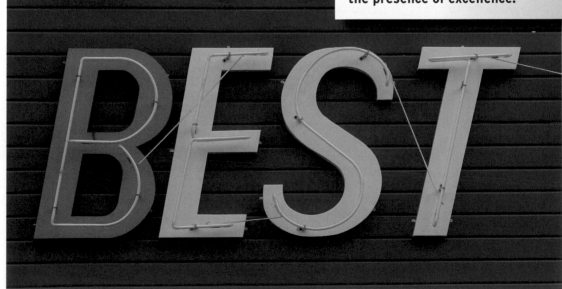

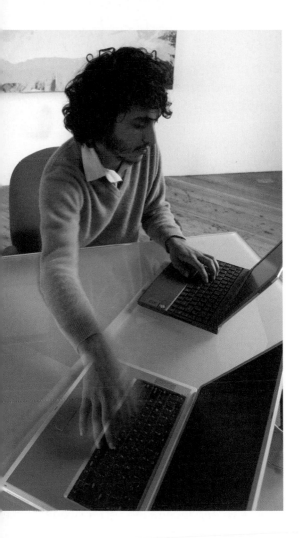

When establishing accountability, it is always wise to pursue the Individual and the team's understanding of what that means and its application in their work. General definitions and attributions to accountability do not have meaning for individuals unless they can associate it with their own work. The leader always works to ensure individual and team clarity with regard to performance expectations.

Accountability Points to Remember

- Accountability must always be experienced within the role.
- Accountability cannot be externally directed or controlled.
- Accountability must be owned by those who do the work.
- Accountability must be directed to outcome, not process.
- Accountability is represented by team commitment to goals.

Clarity

- Simple
- Straightforward
- Understandable
- Brief
- Generalizable
- Role based
- Mutual
- Helps performance
- Principle based
- Supports outcome
- Renegotiated
- Reflects value

The Leader's Role

- Create the environment for excellence.
- Monitor team performance.
- Provide access to needed tools.
- Evaluate problems and progress.
- Expand techniques for problem solving.

Signposts of Personal Accountability

- Individuals have a sense of personal ownership of their own work.
- Individuals have strong team-based relationships with others at work.
- Blame is eliminated from work and relationships.
- Personal advantage over others is eliminated.
- Individuals understand their specific role expectations.
- Individual and team actions have a strong goodness-of-fit.
- Outcomes drive individual performance processes.

LEADER APPLICATIONS ENSURING ACCOUNTABILITY

■ The leader makes no unilateral decisions about the content of an individual's work. Individuals influence and control the elements of their work.

■ Decisions concerning the application of resources and the content of work are rendered to the team process. Achieving consensus demonstrates agreement about required performance.

■ The leader ensures that the decisions of the team are implemented as decided and that the outcomes the team has agreed to are evaluated systematically with regard to whether they were achieved.

■ The leader in a work team helps focus the team on issues related to role, obligation, and achievement of outcomes. The leader's developmental role is to enhance leader effectiveness and provide it with sufficient content to be successful.

■ The leader focuses an accountable team on the necessary linkages between the decisions made and the support necessary from the organization. In this way, the leader ensures a good fit between team decision making and organizational support for the work.

■ The leader focuses on the milieu within which the work is unfolded by team members. The leader always remembers that the positive interaction between system and work provides the frame for achieving successful outcomes.

Accountable Self-Management

- Personal sense of ownership
- Role self-confidence
- Good role fit with others
- Clarifies ambiguity
- Good problem-solving skills
- Relates well with others
- Strong communication skills
- Doesn't seek permission
- Tolerates differences
- Easily explores alternatives
- Questions rituals for relevance
- Good self-evaluation skills

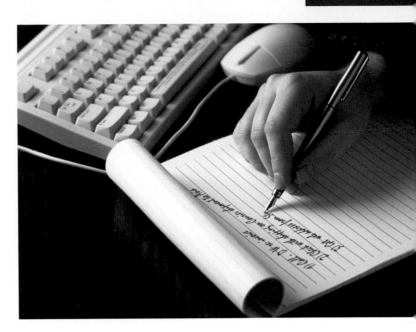

Leader Role Accountability

- Establishing the parameters for teamwork
- Gathering the resources necessary to support teamwork
- Ensuring role expectations are understood by all team members
- Noting anything that is absent from the team resources necessary for work is addressed quickly
- Mechanisms for problem identification and solution seeking are available to team members
- Individual and collective skills necessary to advance competence are always available to team members
- Evaluating process, relationships, methods, ensuring the team moves seamlessly toward its goals

Supervision and Control

Traditional views about supervising and controlling workers need to be challenged by the leader. Included in this set of challenges is whether work will be done unless it is carefully and closely supervised and controlled. As well, there are many challenges related to collective decision making in team-based action, especially as it eliminates the unilateral and "hero" rule of the leader. The understanding that group decision making is inefficient, or not fast, or simply not the most effective way of making decisions is simply untrue. Sustainable and viable decisions having an impact on positive outcomes always depend on the aggregation, coordination, and integration of the work efforts of many (Wiener, 2000). Unless that is supported and advanced in the workplace, problems increase, integration fails, and the quality of both work processes and product is negatively affected. The key to effective decision making is to ensure that the right people are making the right decisions using good skills and acting in concert toward mutually beneficial goals.

SPECIFIC LEADER ACCOUNTABILITIES

Managers and Accountability

The role of leader as manager suggests specific accountabilities that attend to the role. Because of its expectations, performance, and positioning in relationship to the work of the team, managers have what can be called "contextual accountability." This simply means that managers have a fundamental obligation to provide the environment, the frame, and the context for work, rather than for doing the work itself. Perhaps, one of the most difficult aspects of good management leadership is separating the role of the manager from the role of the staff. Managers should not be "super staff." Management is an accountability all its own. It requires full-time commitment and energy and has in it expectations for performance that are specifically different from those of the work. The work of management should be viewed as separate from the work of staff (ANCC, 2005). Even clinical or "working" managers, while performing the management function, are meeting different accountabilities than those found in the performance of their clinical work. These accountabilities are resource driven and specific to addressing issues of how the work is supported with the five fundamental resource categories necessary to ensure effective and sustainable work outcomes.

Note:

Management work is driven by contextual accountabilities. Managers should not be viewed as "super staff." Management must always provide support to the work of the staff; it must never be the work of the staff.

The Five Manager Accountabilities

1. Human resources
2. Fiscal resources
3. Material resources
4. Staff support
5. Systems support

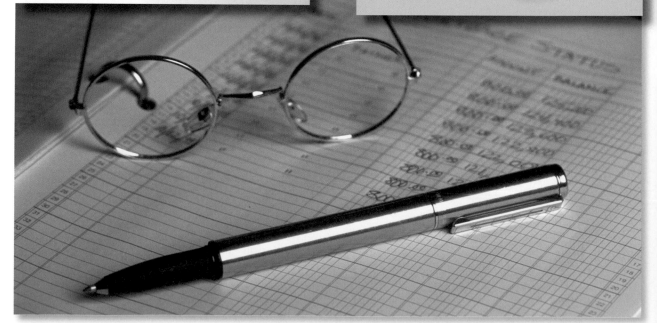

THE MANAGER'S HUMAN RESOURCE ACCOUNTABILITY

The traditional human resource accountability for the manager is that which relates to providing the right people for the right work in the right place at the right time with the right configuration. This human resource task provides support to the staff in matching human effort with appropriate human energy. Here the manager is accountable for ensuring that there is an appropriate number and kind of staff available to balance work demands with resources, and that this balance reflects the appropriate skills, talents, and relationships necessary to advance and sustain the work and the work relationship. This does not necessarily mean that the manager makes these decisions unilaterally or out of context of the relationship with the staff. A large number of organizations fully engage staff in hiring, evaluating, scheduling, and assigning resources based on the staffs perception of the need and distribution of those resources. Whereas the methodology of staff engagement is an effective way of building stronger connections to the human resource accountability, it does not shift the ownership of that accountability from manager to staff. The obligation to achieve the outcomes of appropriate balance between work demands and resources available always remains a management accountability regardless of the techniques and methodologies used to undertake it. Therefore, the manager always has the accountability to ensure the following:

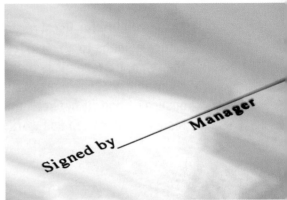

> ## Note:
> The accountable manager never transfers accountability to the staff for expecting them to fulfill the obligations of management. Although accountability may be shared with the staff, the outcomes of that accountability always belong to the manager.

- An organized and systematic approach to matching work demand and human resources operates as an effective process within the context of the work team.

- The manager is constantly engaged in a systematic dialog and interaction with the organization to continually advocate for the right match and mix of resources based on process needs and outcome demand.

- A specific and effective work productivity system evaluates the goodness-of-fit between the staffing, scheduling, and assigning system and the demands of work.

- Adjustments and accommodations in resource needs, skill levels, staff numbers, and work design fall within the resource accountability and must be adjusted as changes in work occur.

- The manager may share the process of resource allocation with staff but is always accountable for human resource outcomes.

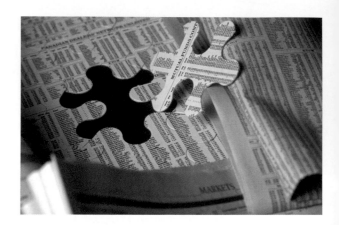

> ## Note:
>
> Responsibility for fiscal performance belongs to all members of the team. However, it is the accountability of the manager to ensure a good fit between financial resource allocation and work needs.

FISCAL ACCOUNTABILITY AND THE MANAGER'S ROLE

The construction, use, management, and evaluation of the application of fiscal resources in the organization is one of the central roles of the manager. The purpose here is to be able to match fiscal and service realities with operational processes and work goals. This effort to match financial resources and to dedicate them to achieving the organization's purposes is a critical cornerstone for effective work. Here it is essential that there be a very strong relationship between fiscal resources and work represented by a goodness-of-fit between the resources applied and the work outcomes achieved.

Managers budget dollars, but rarely spend them. Essentially, it is the work of the team to use resources appropriately and to produce outcomes that ensure the viability and financial health of the organization. Within this context, the manager makes sure that fiscal resources are applied effectively and used judiciously. The manager ensures that the financial system that structures the relationship between dollars and work does so accurately and relates specifically to the expectations for performance. The infrastructure necessary to do this includes good cost center budgeting, staff-driven financial planning, good fiscal control mechanisms, cost evaluation and productivity measures, and cost-benefit analysis. Here again, it may not be the obligation of the manager to undertake all of the activities associated with this accountability. It is, however, the accountability of the manager to see that all the processes in place are used to responsibly allocate, align, and manage fiscal resource work effectively, accomplish their purposes, and facilitate and sustain supportable and viable outcomes.

Elements of Good Financial Accountability

- A fiscal plan that balances work demands with resources available
- Staff engagement and ownership of resource applications to work
- A systematic and effective process of applying financial resources
- A mechanism for variance accommodation in use of dollars
- A regular reporting format and time frame for good cost control
- The method of evaluating and adjusting based on financial performance factors

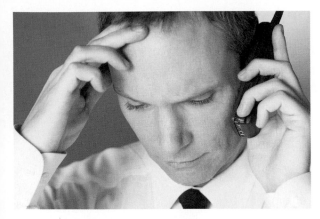

Managers and Capital

Capital planning is a critical element of the manager's role and vital to the success of any work enterprise. Staff have a right to expect that materials planning will accurately reflect the equipment and systems needs support necessary to advance the quality and competence of the work in light of anticipated goals. Increasingly, facility in capital planning includes the role of the staff and facilitates staff ownership and participation decisions that affect equipment priorities, purchases, and utility. Capital planning should at least include:

- A capital priority planning process that matches resource allocation and work priorities
- A good fit between material resources and work demands.
- An ability to adjust the capital plan based on changes in process, environment, circumstances, and goals.
- A mechanism that allows capital planning to match the strategic goals of the organization and the functions and processes necessary to achieve them.
- A new equipment and new technology acquisition process that incorporates state-of-the-art equipment and material into the work process.

Material Support

This is a resource accountability very much like the leader's accountability for fiscal resources. Here the appropriate materials and supplies necessary to undertake the work must be available to the staff in an appropriate manner of distribution and utility. Predominant elements of material resource support are:

- The proper equipment and supplies readily available based on demand and need.
- Continual evaluation of changes in supply needs based on work processes.
- Evaluation of the effectiveness of material support and its goodness-of-fit with work demands.
- The ability to adjust material and equipment support for better facilitation of work.
- Evaluation of the effectiveness of the material supply and support system in support of work.

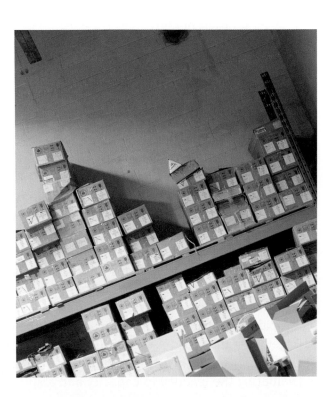

THE LEADER AS A SUPPORT SYSTEM

Creating an environment that results in a desirable workplace for all involved is certainly a critical task. The struggle for the leader is to recognize the complexities involved in creating a safe, productive, happy, and meaningful workplace. This often means the leader must always be attentive to the realities both individuals and teams confront in maintaining high levels of commitment, energy, and motivation. Often, rituals and routines simply suggest that merely doing the work can create a level of boredom and mindlessness that can ultimately decrease motivation and energy in the workplace (Dlugacz et al., 2004).

The leader is fundamentally a storyteller—a journey maker. In this role he or she creates a framework that is supportive of an individual's work behavior and relational, emotional, and interactional dynamics in a way that keeps people stimulated, encouraged, and motivated. In order to do this the leader must always focus on the following.

- Individual needs of staff
- Creating a culture of inclusion
- Providing sufficient variety in the work
- Making sure the staff has the right information
- Celebrating staff accomplishments
- Changing the ritual of work
- Problem solving conflicts immediately
- Creating options to change work routines
- Providing opportunities for staff to grow
- Creating an environment that makes it safe for staff to risk and experiment
- Helping meet the needs of staff members specifically and personally
- Anticipating the challenges ahead and prepare staff to meet them
- Making support, systems, and resources easy to access in a timely fashion
- Making sure the staff develops the skills necessary to personally advance and grow
- Removing the barriers to work effectiveness and team relationships
- Advocating on behalf of the staff, increasing staff opportunities for satisfaction
- Anticipating challenges and difficulties in their earliest stages for better problem solving
- Developing the self-directed skills of the staff to manage their own work and life
- Engaging the staff in evaluating support systems and adjust as required
- Evaluating the leadership capacity and ability to adequately build a support system for staff

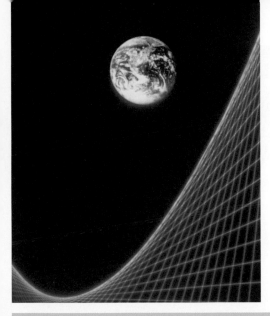

SYSTEM SYNTHESIS

If systems are to be effective they must link, integrate, and coordinate all work effort in a dynamic mosaic that supports and advances the work effort. All elements of the system must ultimately synthesize so common efforts and aggregated work of each component of the system merge to create a dynamic that results in an effective "dance" between each element that moves the whole system toward fulfilling its purpose and meaning.

Providing Good System Support

Tying all elements of the work system together in a cohesive whole that facilitates the work is the coordinative and integrative function of good managers. Leadership requires that all systems resources such as experts, service supports, organizational structure, quality indicators, and data management and generation, outcome facilitation, competence enhancement, and fiscal and system support all work together to create an infrastructure that accelerates the opportunity for worker and work to be successful. In order to accomplish this, the manager is accountable for the following:

- The information system generates data that are relevant, effective, and specific to the role of the team in its performance and its effort to achieve outcomes.
- Available experts are accessible in the right time and with the information and supports necessary to advance the work of the staff and to improve the quality of their processes and the value of their outcome.
- The support systems of finance and materials management and the capital planning process work seamlessly to make sure that the adequate array of goods and services necessary to support the work is readily accessible and in a form that can be used.
- Role descriptions, performance expectations, performance evaluation systems, organizational structure, and role expectations are specific and clear and integrate well in a way that advances the opportunity of the workers to perform effectively and to achieve work expectations.
- The information management and data systems provide an effective framework for documentation, access, application, and evaluation of work and workers in light of expectations for performance and anticipated goals.
- All infrastructure and systems synthesize with work effort in a way that supports it, adjusts it, and evaluates it within the context of defined outcomes, with the expectation that the interface of all systems ultimately advances the productivity of the worker, the effective design of the workplace, and the sustainable achievement of work goals.

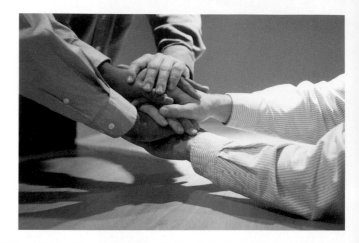

SUMMARIZING THE FIVE MANAGEMENT ACCOUNTABILITIES

1. HUMAN RESOURCES
- The right person is in the right place at the right time doing the right work.
- The number of resources and the budget allocation for them match well.
- The work needs and the human resource numbers and skill level match.

2. FISCAL RESOURCES
- Financial planning is effective.
- Actor and operational budget match work expectations and demand.
- A strong and effective financial monitoring system is in place.
- There is a good system for variance analysis and budget correction.

3. MATERIALS RESOURCES
- There is a renewable, flexible, customer-oriented material supply system.
- Supplies and equipment are matched with the need.
- A viable, inclusive, accurate capital planning process is in place.
- Materials supply variance analysis system works effectively.

4. SUPPORT STRUCTURES
- An empowered and inclusive organization exists for staff and teams.
- Good problem-solving technology and processes are available within teams.
- Leaders provide good personal, relational, and process support to staff.
- Leaders work hard to make sure that form always follows function.

5. SYSTEMS STRUCTURES
- An effective information and data management system exists.
- Strong and meaningful quality control mechanisms help support staff.
- Synthesis and linkage between structures and systems operate well.
- A strong strategic tactical process ensures achievement of work goals.
- Effective education and development program improves staff work.

References

ANCC. (2005). *Magnet recognition program application manual*. Silver Spring, MD: American Nurses Credentialing Center.

Dlugacz, Y. D., Restifo, A., & Greenwood, A. (2004). *The quality handbook for health care organizations: A manager's guide to tools and programs*. San Francisco: Jossey-Bass.

Malloch, K., & Porter-O'Grady, T. (2005). *The quantum leader: Applications for the new world of work*. Sudbury, MA: Jones and Bartlett.

Peters, T. J. (2003). *Re-imagine! (business excellence in a disruptive age)*. London: Dorling Kindersley.

Porter-O'Grady, T., & Wilson, C. (1999). *Leading the revolution in healthcare: Igniting performance, changing systems*. Gaithersburg, MD: Aspen.

Wiener, C. L. (2000). *The elusive quest: Accountability in hospitals*. New York: Aldine de Gruyter.

Suggested Readings

ANCC. (2005). *Magnet recognition program application manual*. Silver Spring, MD: American Nurses Credentialing Center.

Fottler, M., Ford, R., & Heaton, C. (2002). *Achieving service excellence*. Chicago: Health Administration Press.

Malloch, K., & Porter-O'Grady, T. (2005). *Introduction to evidence-based practice in nursing and healthcare*. Sudbury, MA: Jones and Bartlett.

Vaill, P. (2002). *Learning as a way of being*. San Francisco: Jossey-Bass.

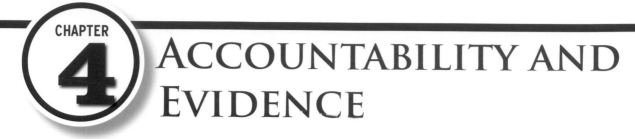

CHAPTER 4 ACCOUNTABILITY AND EVIDENCE

Work is not inherently valuable simply because one does it. Work is valuable when it is informed by purpose and when all are consciously committed to fulfilling that purpose.

ACCOUNTABILITY AND IMPACT

One of the most critical issues regarding accountability relates to whether work performance has any effect. Lots of energy can be expended in undertaking work, and even doing the work well, yet still not make a difference and having an effect is increasingly important in doing work (Malloch & Porter-O'Grady, 2006).

> ### Note:
>
> **Evidence relates to the difference one makes in the exercise and action of work and is the indicator of the sustainable impact of the work.**

At a time when value is becoming increasingly important, it is vital that a goodness-of-fit exist between the work done and the effect of work. Quality of work relates not only to how well the work processes unfold and work activities are carried out but also to whether the outcome or the products of that work were precisely as expected. Embedding the elements of quality within work processes and directly relating them to work outcomes is perhaps one of the most important variables related to accountability.

Every individual, expressing accountability, owns his or her own work effort. This effort represents not only what the person does but also who the person is. The energy, commitment, and investment individuals make in their work effort tell others as much about them as about their work. Accountable individuals seek to have themselves best represented and demonstrated through the quality of their work effort. The accountable individual demonstrates the pride and ownership in the outcomes of work that reflect a detailed effort and a full engagement of the activity essential to creating excellent results. These results are the evidence of the range of personal characteristics, behaviors, and processes that, when aggregated, produce excellent outcomes.

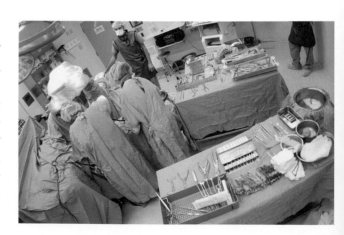

TECHNOLOGY AND THE ROAD TO EVIDENCE

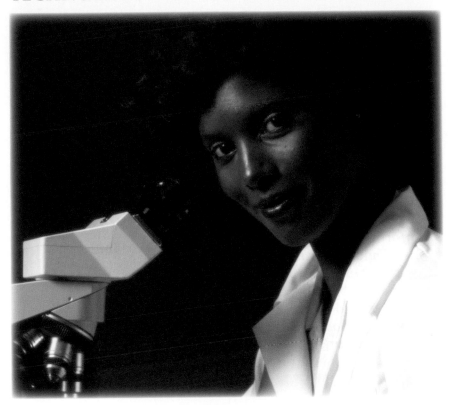

Information is highly mobile and will follow the user everywhere that person goes. Because of its mobility, the individual will be continually connected to information.

The tools of information management will guide action and implementation. These tools will inform the practitioner constantly as the work is being done.

Access is a critical element related to the management and use of information technology. For the practitioner, access to knowledge will be more important than how much knowledge is possessed.

The use of computerized and electronic information will ultimately reduce the amount of human error and variables in action, improving all work outcomes.

Through the use of data systems, work will be evaluated continually and dynamically, rather than simply waiting for evaluation at the end of a process cycle.

Real-time information can alert the worker to variances in process and performance in real time, allowing the worker to alter performance while in the middle of the work process.

Evaluation of the goodness-of-fit between individual work activities and the aggregate of those activities must occur in real time, helping the worker to understand the congruence of work effort.

INTEGRATING TECHNOLOGY INTO ACCOUNTABILITY

Work is constantly moving across work spaces, calling workers to be increasingly fluid and mobile with their work processes.

Information must constantly be shared among team members in order to integrate their activities and coordinate work.

Information can be linked and integrated with other data to create a broader database to inform the individual and teamwork.

Accountability requires that information be accurate and relevant, having a direct relationship to the work.

Information is not permanently relevant or meaningful. Workers change and adapt to new information affecting their work.

The work itself must change as the information about its value and relevance shifts its importance and alters the application of content.

Information should assist the individual in "raising the bar," ultimately improving the processes, outcome, and value of the work.

Information affects accountability in shifting role expectations and performance, affecting process and outcome.

KEY FACTORS AFFECTING
ACCOUNTABILITY AND EVIDENCE

Information Factors Affecting Accountable Performance

- The ability to generate the right information
- The quality of the information gathered
- The willingness and ability to share the right information
- The technology and hardware supporting the use of information
- The accuracy with which the information is translated
- The applicability of the information to the work
- The competence of the worker in using information
- The ability to evaluate the effectiveness of information

Work Factors Affecting Accountable Performance

- The competence of the individual to do the work
- Staffing and scheduling arrangements supporting the work
- The goodness-of-fit of individual work effort with collective effort
- The team's ability to understand the contribution of each member
- The work tools affecting the ability to do the work
- The utility of managing and applying information
- The clarity of expectations with regard to performance
- Time or workload affecting the ability to accomplish the work

Factors related to the supporting infrastructure that affects the ability to do the work is as critical as any other factor. Information and workload issues perhaps have one of the most significant influences on accountability and the achievement of outcomes. A poor fit between the work expectations and the supporting infrastructure that makes the work possible is one of the most critical factors that support work effort, accountability, and the achievement of outcomes. Failure to create the appropriate balance between these factors ultimately ensures failure to achieve sustainable outcomes (Porter-O'Grady, 2004)

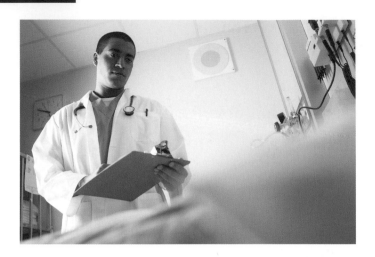

Note:

Error and evidence are not incompatible; in fact, evidence of best practices is the product of good error management and demonstrates the fact that error was acted on positively.

ERROR, ACCOUNTABILITY, AND EVIDENCE

Although error is a tool of learning and adaptation to work processes and of creating good fit between them and performance expectations, it must be carefully managed, reducing the impact on performance and product while accommodating the learning error generates.

Accountable individuals embrace the elements of error and the effort of error to teach as well as express the difference between current performance and expectations. Incorporating error into the work process makes it an acceptable condition of performance improvement.

Evidence of best practice reflects the adjustments that occur in the appropriate assessment and accommodation that are a part of good error management. Best practice is not evidence of the absence of error; it represents how well error was managed.

BARRIERS ON THE ROAD TO EVIDENCE

Barriers	The Issues
Competence	Individual abilities and skills necessary to translate them into action are critical factors with regard to great performance. Preparation for the role needs to be consistent among all participants.
Knowledge	A basic and agreed-upon set of performance requirements with the insights and knowledge necessary to apply them affects achievement and affects the ability to undertake work processes.
Information	Two elements related to information affect the achievement of good practices; one relates to the availability of the information, the other relates to the ability to access it.
Complexity	Integration and coordination of broad-based data components are essential to link the performance and quality information necessary to make good decisions and undertake appropriate action.
Relationships	Evidence of good practice is the confluence and intersection of the actions and contributions of various participants. The ability to relate and tie their work together is critical to good outcomes.
Resources	All resources are finite. Creating a goodness-of-fit between resource availability and work methodology defines whether those performances can be maintained and outcomes sustained.
Technology	Evidence-based practice requires a digital infrastructure to support its complexities and interfaces along the continuum of service requiring good hardware and software integration.
Support	Problems with creating sustainable best practice relates more to inadequate support structures than to almost any other factor. The failure to provide adequate support for work always compromises it.

MASS CUSTOMIZATION MEANS "USER" VALUE

User-Driven Characteristics

- Specific to individual needs
- User-defined expectations
- User participates in design of work
- User-defined specifications
- Work is individualized, not generalized
- Evidence of good practice and great outcome

The contemporary term for consumers is now "users." The definition of user is just as it appears; an individual who makes use of some process or product. The contemporary age is a user-driven time. Because of the effect of the Internet and other personal technologies, decisions and outcomes are now more user driven than provider driven (Porter-O'Grady & Wilson, 1999). In the 20th century, the reflection of the industrial age was a much stronger provider- and producer-driven frame of reference. Work was mechanized, products were predefined and developed, and users were marketed to purchase the products as presented.

Through technology it has become possible for the user to customize almost every product and service desired. As a result, this user-driven world creates a different set of relationships among worker, work process, and outcomes. Often, organizations produce products designed by users and customized to fit their specific needs. As a result, these users generate a pattern of demand and expectation that changes their relationship to the provider. For example, in health care, users now specify the particular needs or demands they have from their providers in a way that represents their unique needs and differentiates them from the needs of others. In the past, the provider's attitude was that the consumer received the same level of high-quality care as all other consumers. In a mass-customized frame of reference, the user receives the service that meets the specific needs and demands of the individual regardless of the service provided to another.

Value is now invested in how well the service fits the needs of the individual rather than broader definitions of "same quality for all." This customized notion of service design changes performance, expectations, and results. Evidence of fitting and fulfilling the individual's particular needs with a set of practices that best accomplishes that, is a critical element of work. Outcome is no longer generalizable and satisfaction is rarely generic. Value is directly related to how specifically the individual has been satisfied and how the balance between cost and return has been advanced in so doing. Individual workers are accountable for giving evidence of how well they customized service to the particular needs of individuals.

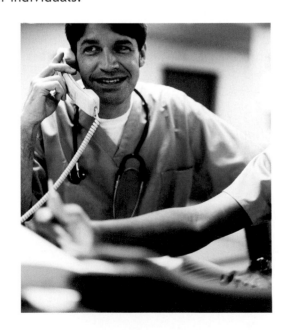

MEETING INFORMATION-SEEKING NEEDS

If there is to be any evidence of the goodness of fit between work process and product, information will be the key variable. Information is the seamless connection of all resource elements necessary to inform decisions and undertake action. Therefore, it is important to examine and understand the information-seeking needs of those using information for specific purposes in the process of achieving sustainable outcomes. The following issues must be addressed in responding to user-driven information needs in an evidence-based framework:

- The kind of hardware and software support at the point of service must be readily accessible to the user in a format that can be readily and easily used.

- Information takes the form that can be readily understood and easily used at the point of service in a way that has direct impact on the user and the work to be performed.

- Although information integration is complex, its presentation needs to be simple and straightforward, such that it can be quickly accessed and both easily translated and immediately applied.

- There is no doubt that information is valuable, but too much information ceases to be of any value if the user must sort through unrelated or useless information in order to find helpful data.

- Relevance is critical to good information management and utility. Accuracy and efficacy of information obtained are essential if information is to be trusted and depended on for making meaningful decisions.

- Obstacles must be removed, making it possible to access information directly at the point-of-service, where the provider works, at the center of the place where the specific work and activities are carried out.

- The more portable the means of delivering and managing information the more flexible and useful it is.

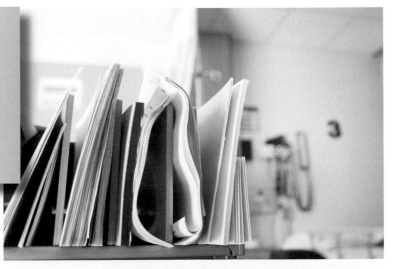

Note:

Evidence-based practice cannot build in a manual information management environment. A digital information environment is a requisite for effective evidence-based practice approaches.

SCENARIO

Evidence-Based Practice

Michael, the nurse manager on the medical-surgical unit, has been experiencing significant staffing problems for the past year. What was difficult for Michael has been trying to find a match between the needs of patients and the availability of professional nursing staff. The problem wasn't so much a shortage of nursing resources; instead, it was that a wide variability in patient acuity and census created difficulty in scheduling and staffing.

Michael recognizes the need to blend financial, administrative, and clinical realities and create a framework for appropriate staffing at a level that would meet the needs of the patients but still operate within specified financial constraints. Furthermore, he wanted to engage the professional staff in a way that would help bring ownership to the processes developed and to the standards created in designing and organizing an evidence-based approach to resource use. Michael discussed these issues with Nancy, the clinical nurse specialist for the unit. They have laid out a grid related to labor productivity, clinical nursing work, productivity measures, workload issues, patients and staff variances, and value and quality issues related to the delivery of nursing care. They realized that all of these elements would need to be included in a systematic plan directed to meeting patients' needs and defining specific nurse staffing—patient care delivery relationships.

Michael and Nancy were challenged with clarifying the next steps in initiating an evidence-based approach to nursing patient care workload management. They both recognize that each of the elements would need to be explored with regard to existing information, best practices, research-based information resources, and experiential data generated out of the practice environment. They have called on you as their practice consultant to help them organize a systematic process for workload management using evidence-based approaches. They formulated the following questions to initiate this process:

1. How does the unit create a model that integrates the elements identified above and establishes a framework for planning?
2. How can we engage the staff in the process of planning and implementing an evidence-based model so that there are higher levels of ownership from each of the practitioners?
3. Can we link patient needs, workload measurement, staffing skills and competencies, acuity needs, and resource parameters in an ongoing dynamic application that adjusts to the reality of a highly variable census

As the consultant to this process, your obligation is to help gather information necessary to address these questions and help management and clinical staff develop a partnership around building an evidence-based format to address practice, resource, and quality issues on the nursing unit. Where might you begin and how can you help them through these initial steps based on information already covered in this chapter?

COMPETENCY, CURRENCY, AND EVIDENCE

In an environment of great change, the ability to remain competent is seriously challenged. With the pace of knowledge generation and the increasing aggregation of data, it is virtually impossible to remain fully competent and have all the knowledge necessary to do work well. The old industrial notion of knowledge as a capacity is no longer adequate when knowledge accelerates at a rate where the individual no longer can keep pace. Therefore, the ability to access information and to manage the information technology is of greater importance than the capacity associated with having the information and knowing it all (Malloch & Porter-O'Grady, 2005). This transfer in the locus of control from knowing information to accessing it creates a challenge in the role of providers and users. Access skills are now essential to remain competent and to aggregate practices and data that will result in a growing data-driven evidence base for best practices.

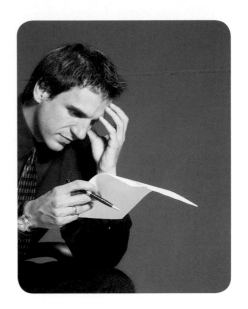

"Proximity" of information is as important as the relevance of the information. Information that exists other than in the place where it needs to be used or is not easy to access makes it irrelevant. Making sure that information can be readily obtained and managed at the point-of-service, by the service providers, is as important as what information is available to them. Access means more than competence; it also means ease in obtaining it and using it as a regular and ongoing part of the work.

"Accessibility" of information means more than the ability to get the information. It also means the ability to use that information and apply it with facility and effectiveness. Information generated in a form and framework that does not make it fluid and flexible in its translation to application or its informing of practice has no value to the practitioner. Accessibility of information has no value if it is not translated into action in a way that makes a difference in the practices of the provider and in the demonstrable process of providing service.

"Reliability" of information means the level of trust that can be applied to it as the practitioner uses it to inform and guide action. Confidence regarding the information decreases to the extent that the information is either incorrect or not relevant to the current work activities of the user. The value of the information declines directly in relationship to the distance between its viability and its accuracy. Practitioners will retreat from use of data that reflects the wrong information.

EVIDENCE-BASED DECISION SUPPORT

Evidence-based practice requires a complex infrastructure that matches a wide variety of data, links it, integrates it, and synthesizes it so the practitioner can use it (Freshwater & Rolfe, 2001). Furthermore, the data are sorted and matched and tied together with algorithms that provide a knowledge framework that refers to a composite of knowledge but generates it in a simple useful form.

Decision support systems are active knowledge management processes that manage and generate knowledge and information in a way that can be immediately used. Further documentation of the action based on the information used adds to the knowledge base and aggregates the data in a good decision support system for the user. The clinical decision support system should provide a range of elements and services that make it useful for the translation and application of the information in individual practices and work processes. Some examples of the elements of good decision support for practitioners are:

- Providing—making sure the right data in the right form are available to the right person at the right time and can be applied immediately.

- Alerting—highlighting or pointing out specific elements of the data that had use and value at any given moment in time and reflect the needs and priorities of the information user.

- Interpreting—providing relevant translation and interpretation of data in a way that has implications for current practices and can be applied to specific practice circumstances.

- Critiquing—determining value of information and providing evaluation of the significance, veracity, and relevance of the data to the specific clinical situation to which they are applied.

- Suggesting—recommending which elements of the data presented have greater applicability, timeliness, or importance to the specific work process or clinical situation to which it is being applied.

- Predicting—determining the likelihood of a specific impact or outcome related to the application of data, which can then be generalized as likely or probable from the application of the data.

- Assisting—providing support information, recommendations, or priorities that guide a person in making choices and applying these choices to the specific circumstances for which they are used.

- Evaluating—suggesting a format or template for linking and integrating data generated from a new situation or application in a way that adds to the aggregated value of the data subsequently applied by future users.

EVIDENCE AND CHOICE

Clinical choice making has not always been based on best practice or scientific foundations. With the introduction of digital systems, the ability to integrate and collate large amounts of data has resulted in a growing interest in building an evidence-based practice system. Clinical choices would be based on the aggregate of available information. That information would be portable and mobile and readily available to inform and influence decision making and choice making. The challenge, however, is the demand to bring discipline and common frames of reference to practice so that dependable and correlated information would be generated and used consistently by decision makers as a way of doing the business of practice. Unilateral and nonaligned individual actions that didn't represent the evidence of best approach would be avoided in favor of the valid and substantial database enumerating and forming the foundations of best practice in the clinical environment.

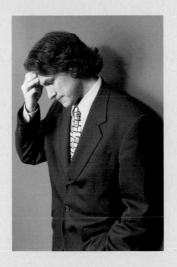

Choice and Error
- How rational?
- What data are used?
- When did error occur?
- Nature of the error?
- Circumstance of error?
- Lesson of the error?
- What corrective action?

Evidence and Error
- What information base?
- How available are data?
- What is past error?
- What were past practices?
- How is data used?
- How is error documented?
- What learning occurred?

Evidence-Based Corrective Action

Error must always be placed in a broader context in order to determine value and impact on practice. Although there are certainly egregious errors, it is important to know the circumstances and context for an error to fully comprehend its implications and to explore its resolution. Too often the error is looked at in isolation of its history and circumstances, both of which may have a dramatic effect on the intensity and interplay of forces that resulted in the error. In fact, when tied to a broader database related to the error, the actual error may be of less concern than the context out of which it flowed. Poor or inadequate training for a specific practice, for example, may have a greater impact on the commission of an error than limited resources might. Focusing solely on the error, in this case, simply misses the point.

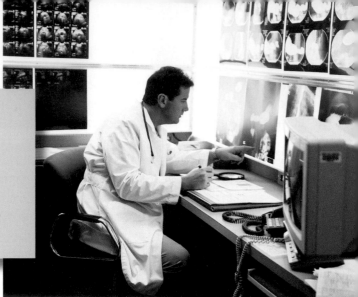

> ## Note:
>
> Evidence of best practices is a system, not an event. The structure constructed to support and sustain it is as important as the practices that reflect it. Evidence of good practice is the culmination of an entire system's commitment to good practice.

GOOD SUPPORT INFRASTRUCTURE AND CLINICAL EVIDENCE

To ensure that good clinical decision systems are in place, it is critical that the information infrastructure is developed in a way that ensures support for good clinical process (see below). A series of steps and processes must be in place in order to ensure good evidence-based practices operate as a clinician's way of doing business.

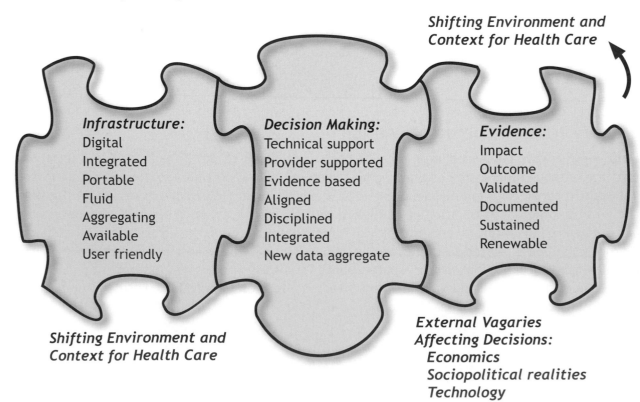

Shifting Environment and Context for Health Care

Infrastructure:
Digital
Integrated
Portable
Fluid
Aggregating
Available
User friendly

Decision Making:
Technical support
Provider supported
Evidence based
Aligned
Disciplined
Integrated
New data aggregate

Evidence:
Impact
Outcome
Validated
Documented
Sustained
Renewable

Shifting Environment and Context for Health Care

External Vagaries Affecting Decisions:
Economics
Sociopolitical realities
Technology

ACCOUNTABILITY, EVIDENCE, AND TECHNOLOGY

Integration

The best of clinical experience, knowledge, and research are integrated in an evidence-based and accountability-driven system. It is not any one of these elements of clinical decision making that drives the search for solid foundations for practice; it is all three.

Technology

The means of good evidence-driven decision making is grounded in the digital systems necessary to correlate, integrate, and synthesize large aggregates of data and make them available to the practitioner in a form and format that can be easily and readily applied in the clinical practice setting in real time.

Evidence

The results of good decisions, the integration of data, and the impact of excellent practice create the frame for an evidence-based approach to practice and evaluate the value of clinical work from the perspectives of desirable outcomes and the best practices that lead to them.

The integration of clinical processes based on best past practices, research, and expert application creates the foundation for building effective accountability. Practitioners want to make a difference in the lives of people served and apply the best in critical process to achieve that end. Good models of evidence-driven processes demonstrate the need for good interface of data sources related to practice (Higgs et al., 2004). They understand that in order to advance the clinical work there must be a strong relationship among work processes, functions, and actions and the outcomes they produce. Furthermore they must be desirable and translated into a language that can be generalized for both provider and person, and they must be replicable. Most practitioners are caught in a web of ritual and routine that is so habit-driven that the work has become an end in itself. Evidence-driven accountability calls providers to refocus their work and attention on the value of their work and the potential difference it makes in the lives of others. In this framework, providers can build a body of evidence for particular practices and work patterns that better fit the expectations for them. In this way they can be aggregated with other similar data points to generate a best practice foundation that all providers can use (McNamara, 2002).

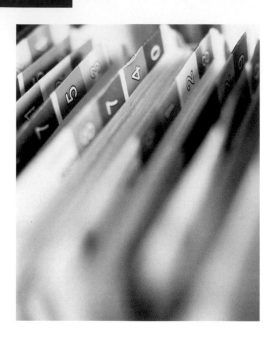

The ability to tap both external and internal sources of knowledge and information related to practice is a central component of the supporting structure of evidence-based accountability. The format for managing information critical to practice is built on the availability and integration of data in a way that the provider can use. Also the design must link well with the methods of practice and the setting where provider and patient meet and within the circumstances of clinical need (see model below). The utility of the system must reflect speed, accuracy, simplicity, and an internal logic that get at obtaining and documenting clinical information.

Filtering and Abstracting to Affect Accountability

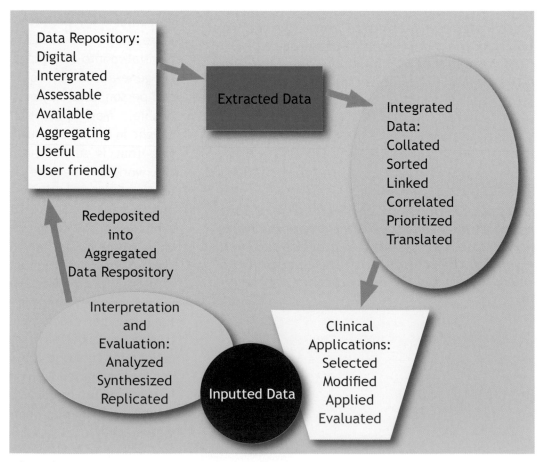

Data Repository:
Digital
Intergrated
Assessable
Available
Aggregating
Useful
User friendly

Extracted Data

Integrated
Data:
Collated
Sorted
Linked
Correlated
Prioritized
Translated

Redeposited
into
Aggregated
Data Respository

Interpretation
and
Evaluation:
Analyzed
Synthesized
Replicated

Inputted Data

Clinical
Applications:
Selected
Modified
Applied
Evaluated

ACCOUNTABILITY AND THE CLINICAL ELECTRONIC HIGHWAY

Develop a rationale for designing and structuring technology and support for evidence-based practice that reflects the programmatic needs of the approach and the resource needs that drive choice and design.

Select the technology that most reflects need and supporting infrastructure and hardware that best actualize the clinical approach desired. Engage stakeholders in designing and selecting the technology they will use.

Adapt clinical behavior patterns to reflect a new way of "doing business." The change in thinking, acting, and evaluating clinical process will be significant. Organization resources must support the developmental learning.

Developing a technology infrastructure to support evidence-based practice is planned and staged methodology. Each stage must be timed and carefully linked and integrated with activities at the point-of-service.

Constructing real-time support system is as important as successful application. As with any technology, there are problems that need immediate resolution. Assistance should be easy to obtain and understandable to apply.

THE ARCHITECTURE OF E-LEARNING FOR EVIDENCE ACCOUNTABILITY

Skills in building evidence-based competence are as difficult to learn as are any other learning processes associated with new conceptual and behavioral skills. The learning process should be well developed before performance expectations change in the system. Access, utility, and evaluation skills need to be inculcated in the practice patterns of professionals before evidenced-based approaches can be effective (McNamara, 2002). The evidence-driven learning model (see above process model), must be inculcated into the system's way of doing its clinical work before meaningful outcomes and cost-benefit can be clealy determined. The e-learning process must be designed much like the work orientation process for new employees. Expectation, behaviors, skills, and value must be articulated with practice before effect will be clear.

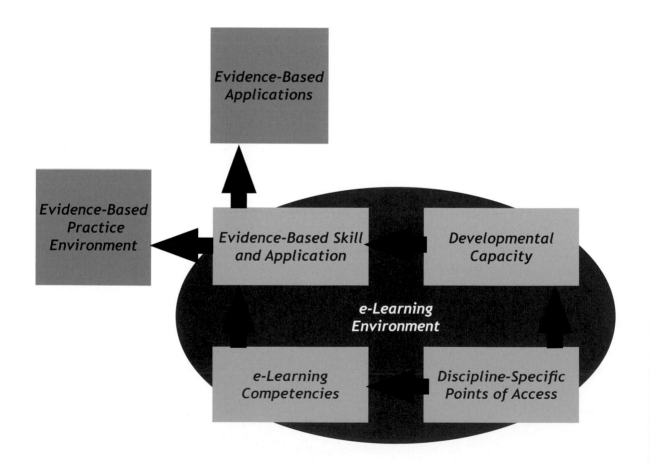

Building the Culture or Evldence and Accountability

The leader has an obligation to build the culture that supports the development of efficient and effective practice (Hamer & Collinson, 1999). In an environment increasingly defined by the focus on the value rather than the volume of work, an entirely different approach to doing the work of care emerges. The manager must be able to create this context before changes in behavior from the staff can be seen. The expectation for change in practice calls the manager to deliver a different message about what clinical work is becoming and what the work effort must focus on and produce.

The innovations in technology affecting clinical practice boggle the imagination. It is vital for the leader to press upon the clinical staff how time is of the essence and that engagement of the vagaries affecting the future of practice must occur in the short term. Relevance in practice demands a reconfiguration of the clinical competencies and performance expectations. Staff simply cannot do clinical work the same way and expect different outcomes from it. A number of factors must be incorporated into this dialog and response:

1. Practice based on length of stay no longer reflects the technology of patient care and the movement of therapeutics from inpatient to outpatient.

2. Portability of therapeutics creates the conditions of portability in practice. It is expected that this portability of technology will further refine clinical services for the next century.

3. The mobility of the patient will be a cornerstone of the future of health service. Increasingly noninvasive therapeutics will create the conditions that will change the institutions of clinical service in order to better service this mobility.

4. Practitioners must be more flexible and fluid in their orientation to clinical work. The work will continue to transition at a rapid rate, calling for quick accommodation and response from health care providers.

5. In a user-driven world, the choice and options for exercising them change the consumer's relationship to the health system and the service model applied to address them. Including the user in design and evaluation will no longer be an exception.

6. Evidence-driven accountability will exact from the provider a focus on value and the goodness-of-fit between the actions of the caregiver, the values and expectations of the patient, and the viability (cost-benefit) of the entire clinical experience. Data-driven supports will provide information regarding expectation, value, and satisfaction.

INTEGRATING TECHNOLOGY INTO EVIDENCE AND PRACTICE

Building an effective frame for continual evidence-based practices requires a strategic commitment that is inclusive of financial, technological, and practice planning (Porter-O'Grady, 2004). Compartmentalization of these efforts is not an acceptable way to build the integration and infrastructure necessary to make evidence a way of life and a frame for practice. Every level of the organization must be fulfilling the stages of development and processes associated with making the approach a success. The context for evidence is as important to sustaining it as are the processes in place.

The major commitment of the system is to the resource outlay for the technological infrastructure necessary to support the digital environment that underpins the practice frame for evidence. This technology must be fluid and flexible enough to incorporate a large number of practitioners and clinical approaches and still aggregate the data generated from each of them in a way that produces meaningful and useful data for effective clinical decision making.

Careful technology assessment and planning must result in a system that can work across the system and be refined and adjusted as well as grow with the success of an evidence-building approach.

Integration with Mission

Evidence-based practice should not be separate from the central strategies and purposes of the system. It is critical to the effectiveness of the organization that its core service deliver what is expected and raise performance to meet a growing expectation for excellence and quality.

Establishing Specific Goals

Priorities regarding the focus of excellence and quality are critical elements of goal-setting for the system and the clinical providers. Evidence-based accountabilities cannot be met all at once. The implementation is progressive and continually building inexorably toward a system of evidence as a clinical way of life.

Making Evidence the Core Practice

Excellence and quality demand that an evidence-based framework be inculcated into the life of the health agency and its clinicians. it cannot be marginalized or collateralized when other fashions or priorities emerge. Effectiveness and advancing clinical quality require everyone's constant energy.

THE ELECTRONIC MEDICAL RECORD AND EVIDENCE

Leaders must be clear about what needs to be in place regarding building the documentation system that supports evidence-based accountability. The record cannot be fully established unless a system has unlimited resources. Even if it did, the progress of documenting for the electronic medical record (EMR) must be based on the progress of the development and the needs that arise from its development. What best fits for the practitioners and the environment of practice is a critical concern in the effective development of the EMR. Clinical leaders must make decisions about what priorities drive the development and what applications are needed and when they are required. The following is a partial list of the elements that must be considered to fit into the logical flow of development based on need and timing:

- Document scanning/imaging systems
- Order communication/results retrieval systems
- Clinical messaging systems
- Charting patient care processes
- Physician order entry systems
- Clinical support systems
- Provider-patient portals
- Personal health records
- Population health records
- Business/payment records
- Interface with clinical data repositories
- Research databases
- Best practices data
- Aggregated clinical applications data
- Quality improvement records and data
- Critical incident and error management documentation
- Patient experience and satisfaction data
- National standards of practice repositories

Note:

The accountability for producing evidence that clinical practice has made a difference depends on the quality and completeness of the data upon which it is based. It cannot be sustained if the infrastructure is inadequate and fails to support the activities that depend on it.

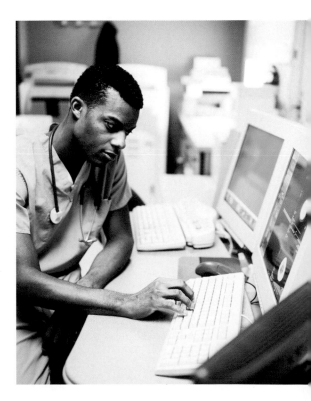

BUILDING CLINICAL PARTNERSHIP FOR EVIDENCE

Evidence-based practice is built on the integration of clinical effort and the aggregation of the information that each provider generates in a way that produces an accurate picture of the impact and value of clinical effort for the patient. It is this integration of effort that is the cornerstone of good clinical evidence. Building that partnership is the centerpiece of a viable and sustainable evidence-based clinical system.

The disciplines must be willing to share clinical processes and data that generate out of their work and represent their contribution to the patient's clinical outcomes.

Models of clinical partnership must provide a vessel for sustaining partnerships that are built. These models must provide a framework and a format for partnering and establishing the common ground for evidence.

Behaviors and performance expectations for the partners need to be identified and developed at the outset so that the parameters for relationship and performance are clear to all.

Developmental programs and processes should be built into the development process. Learning about extinguishing past behaviors is as important as learning about new ones.

Technology competencies should be expected of every partner, equally. No one partner should have to bear the burden of nonperformance by another. Partnership means partnership.

References

Freshwater, D., & Rolfe, G. (2004). *Deconstructing evidence based practice*. London: Routledge.

Hamer, S., & Collinson, G. (1999). *Achieving evidence-based practice: A handbook for practitioners*. Edinburgh; New York: B. Tindall.

Higgs, J., Richardson, B., & Dahlgren, M. A. (2004). *Developing practice knowledge for health professionals*. Edinburgh: Butterworth-Heinemann.

Malloch, K., & Porter-O'Grady, T. (2006). *Introduction to evidence-based practice for nursing and health care*. Sudbury, MA: Jones and Bartlett.

Malloch, K., & Porter-O'Grady, T. (2005). *The quantum leader: Applications for the new world of work. Sudbury, MA: Jones and Bartlett.*

McNamara, 0. (2002). *Becoming an evidence-based practitioner: A framework for teacher-researchers*. London: Routledge/Falmer.

Porter-O'Grady, T. (2004, January-February). Accountability and action. *Health Progress,* 44-48.

Porter-O'Grady, T., & Wilson, C. (1999). *Leading the revolution in healthcare: Igniting performance, changing systems*. Gaithersburg, MD: Aspen.

Suggested Readings

Malloch, K., & Porter-O'Grady, T. (2006). *Introduction to evidence-based practice in nursing and health care*. Sudbury, MA: Jones and Bartlett.

Malloch, K., & Porter-O'Grady, T. (2005). *The quantum leader: Applications for the new world of work*. Sudbury, MA: Jones and Bartlett.

McSherry, R., Simmons, M., & Abbott, P. (2002). *Evidence-informed nursing: A guide for clinical nurses*. New York: Routledge.

Melnyk, B. M., & Fineout-Overholt, E. (2005). *Evidence-based practice in nursing & healthcare: A guide to best practice*. Philadelphia: Lippincott Williams & Wilkins.

Porter-O'Grady, T., & Malloch, K. (2002). *Quantum leadership: A textbook of new leadership*. Sudbury, MA: Jones and Bartlett.

Smith, P. (2004). *Shaping the facts: Evidence-based nursing and health care*. New York: Churchill Livingstone.

UNIT 4:
STRUCTURING FOR EXCELLENCE:
BUILDING A CONTEXT FOR RETENTION

1. STRUCTURING FOR EXCELLENCE: WHAT IS STRUCTURE?

2. SUPPORTING THE STRUCTURE

3. STAFF LEADERSHIP

4. ADVANCING THE PRACTICE OF NURSING

5. SUSTAINING EXCELLENCE

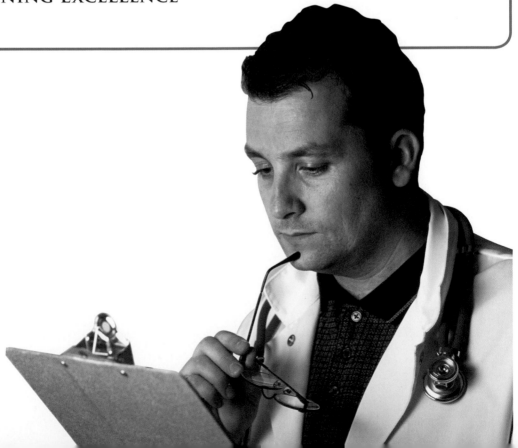

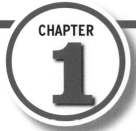

CHAPTER

1

STRUCTURING FOR EXCELLENCE:
WHAT IS STRUCTURE?

Structure is the sum total of the ways in which labor is divided into distinct tasks and then how coordination is achieved among those tasks (Mitzenberg, 1983). Structure demonstrates the relationships among an organization's components and presents us with its design.

In this section, considerations for both the foundation and the elements of organizational structure are discussed. Leaders need to be clear about the work of health care, the individuals needed to do the work, and the framework or delivery model of care in which the work occurs. Creating an organizational structure begins with a clear vision, an understanding of the work to be done, the values to be embraced, and the desired outcomes of the defined work.

The structure best supportive of health care leadership is one that requires role clarity, autonomous role performance, shared decision making and the means to get the work done in the most timely and effective manner that is consistent with the mission and vision of the organization. The structure must also embed the expectation for ongoing evaluation of the work and modification of the work and the structure to support the changing work of health care.

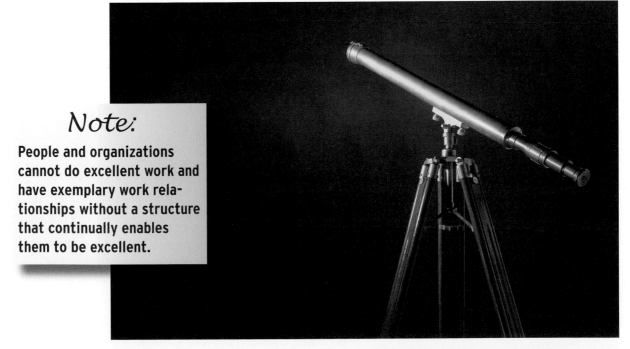

Note:

People and organizations cannot do excellent work and have exemplary work relationships without a structure that continually enables them to be excellent.

FOUNDATIONS FOR ORGANIZATIONAL STRUCTURE

Once the vision and values are articulated and agreed upon, the structure will begin to evolve. Whereas some leaders believe that form or structure follows function, the reality is that both structure and function are dynamic and continually affecting each other. The only time it is difficult, if not impossible, to achieve the mission of the organization is when structure or form is the sole determiner of the work of an organization. When structure dictates work processes, flow of activities, and communication, operational efficiencies can be compromised, work satisfaction decreases, and productivity declines.

Effective structure evolves and is re-created to adjust to changes in the environment. The allocation of power and authority for decision making, the span of control, number and types of roles, delivery models, the supporting policies, skill mix, and core staffing levels can be determined. The structure for contemporary health care organizations must necessarily consider the work of healing and the fundamental role of professional nursing, which provides the largest amount of direct patient care. All caregivers need to be able to assess, intervene, and put patients in the best condition for nature to act on them, primarily by altering the environment. Structure that supports collaboration and therapeutic relationships is essential.

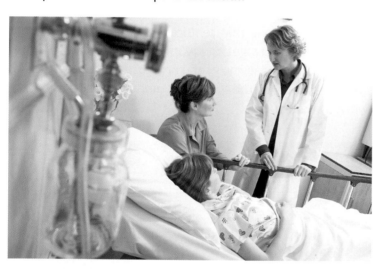

The Work of Nursing

The structure for contemporary nursing considers not only the work of healing but also the role of professional nursing. The goal of nursing, to put patients in the best condition for nature to act on them, primarily by altering the environment, requires a structure supportive of collaboration and therapeutic relationships within the defined scope of nursing practice.

The International Council of Nurses (ICN) defines nursing as work that encompasses autonomous and collaborative care of individuals of all ages, families, groups and communities, and sick or well in all settings. Nursing includes the promotion of health, prevention of illness, and the care of ill, disabled and dying people. Advocacy, promotion of a safe environment, research, participation in shaping health policy and in patient and health systems management, and education are also key nursing roles.

SOCIETY: A MANDATE FOR HEALTH CARE

Health care's unique contribution to society transcends all caregiver roles, functions, and settings in working with individuals to improve health in ways appropriate for each individual's situation. Leaders have the distinct accountability to design, facilitate and manage patient care delivery that ensures social accountability to the public. It is this work that the caregivers must continually evaluate and affirm commitment to—not only to themselves, but also the organization and society.

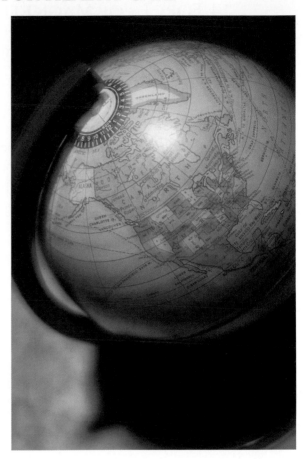

A philosophy of caring must necessarily pervade the structure of the organization. Caring must be more than mere sentiment; it must be a defined way of being, or state of natural responsiveness to others that includes personal involvement, knowledge of how to improve situations, and intention to help based on what is good for the patient. The work of healing must be inexorably embedded into the structure; it is work that is not about perfection but about identifying patient health needs, creating plans to manage health care needs, and providing service of the highest level of quality that improves the status of the patient's health.

> **Best practices are lessons learned. As suggested by Henry Ford, they need to be shamelessly borrowed and adopted.**
> **(Havens, 2001)**

Evidence for Health Care Structure

Evidence for health care excellence has emerged from the Magnet program that identifies those organizations most supportive of nursing excellence and high-quality patient care outcomes. Specific guidelines for organizations are integrated into the 14 Forces of Magnetism (FOMs) (see next page) that identify the preferred characteristics of the contemporary organization committed to excellence. Research results continue to emerge that support the adoption of Magnet characteristics. The 14 FOMs identify key characteristics of organizations able to achieve high levels of excellence in patient care quality, nurse satisfaction, and organizational viability. These forces, based on evidence, guide the development of an effective, sustainable structure.

THE BEACON FOR EXCELLENCE:
14 FORCES OF MAGNETISM

1 *Quality nursing leadership*: the voice for nursing.

2 *Organizational structure*: flat, decentralized organizational structure to support functional and operational partnerships.

3 *Management style*: participative management style to include those involved with and affected by care processes.

4 *Personnel policies and programs*: policies and systems involve staff to ensure that accountability is the cornerstone of professional practice.

5 *Professional model of care*: nurses have responsibility, accountability and authority in their patients' care. They coordinate their own care with support and proper resources from the organization.

6 *Quality of care*: nurses believe they are giving high-quality patient care consistent with the needs of the patient and that their organization sees high-quality care as a priority.

7 *Quality improvement*: staff nurses participate in the quality improvement process and believe that it helps improve patient care within the organization.

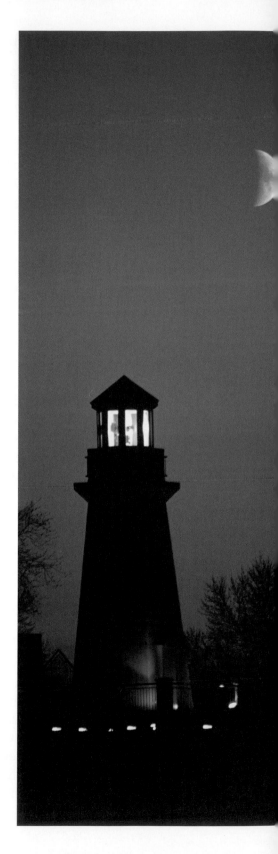

8 *Consultation and resources*: consultation, including advanced practice nurses and peer support, is available and used.

9 *Autonomy*: independent judgment supported. Nurses are allowed and expected to work autonomously, consistent with professional standards and members of a multidisciplinary team.

10 *Community involvement*: hospitals maintain a strong community presence that includes a variety of long-term outreach programs.

11 *Nurses as teachers*: nurses teach in all aspects of their practice; teaching is a basic role of the nurse and is an expectation, not an option.

12 *Professional image of nursing*: nurses are seen as essential to the hospital's delivery of care model.

13 *Interdisciplinary collaboration*: physicians, nurses, pharmacists, therapists, social workers, nutritionists, and all other members of the health care team treat each other with respect.

14 *Professional development*: the organization emphasizes orientation, inservice education, continuing education, formal education, and career development.

WHY MAGNET ACCREDITATION?

Some leaders may wonder if Magnet recognition is another fad like MBO, CQI, TQM, or quality circles and are reluctant to join the Magnet bandwagon. Leaders wonder if the Magnet characteristics and behaviors are merely good practices that should be practices of all leaders without the need for an additional label and cost of the Magnetism credential. Other designations from Joint Commission and the Industrial Standards Organization (ISO) also provide templates for quality that some organizations rely on. The Magnet credential is more appropriate for several reasons.

1 The focus is on quality patient care from the nursing perspective—the perspective of the largest group of caregivers within the patient's experience of care. Note: these characteristics are applicable and supportive of the work of all caregivers.

2 It is a framework of characteristics that has been examined and validated as indicative of the best practices for patient care quality.

3 The development of the professional nurse role within the standards reflects best practices that are comprehensive, documented, and proven. Four areas are emphasized; management philosophy and practices, adherence to standards for improving the quality of care, leadership behaviors supporting professional practice, and attention to the diversity of needs of staff and patients.

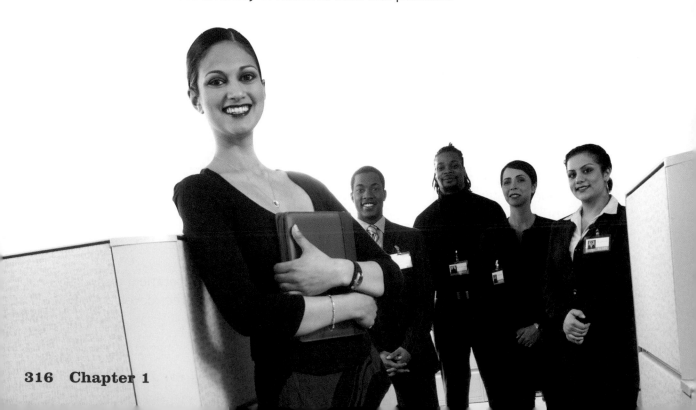

FOUR KEY ELEMENTS OF STRUCTURE

The characteristics of an organization's structure have been identified as indicators of the quality of work life in health care settings (Hall, 2005). In this section four of the key elements of structure are discussed.

The interrelationships among the elements of the organizational structure are undeniable. Consistency and congruence between the levels of authority, job descriptions, communication channels, and the delivery model are required to create effective processes. Failing to examine and ensure congruence between the expectations for performance, values, and the desired outcomes will result in organizational inefficiencies and less than desired levels of quality. For example, allocating power to an individual on the organizational chart without the supporting job role and accountabilities creates confusion and mistrust among employees.

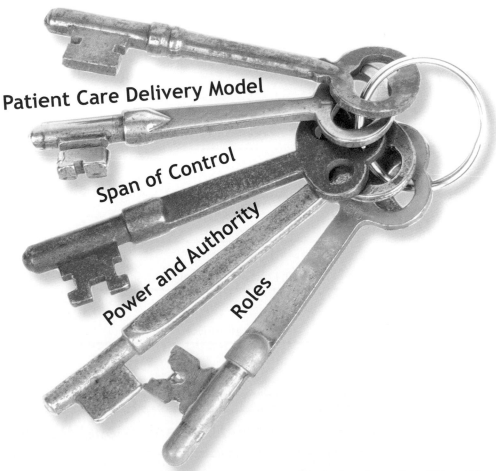

Patient Care Delivery Model

Span of Control

Power and Authority

Roles

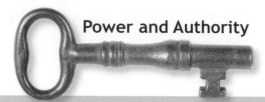

Power and Authority

The framework for excellence begins with structure that supports work processes that are fluid, flexible, and supportive of practice excellence in the organization. Building excellence into the fabric of an organization requires a supportive structure for caregivers as well as the commitment and engagement of individuals to the work of healing. Todays nurses are seeking work environments in which excellent patient care is supported, effective communication occurs, caregivers are acknowledged for their positive behaviors, and negative behaviors are addressed quickly.

A structure that allows for change and supports efficient work processes and satisfaction is essential to achieve the desired excellence. A flat, decentralized structure is the hallmark of organizations that have achieved Magnet accreditation and high levels of excellence (ANCC, 2004).

Models

Organizational structure models vary from the traditional top-down pyramid to matrix-like, flexible relationships with multiple linkages based on functional collaboration.

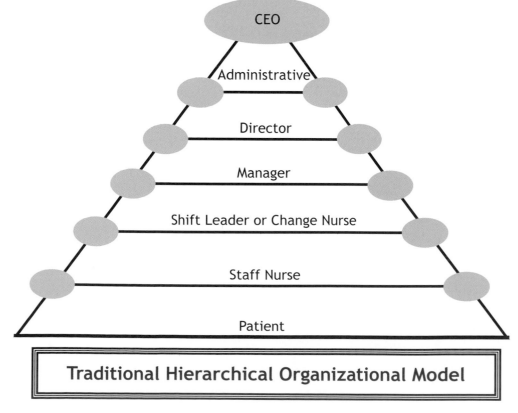

Traditional Hierarchical Organizational Model

FLAT, DECENTRALIZED STRUCTURE

The Magnet structure for excellence is flat, decentralized, and supportive of shared decision making, The structure is dynamic and responsive to change. Nursing is present and actively involved in organizational committees. The CNO reports to the CEO and executive level nursing leaders serve at the executive level of the organization.

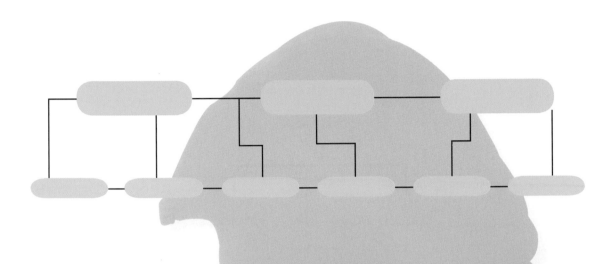

Determining the Appropriate Structure for Your Organization

Creating and sustaining the ideal organizational structure is an ongoing responsibility of the leadership team. Multiple factors influence the structure of an organization; the relationships between workers, the value of the work to be done, availability of competent and skilled workers, innovations in work processes, available technology to support the work, and adequacy of resources.

No single structural model is appropriate for all organizations. Each organization must assess the work to be done, who can do the work, beliefs and values, and resources available to achieve the desired goals.

Decision Making

A participative management style in which all employees work collaboratively to accomplish the best patient care is pervasive in a Magnet organization. The optimal structure supports and encourages staff feedback, values contributions, and encourages involvement in decision making. Nursing leaders are visible and accessible and communicate effectively with staff. These behaviors in Magnet organizations are expectations rather than options or intermittent activities. Collaborative relationships of mutual respect are evident throughout Magnet organizations as all members of the health care team contribute to achieving clinical outcomes.

ORGANIZATIONAL STRUCTURE: MATRIX MODEL

The matrix model supports open communication, minimal reporting layers, and cross-functional-teamwork. Unnecessary layers of reporting and communication channels dilute the effectiveness of the communication and marginalize the role of the professional nurse. A structure that supports and expects direct communication between the caregiver and the physician is fundamental to empowered and autonomous practice.

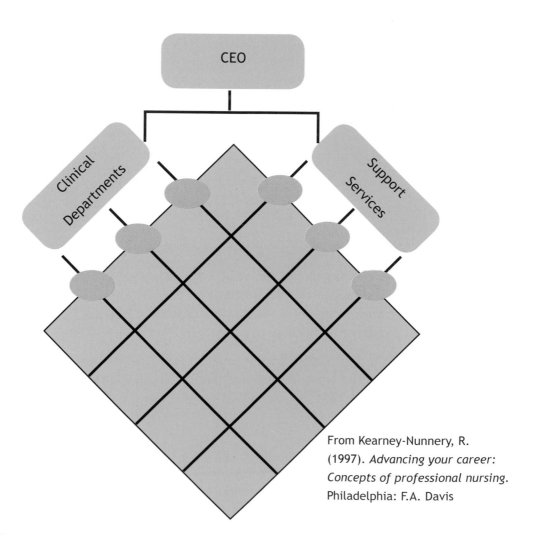

From Kearney-Nunnery, R. (1997). *Advancing your career: Concepts of professional nursing*. Philadelphia: F.A. Davis

ROLES AND RESPONSIBILITIES

Defining and describing the nursing work to be done is an essential step in creating an organizational structure for excellence. The role of nursing by its very nature is embedded within a complex system that includes multiple autonomous health care disciplines. Role definitions that reflect the mission and goals of the organization and integrating the desired behaviors and competencies are essential to create and sustain a culture that fosters commitment to the defined work of the patient care team.

Roles

Role Definitions

The context for excellence requires clear role descriptions to support focused work processes, to minimize redundant work, and that include the expectations for results. Roles in an environment dedicated to excellence require knowledgeable strong leaders willing to take risks and advocate for their staff. Caregivers must be licensed or credentialed, clinically competent, skilled in developing therapeutic relationships, and able to integrate their work into the system in which they work.

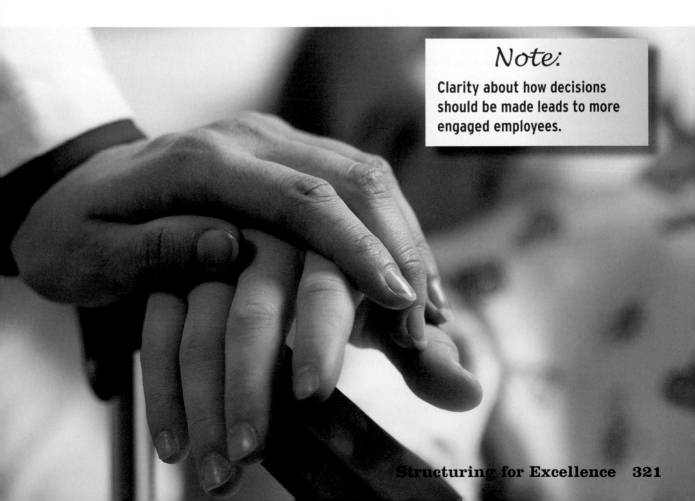

Note:

Clarity about how decisions should be made leads to more engaged employees.

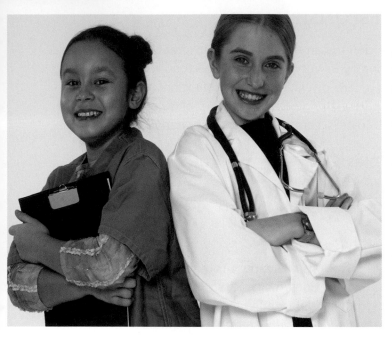

THE EMPOWERED NURSE

Many people still view a nurse's job as a primary caretaker. But the health field has evolved immensely since 1859, when Florence Nightingale described the work of nursing and included tasks of housekeeping, meal preparation, and patient hygiene. Today's nurse does things that were done by only doctors less than 40 years ago: taking blood pressures readings, changing dressings, performing physical examinations, giving injections, and handling machines and sophisticated monitors.

Empowered employees are always optimistic, able to lead by example, and share information respectfully and appropriately.

CAREGIVER ROLE: ADVANCED PRACTICE NURSE

The structure and delivery model for patient care must include the role of the advanced practice nurse. The nurse with advanced education is vital to the ever-expanding knowledge and work of the registered nurse. Both the clinical nurse specialist and doctorally prepared nurse play critical roles in developing and sustaining excellence in practice and decision making. Examples of the roles of the nurse with advanced education include:

- Coach, mentor, and provide expertise that will advance the practice of nursing and ensure the best possible patient care.

- Provide consultation with other disciplines.

- Assist in identifying resources to achieve excellent patient care.

- Serve as a role model for the nurse as teacher.

- Identify and develop research projects to test and validate the evolving work of nurses.

In Magnet organizations, education is a high priority and includes orientation, inservice programs, continuing education, formal education, and career development.

The advanced practice nurse provides on-the-spot consultation and education of nurses—often a more effective approach that is retained by nurses than the traditional classroom approach.

One of the most significant challenges for the advanced practice nurse is to practice the three roles of consultant, educator, and researcher. Often with the rapidly changing nurse workforce, clinical nurse specialists become a nurse educator, focusing primarily on orientation rather than all of the dimensions of the role.

CAREGIVER ROLE: TEACHER

Teaching is the hallmark of nursing practice. The nurse's role as a teacher begins with the patient, moves to the role of coach and mentor for the novice graduate nurse, support for student nurses, and on to other members of the health care team.

Nurses also provide health care information to community organizations, particularly schools and churches. Publishing new knowledge, providing workshops, and teaching nursing courses are other ways that nurses share their health care wisdom.

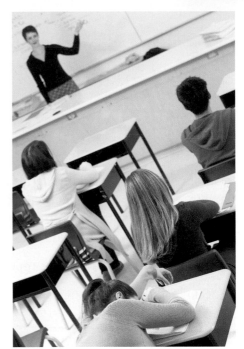

CAREGIVER ROLE: COLLABORATOR

No longer is the nurse the only caregiver with the physician; therapists, pharmacists, technicians, and assistants comprise the team of caregivers. The infrastructure of the contemporary organization must support both communication and relationships to achieve excellence in patient care. In addition, as the responsibilities of the nurse continue to grow and as innovations abound in genome therapy and technological advances in clinical and management systems, the quality of the communication is of the utmost importance. All caregivers must be able to evaluate, reconsider, and modify roles when needed.

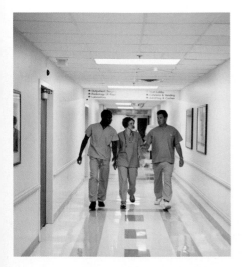

Roles and Responsibilities: Communication and Teamwork

The caregiver-physician relationship is the most important relationship in an environment that supports professional practice. Mutual respect, interdependency, concern for patients, and good communication are the descriptors of quality collaborative practice. In contrast, poor physician relationships account for patient dissatisfaction and caregiver emotional exhaustion, which is a component of burnout, leading to resignation from the organization. Each member of the team—caregivers and physicians—contributes to positive relationships through regular discussion of role expectations and licensure requirements.

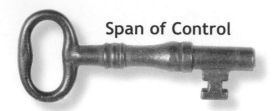

Span of Control

Span of Control:
The number of people who report directly to a single manager, supervisor, or leader and includes the functions of planning, organizing, and leading.

Span of control is a key consideration in ensuring that participation and collaboration are fluid and flexible, allow for timely decision making, and are supportive of practice excellence in the organization. The appropriate number of individuals in one's span of control depends on many variables and includes the following considerations:

- Number of staff categories reporting to the manager
- Similarity or complexity of functions supervised
- Geographic proximity
- Degree of direction, control, and coordination required by those supervised
- Planning and evaluating time required
- Number of units the manager is responsible for
- Level of unit unpredictability
- Technology
- Type of unit
- Number of support staff for the unit or organizational assistance available

Evidence for Span of Control

No studies have been published linking the manager's span of control to patient outcomes.

Span of control studies are related to the effect on staff performance:

—A higher level of support from managers decreases nurse frustration.

—Wider spans of control result in communication that is more distant, less frequent, and more formal, thereby decreasing nurse satisfaction.

DESCRIPTION

A patient care delivery model is the method or system of organizing and delivering nursing care; the manner in which nursing care is organized in order to deliver the care necessary to meet the needs of the patients. The delivery system encompasses work delegation, resource utilization, communication methodologies, clinical decision-making processes, and management structure (Hall, 2005).

Traditional Delivery Models

- Functional
- Total patient care
- Team nursing
- Primary nursing
- Case management
- Patient-focused care

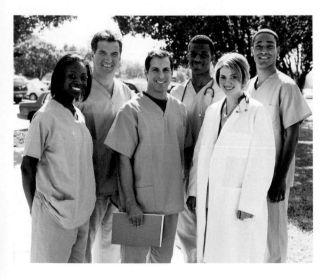

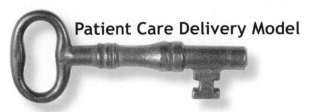

Patient Care Delivery Model

Putting It All Together: The Patient Care Delivery Model

The professional practice model for patient care delivery emerges from the roles, power, authority, and span of control defined by the organization. The model has a direct and significant effect on staffing levels. Current systems for the provision of patient care or patient care delivery models are dynamic due to the continually changing health care environment that affects goals and resources. What remains stable is the need for congruence with the mission vision and values of the care providers and the organization. An effective care delivery system must ensure that the needs of patients are appropriately matched to resources, quality care provided contributes to the outcomes, and documentation is created to reflect the care provided and outcomes obtained. A comprehensive model also requires having the right caregiver with the right patient at the right time and is therefore linked to a valid and reliable patient classification system, which is essential in the planning and evaluation of the selected patient care delivery model.

Creating innovative patient care delivery models is an exemplar for the leadership Force of Magnetism in which nurse leaders are expected to be knowledgeable and strong visionary risk takers. Leaders advocate for and support staff and patients using a clear well-articulated philosophy that guides day-to-day operations of nursing services.

Organizations frequently change delivery models depending on patient needs and the availability of staff. New patient care delivery model research noted that in many organizations, the model for care delivery varies from shift to shift and from hour to hour (Kramer and Schmalenberg, 2005). What remains constant is the philosophy of primary nursing; the registered nurse is responsible and accountable for the care of all patients at all times.

A Final Thought on Structure

Leaders are often challenged with the changes in organizational structure: too many, too few, or changes to manage poor performers rather than the changing work of the organization. Some leaders are reluctant to modify organizational structure, whereas others may modify structure too quickly and without good rationale.

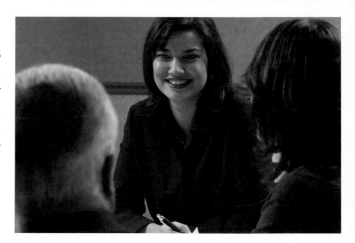

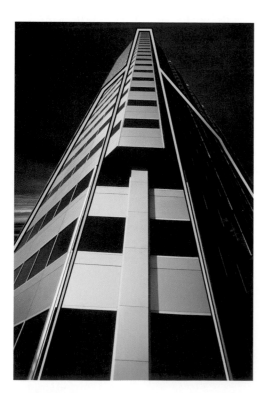

As noted, organizational structure is dynamic. No structure can remain constant and still meet the changing needs of the environment. New technology, new therapies, new regulations, and new financing models are continually changing and creating new expectations and new limitations.

The challenge for leaders is to create a structure that not only supports excellence but also is dynamic and sustainable. Only when the defined purpose, work, or vision of the organization is changing should leaders consider modifying the organizational structure.

INNOVATIONS IN PATIENT CARE DELIVERY

Banner Estrella Medical Center (BEMC) in Phoenix, Arizona, used the opportunity of building a new facility to create a model of care that would address many of the shortcomings of current models and integrate the forces of magnetism. The innovative delivery model integrates the cultural expectations of interdisciplinary collaboration, the availability of clinical experts, and optimal use of registered nurses, licensed practical nurses, and nursing assistants. The essence of the desired patient care is found within the energetic relationships among all members of the health care team who facilitate healing, self-actualization, and empowerment, and provide appropriate patient care interventions. The model embeds a culture of competence and core values that not only encourage but also expect excellence in patient care processes that are multidisciplinary in nature, evidence based, and timely.

The accountability-based model requires that all members of the team participate in the work of patient care to their fullest capacity. In this learning environment, decision making embodies the beliefs and values of shared leadership, multidisciplinary teamwork, and an orientation to achieving and continually improving results (Drexler & Malloch, 2005).

Although many delivery models have emerged over the years, including functional, team, primary, and case models, the goals remain constant. According to Hall (2005), the model that emphasizes input of patients, nurses, and the organization, the throughput factors of communication, coordination, and environmental complexity, is well positioned to transform the interactions into outputs of effective patient care processes.

Key Points

- A patient care delivery model enables the conceptual link between resource utilization, nurse measures of quality, and patient outcomes.

- A patient care delivery model gives nurses the responsibility and authority to provide, coordinate, and ensure continuity of care across the continuum.

- A patient care delivery model is designed to ensure that patients' unique needs are addressed and the desired outcomes are achieved.

- The challenges of a dynamic health care environment include:
  — Changing skills needed.
  — Changing expectations of patients.
  — Technology advances.
  — New therapeutics.

The BEMC model (see next page) integrates and supports the beliefs that will transform the health care experience and include the following:

- Heal and nurture all those we have the opportunity to serve.
- Value people first and foremost, which fosters our ability to achieve true excellence in all categories, and supports the core values of Banner health.
- Embrace the diversity of the community into our work environment Create innovative and sustainable patient care practices that exemplify best value care.
- Support a model of integrative health care therapies.
- Provide flexible and adaptable physical space that meets the health care needs of today and tomorrow.
- Incorporate evidence-based research to continually evolve and improve in all categories.

Circles of Staffing Support

The BEMC model is designed to create stability at the core level of patient care for the predictive portion of patient care. The oversight team is a second level or circle of support to unplanned and complex work of the patient care unit.

Core staff:
This level of staff—registered nurses, licensed practical nurses, and nursing assistants present 24 hours a day—provides approximately 80% of the care of the designated area, care that is planned and somewhat predictable.

Oversight team:
This level of staff is designed to provide stability to the core staff, support timely work processes, and provide support for the unpredictable work of patient care. Processes that are included are the completion of the patient admission assessment within 2 hours, support for patient emergencies, and break or meal relief. The clinical nurse specialist is a key member of this team, providing real-time expertise in complex patient care situations, discipline-specific education for staff, and use of research as well as creation of new research studies.

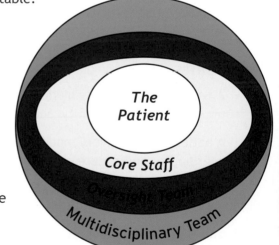

Multidisciplinary team:
These staff members comprise all other professionals, providing care at intermittent times during the day.

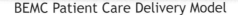

Innovative Model of Care: Circles of Support
Banner Estrella Medical Center

BEMC Patient Care Delivery Model

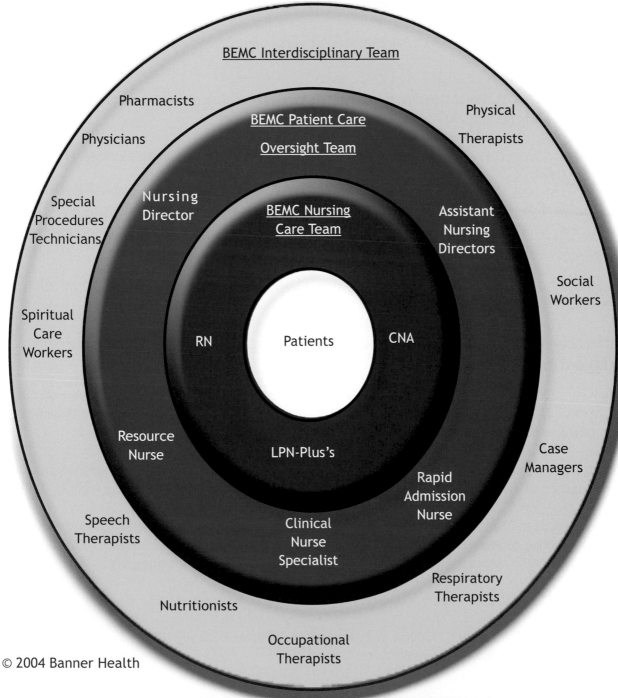

BEMC Interdisciplinary Team

BEMC Patient Care Oversight Team

BEMC Nursing Care Team

Pharmacists

Physicians

Physical Therapists

Special Procedures Technicians

Nursing Director

Assistant Nursing Directors

Spiritual Care Workers

Social Workers

RN

Patients

CNA

Resource Nurse

LPN-Plus's

Case Managers

Rapid Admission Nurse

Speech Therapists

Clinical Nurse Specialist

Nutritionists

Respiratory Therapists

Occupational Therapists

© 2004 Banner Health

References

American Nurses Credentialing Center. (2004). *Magnet recognition program application manual.* (2005 ed.). Silver Spring, MD: Author.

Drexler, D., & Malloch, K. (2005). Cultural transformation, computerized documentation. *Nurse Leader: From Management to Leadership*, 3(4), 32-36.

Hall, L. M. (2005). *Quality work environments for nurse and patient safety*. Sudbury, MA: Jones and Bartlett.

Havens, D. S. (2001). Comparing nursing infrastructure and outcomes: ANCC magnet and nonmagnet CNEs report. *Nursing Economic$*, 19(6), 258-266.

Kearney-Nunnery, R. (1997). *Advancing your career: Concepts of professional nursing*. Philadelphia: F.A Davis.

Kramer, M., & Schmalenberg, C. (2002). Staff nurses identify essentials of magnetism. In M. McClure, & A. S. Hinshaw (Eds.): *Magnet hospitals revisited: Attraction and retention of professional nurses* (pp. 25-59, 31-34). Washington, DC: American Nurses Publishing.

Kramer, M., & Schmalenberg, C. (2005). Revising the essentials of magnetism tool. *JONA*, 35(4), 188-198.

Mitzenberg, H. (1983). *Power in and around organizations*. Englewood Cliffs, NJ: Prentice-Hall.

Suggested Readings

Aiken, L. (2005, April). Are patients safer five years after the Institute of Medicine report on medical errors? Implications for nurse leaders. Keynote address. Washington, DC: American Organization of Nurse Executives.

Aiken, L., Havens, D. S., & Sloane, D. M. (2000). The magnet nursing services recognition program: A comparison of two groups of magnet hospitals. *The American Journal of Nursing*, 100(3), 26-35.

American Nurses Credentialing Center. (2002). Magnet recognition program. Recognizing excellence in nursing service. Health care instructions and application process manual. (2002-2004 ed.). Silver Spring, MD: Author. Retrieved March 2005 from www.nursecredentialing.org.

Pekkanen, J. (2003, September). Condition: Critical. Reader's Digest, 84-93.

Steinbinder, A., & Scherer, E. (2005). In K. Malloch, & T Porter-O'Grady (Eds.): *Evidence based practice*. Sudbury, MA: Jones and Bartlett.

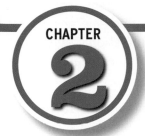

CHAPTER 2 SUPPORTING THE STRUCTURE

Culture is the essence of the organization. Culture is reflected in the behaviors of the organization's members and includes subtle and overt activities common to an organization. Beliefs, behaviors, and the selected system tools bring the structure of the organization to life.

Culture is...

...the standards, techniques, and strategies for dealing with problems.

...the internal psychological environment of the organization.

...the assumptions taught to new members as the correct way to perceive, think, and feel in order to be successful.

...the pattern of basic assumptions that a given group has identified, discovered, or developed in learning to cope with its problems of external adaptation and internal integration, and that have worked well enough to consider valid, and therefore, to be taught to new members as the correct way to perceive, think, and feel as related to these problems (Schein, 1991).

Once the decision-making power and authority expectations, clinical and leadership roles, and evaluation framework are determined, the culture, or essence, of the organization emerges. In this section, the elements of culture, beliefs and behaviors specific to healing, professional autonomy, patient safety, and leader behaviors that support excellence in the practice of nursing and patient care are discussed.

The structure of the organization must necessarily support the work of healing—work that requires caregivers, equipment, technology, processes, reward and recognition programs, and evaluation methods. Leaders work to ensure that the structure serves first and foremost to facilitate patient health and healing.

Health care leaders, as knowledgeable, strong, visionary professionals often take risks to ensure that the context and supporting processes for effective healing do indeed occur. They advocate and support both staff and patients on the basis of a well-articulated philosophy steeped in the spirit of healing that guides the day-to-day operations of patient care services.

In this section, the essential culture that supports excellence in healing services, professional behaviors, autonomy, safety, inherent risks of leadership in sustaining the structure, and considerations for evaluating effective structure are discussed.

Foundational belief: Healing is our work

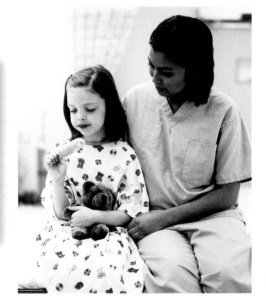

The organizational structure supports the special relationship between the healer and the patient. Behaviors that reflect the belief of the healing nature of nursing are ever present in caregivers. The values and standards of practice that discriminate the ordinary from the out-of-the-ordinary health care make the relationship of patient and healer special. The experiences of caring and healing through comprehension of healing as an experience of a particular kind of human relationship and the intention to create relationships that are caring, compelling, and gratifying distinguish health care workers from any other profession.

A CULTURE OF HEALTH CARE EXCELLENCE

The organizational structure for excellence must support professional behaviors that allow for members of the health care team to assist patients to enhance their ability to manage their health, relieve pain and distress, restore functionality, and/or experience a peaceful death. Professional behaviors emerge from a structure of excellence and result in a sense of satisfaction and accomplishment when a patient experiences relief, a patient's functionality is improved, or a terminally ill patient dies tranquilly.

The culture of health care excellence embodies professional behaviors of autonomy, personal accountability (ethic) for competence, and honesty. Participation in the work of nursing is not optional or embraced intermittently; it is an expectation of professional practice and membership in the organization dedicated to excellence.

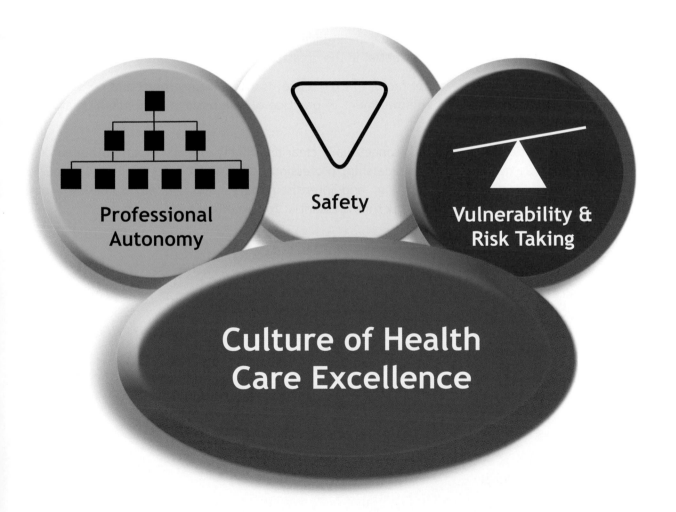

Professional Autonomy

Safety

Vulnerability & Risk Taking

Culture of Health Care Excellence

INDEPENDENT JUDGEMENT SUPPORTED

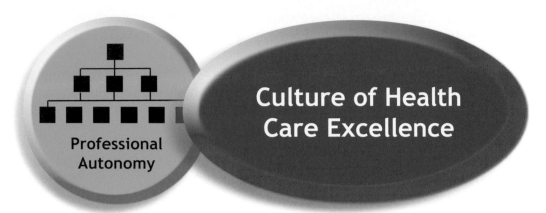

Creating a culture of excellence is a complex and multifaceted process. Healthy authority processes, clear roles, and commitment to healing can only be realized when professionals behave in ways that represent professional accountability and competence. Specifically, clarity of the role and expectations of professional autonomy are essential in the creation of a healthy, healing culture.

Professional autonomy, a key Magnet factor of excellence, is often misinterpreted as personal independence rather than a state of empowerment to practice on the basis of professional clarity and obligation.

The theoretical notion of autonomy is conceptually clear and highly interwoven into other forces of magnetism such as quality nursing leadership, professional models of care, high-quality patient care, the professional image of nursing, and interdisciplinary collaboration. Embedding nurse autonomy within the organizational structure is essential for excellence.

Clinical Autonomy

Clinical autonomy is the freedom to act on what you know, to make independent clinical decisions that exceed standard nursing practice, in the best interest of the patient (Kramer & Schmalenberg, 2002). Clinical autonomy has been identified as a key indicator of quality work environments.

Caveat

No discipline is ever empowered to act in isolation when the work is about healing another individual.

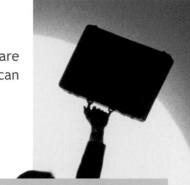

AUTONOMY VS. INDEPENDENCE: A CHALLENGE FOR LEADERS

Development of professional autonomy within traditional cultures that are not structured and supported for participative, shared decision making can be difficult. Creating and sustaining a culture supportive of professional nurse autonomy requires a clear understanding of the notion of autonomy, the expectations for collaboration, and the mutually developed patient goals.

Leaders play a key role in maintaining and transmitting the culture by what they pay attention to; measure and control; how they react in a crisis; and whom they recruit, promote, and fire.

Often leaders are required to take risks and challenge the status quo, which may be ingrained in the existing culture. Taking risks in which the outcome is uncertain requires leaders to be comfortable with the reality that all leaders are indeed vulnerable; no leader can be certain of the outcome when challenging the status quo. Despite the uncertainty of the work and challenges encountered in the creation of an infrastructure to support professional autonomy, competent leaders can make this happen. Competent leaders steeped in the belief of shared decision making see this as nonnegotiable, essential work.

Most leaders are readily able to understand the concept of autonomy and its relationship to patient care outcomes and caregiver satisfaction. It is, however, much more difficult to create and sustain the daily conditions in the workplace that support the empowered, autonomous professional. The major challenge is in building trust for professionals in the clinical setting to take actions that might be risky and adversarial, and might sometimes fail.

Clinical practice autonomy does not imply independence. It implies the right to exercise clinical and organizational judgment within the context of an interdependent health care team and in accordance with the socially and legally granted freedom of the discipline.

Leaders support autonomous practice when they verbally and publicly recognize professionals who have taken the initiative to act on behalf of a patient. More importantly, the leader recognizes unsuccessful efforts with the caregiver when the autonomous act does not achieve the desired outcome. Leaders understand the reality that it requires more time to lead in this manner. The time to learn about the situation, discover lessons, and reinforce autonomous practices requires much more than the time to reinforce a successful intervention, but is perhaps more important in the development of expertise in autonomy, increased trust, and belief that taking action on behalf of the patient is always supported.

Supporting the Structure   335

Critical Attributes of Autonomy

- Professional knowledge and skill

- Defined area of practice

- Desire for autonomy

- Responsibility and authority to make decisions based on professional knowledge and skill and the ability to execute these in practice

- An environment that supports professional practice and respects the professional's individual and collective right to challenge circumstances and decisions

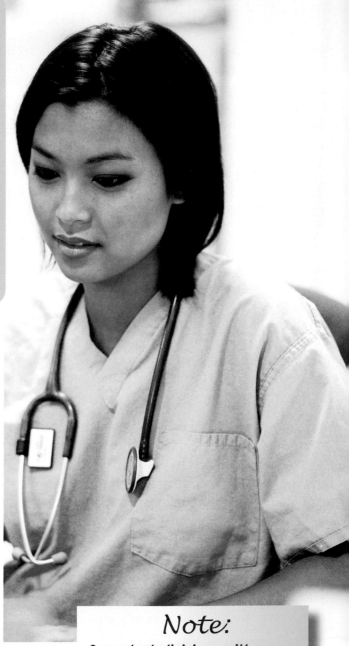

More Definitions:

Structural and work autonomy: the worker's freedom to make decisions based on job requirements

Attitudinal autonomy: the belief in one's freedom to exercise judgment in decision making

Aggregate autonomy: encompasses attitudinal and structural dimensions, the socially and legally granted freedom of self-governance, and control of the profession without influence from eternal sources. Autonomy is viewed as self-determination in practicing according to professional nursing standards.

Professional nurse autonomy: the belief in the centrality of the client when making responsible decisions both independently and interdependently that reflect advocacy for the client

Note:

Competent clinicians, with expertise as autonomous professionals, function most effectively in the context of a team of similarly competent professionals.

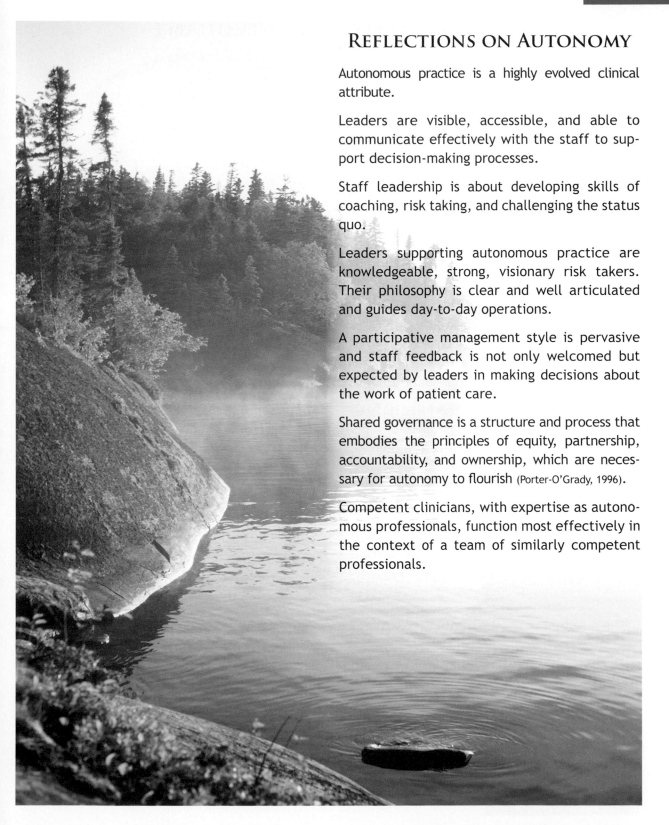

REFLECTIONS ON AUTONOMY

Autonomous practice is a highly evolved clinical attribute.

Leaders are visible, accessible, and able to communicate effectively with the staff to support decision-making processes.

Staff leadership is about developing skills of coaching, risk taking, and challenging the status quo.

Leaders supporting autonomous practice are knowledgeable, strong, visionary risk takers. Their philosophy is clear and well articulated and guides day-to-day operations.

A participative management style is pervasive and staff feedback is not only welcomed but expected by leaders in making decisions about the work of patient care.

Shared governance is a structure and process that embodies the principles of equity, partnership, accountability, and ownership, which are necessary for autonomy to flourish (Porter-O'Grady, 1996).

Competent clinicians, with expertise as autonomous professionals, function most effectively in the context of a team of similarly competent professionals.

PATIENT SAFETY IS NOT NEGOTIABLE

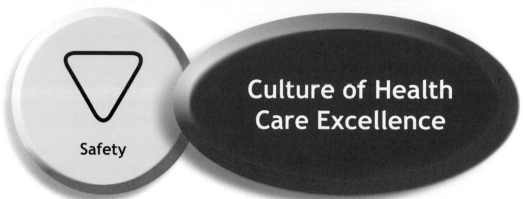

Safety

Culture of Health Care Excellence

Patient safety, error as opportunity, and remediation before discipline are essential priorities in a high reliability organization.

No patient ever expects to be harmed while under the care of a healer, and no healer ever expects to harm a patient. Yet unexpected events and deviations do occur and injuries result. All healers will make mistakes no matter how competent they are. The responsibility accepted by a healer is indeed awesome because patients entrust caregivers with enormous power and authority. It takes considerable spiritual maturity to accept patient trust and understand that mistakes happen.

Health care leaders have much work to do in the area of patient safety. The four Institute of Medicine reports have raised the consciousness of Americans and according to the Kaiser Family Foundation (*www.kff.org*), Americans continue to be concerned about the quality of health care.

• 40% believe the quality of health care has declined over the past 5 years.

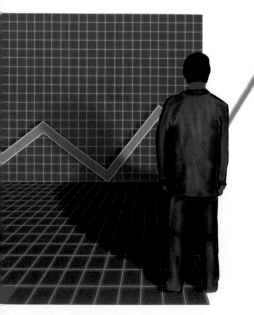

• 50% are worried about medical care safety.

• 33% reported personal or family experience with medical error.

• 55% are dissatisfied with the quality of health care compared to 44% in 2000.

Patients believe quality could be improved by:

• More nurses.
• More physicians.
• Better facilities.
• Better admission processes.

The problem is how many more nurses and physicians are needed and the specifics of the improvements in facilities and admission processes are not identified.

Creating a Culture of Safety

Creating a culture in which safety is paramount requires a new sense of focus and urgency in health care. Current cultures focus on finding the root of the error and attaching blame to an individual. According to Weick and Sutcliffe (2001) intelligent organizational design and management can avert serious errors when four factors are integrated in the system:

1. Safety is a priority.

2. There is high redundancy in both technical and personnel systems.

3. Operations are decentralized.

4. Well-developed trial-and-error organizational learning processes are present.

Key Concept: High Reliability Organization (HRO)

The core belief of this theory, high reliability, is that accidents or errors can be prevented though good organizational design and management. Redundancy enhances safety as duplication and over-lap can render a system reliable rather than unreliable. Continuous evaluation, training, and simulations further support and maintain high reliability operations. And most importantly, trial and error learning from accidents is believed effective and necessary (Weick & Sutcliffe, 2001).

Leaders in organizations with established and successful high reliability systems have identified that distributed decision making, management by collaboration and negotiation, and an eye on both the local issues and the larger system simultaneously help tremendously in supporting a culture of safety. Lessons are learned continually in these high reliability organizations. Further, the lessons are shared willingly with others to assist in avoiding similar missteps. These behaviors are consistent with shared leadership and principles espoused in the Forces of Magnetism.

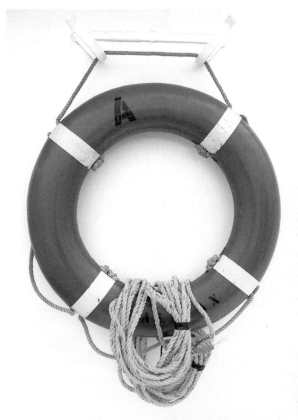

Note:

Organizations that emphasize respect for individuals, team-work, and open communication have greater potential for safe and effective practices.

MOVING FROM ERRORS TO HIGH RELIABILITY

Leaders in organizations focused on excellence work diligently to transform the traditional culture of blame to one in which errors are seen as opportunities for improvement. The shift in behavior begins with the move from a traditional culture of expecting perfection to one of honoring excellence. Integration of high reliability principles into the organization's structure occurs in several ways: policies specific to safety, human resource policies to support a nonpunitive culture, and decentralized decision making. New behaviors to address errors are created that emphasize remediation rather than punishment and emphasize excellence rather than perfection.

Traditional *Expecting Perfection*	Transforming *Honoring Excellence*
• Is unrealistic but expected by many • Creates unrealistic expectations • Fails to consider the wide variability in patient situations • Positions caregivers as scapegoats for lack of success	• Requires trial and error • Evolves to best practices • Supports continual improvement processes • Respects the nature of human interactions

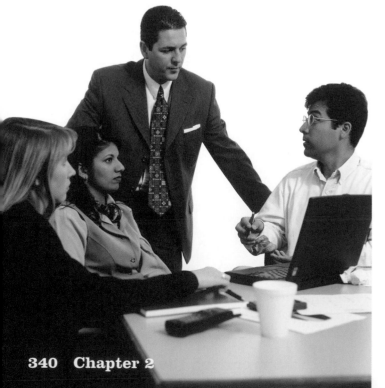

Remediation before Discipline

Traditional society values success and provides winners with recognition, trophies, financial rewards, and promotions. The achievement of goals and best practices receives high recognition whereas leadership failure is more likely to be recognized as a scarlet letter, or worse, is not discussed at all. Along the journey to success, leaders do indeed experience failures or less than anticipated positive results. Failure is bound to occur in every organization and every career.

A new perspective that recognizes and values the information gained in less than successful attempts is needed. Leaders need to reverse many assumptions and learn to embrace situations in which the desired outcomes were not realized. Failures must be viewed as acts of courage and recognized for the incredible insight and dialog that results as essential behaviors that do indeed support a culture of excellence. A positive and realistic interpretation of the failure experience and the resulting lessons provides all leaders with the necessary experiences for a better future.

A perspective grounded in valuing the experience of error begins with the transition from discipline as the initial reaction to remediation in which the human factors are identified as efforts to learn for error events is an expectation rather than an option.

Consider remediation when:

- The potential risk of physical, emotional, or financial harm due to the incident is very low.
- The incident is a singular event with no prior pattern of poor practice.
- The employee exhibits a conscientious approach to and accountability for his or her practice.
- The employee appears to have knowledge and skill to practice safely.

Consider discipline:

- As a matter of last resort.
- When attempts to remediation have failed.
- When there is evidence of incompetence that cannot be rectified.

As leaders work to transform traditional cultures of blame to cultures of tolerance, a sense of caution and uncertainty ensues. Leaders worry about the ability to change behavior without punishment or the fear of punishment, the fear of litigation, and feedback from colleagues as the approach becomes more professional, realistic, and therapeutic. Leaders conceptually understand the need for more healing approaches, yet turning negative events into opportunities for improvement requires more time and greater leadership communication skills than does the punishment process.

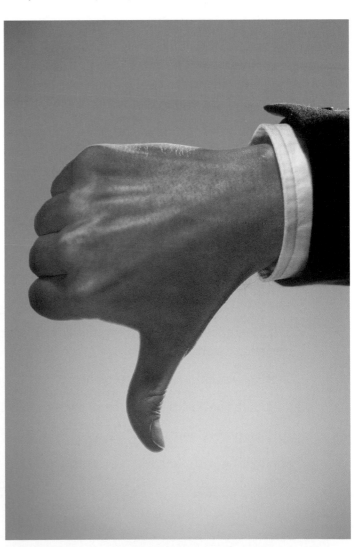

LEADERS ARE VULNERABLE

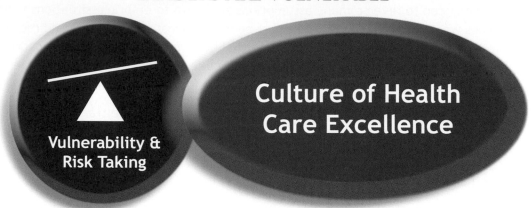

Vulnerability, the emerging leadership characteristic, is an important vehicle to assist leaders in creating cultures of health care excellence.

Professional behaviors include more than promoting and being proactive to advance the profession and practice of nursing. The professional works to promote effective behaviors and takes risks to recognize and alter nonproductive, hurtful behaviors. The expert leader willingly embraces the essence of vulnerability and risk taking to advance the work of quality patient care.

No leader can know everything all the time. In organizations dedicated to excellence, the leadership trait of vulnerability is pervasive and honored (Porter-O'Grady & Malloch, 2003). Vulnerable leaders role model and coach others in the following behaviors:

- Openness to others' ideas

- Openness to new ideas

- Recognition of one's personal limitations and understanding that such limitations are a reflection of one's reality and not the reflection of personal inadequacy

- Self-awareness of one's strengths and willingness to share with others in the development of similar strengths

- Sharing wisdom in a kind, humanistic, and nonthreatening manner

- Collaboration for the creation of synergy and the best outcomes

- Trust in others' motivations as good willed

- Apologizing with flair when missteps occur!

BARRIERS TO LEADERSHIP VULNERABILITY

Often leaders can agree to the reality of vulnerability but are unaware of their behaviors that are inconsistent with the essence of the vulnerable leader. Examples of behaviors that are barriers to achieving an effective level of vulnerability include:

- An attitude of aloofness and arrogance.

- Strong ego; always needing to be right—at any cost.

- Fear of losing control; fear that someone else may be more competent than you.

- Fear of discovery that you don't know everything.

- Believed immunity to anxiety, fatigue, illness, and overwork.

Risk Taking

Being vulnerable requires risk taking, a behavior not viewed as a classical leadership behavior and is seldom welcomed or encouraged. Instead, it is seen as increasing the organization's exposure to unforeseen hazards and increased costs. Risk taking is an essential characteristic of leadership vulnerability; the challenge is to know when and why to take risks. Experienced leaders act on the intuition, facts, and supporting information, knowing that the results are seldom guaranteed. They manage the results whether anticipated or not. Leaders take stock of a situation, often pulling back temporarily (but not too long) while they plan the next steps. The focus is always on the present and the future, both of which offer perils and possibilities, rather than on the past, about which nothing can be done.

Resiliency is the key. Leaders must be resilient in order to manage the uncertainty and inherent risks that are features of the leadership role. They must act with confidence, purpose, and enthusiasm rather than hesitation and self-doubt. To manage risks through resiliency, they must apply determination and energy, inspiring those around them at the same time.

Skilled Risk Taking: Essential for Excellence

Postive Attributes	Negative Attributes
• Encourages creativity	• Avoided by most leaders
• Supports "tinkering"	• Inconsistent with classical leadership behaviors
• Allows for mistakes	
• Requires vulnerability	• Supports the status quo
• Requires resiliency	• Reflects irresponsible behavior

AVOIDING TOXIC CULTURES

Failure to support healing becomes unhealthy and toxic to the healer and the patient.

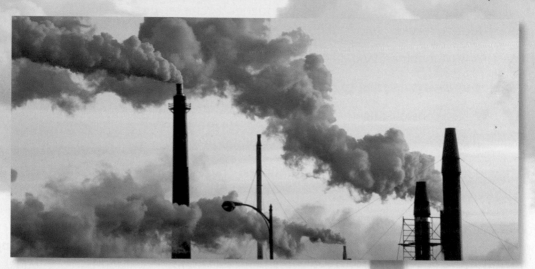

Health care workers further demonstrate professionalism and the essence of the healer as they work to minimize organizational toxicity by confronting negative behaviors and replacing them with the following positive, healthy behaviors. Examples of these behaviors include:

- Avoiding "nontrusting" behaviors such as gossip and partial truth telling.

- Partnering colleagues with others to ensure that others have support and consultation in a timely manner.

- Ensuring breaks and meals occur as well as checking in hourly to remove the fear of physical isolation.

- Recognizing the limitations of each individual by working to communicate and remove the ethic that forbids asking for help; offering assistance to others and assisting others in the completion of the work of the team. When team members are barely surviving or able to get only the minimal work completed, assistance is offered over and over to help the colleague reach a level of accomplishment that can lead to thriving rather than surviving as a health care provider.

- Addressing issues of workload; when the workload is consistently overwhelming, the professional collects data, formulates potential solutions, and works with leaders to solve the dilemma of low staff satisfaction.

These behaviors are essential to support and strengthen the structure and culture of the organization. Failure to address negative or toxic behaviors leads to self-defeating cultures that make it nearly impossible to achieve the desired outcomes. The table on the following page lists common self-defeating organizational behaviors that should be avoided at all costs.

CULTURES GONE BAD: DESTRUCTIVE BEHAVIORS

Organizational culture, or the patterns of behavior, standards, techniques, and strategies for dealing with problems, can be healthy, flexible, and appropriate. Also, cultural behaviors can be self-defeating when these behaviors fail to anticipate changes in the environment, refuse to innovate in the face of challenge, and continually deny the core beliefs that form the basis of earlier success. The work then shifts to putting out fires, quelling internal rebellion, and assigning blame for less than optimal performance. The emphasis is on damage control and survival rather than on the work of healing. Hardy and Schwartz (1996) identified five descriptions of organizations with self-defeating behaviors.

Maintenance Crew	Workers go about their tasks with little enthusiasm, hope, or urgency. Petty rituals and procedures are paramount. Control is valued above all else.
Funhouse Gang	There is a hotbed of activity, urgent activity, with workers scrambling frantically to resolve problems caused by prior frantic activity. There is a fear of accountability.
The Pep Squad	Workers rely on theatrics, flamboyance, and relentless high-spiritedness. Smile buttons, enlarged cartoons, and slogans dominate the organization and serve to mask a diminished sense of organizational purpose.
The Alumni Club	Workers dream of the past or fantasize about the future. They distract themselves from the policies, procedures and activities of the present. The prevailing fear is about the future.
The Cargo Cult	The organization justifies ongoing low performance and internal discontent on the grounds that circumstances will change dramatically once a distant goal is achieved. Hope is kept alive and the organization is distracted from the daily performance issues.

STRUCTURE EVALUATION: IS IT WORKING?
A MULITIFOCAL SYSTEMS APPROACH

Organizational structure cannot merely exist without review and evaluation. The selected or evolved characteristics of the structure significantly affect multiple organizational outcomes and must be validated routinely to ensure the appropriate mix of structure variables results in optimal outcomes. Evaluating structure must consider the multiple indicators; not one structure variable can be said to cause one particular outcome. For example, a span of control of five to six individuals cannot be determined to be the cause of high employee satisfaction in and of itself. Multiple variables such as schedule, pay rate, supervisor support etc. all affect employee satisfaction.

Clearly defined processes for effective, timely evaluation to measure the quality of care are essential. Staff nurses must actively participate in these evaluation processes as a means to improve patient care and gain knowledge about changing patient care needs in the process. An approach that includes multiple measures and considerations is needed to evaluate the complex work and impact of nursing care. Five types of evaluations (Buerhaus, 1998) and a comprehensive evaluation matrix are presented.

The five types of analysis are seldom mutually exclusive. Each offers additional information from which to select an option. For example, if the goal is to establish a pain management center, expectations would be to provide pain relief, minimize cost to the patient, and generate revenue. Cost-minimization, cost-effectiveness, and cost-benefit analyses would be required. When only one analysis is considered, the specific intent of the program may not be met. if the center is evaluated solely on revenue generated, the work of the organization is not accomplished.

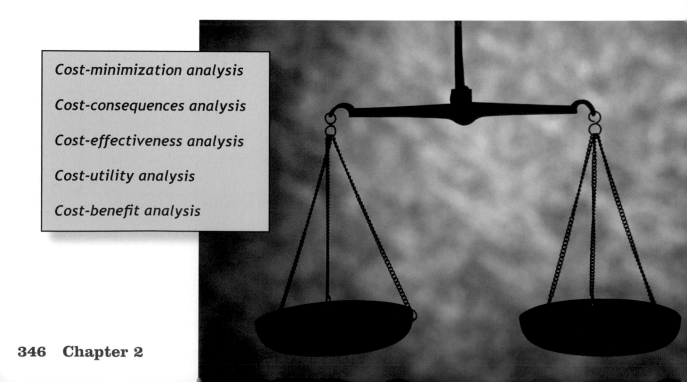

Cost-minimization analysis

Cost-consequences analysis

Cost-effectiveness analysis

Cost-utility analysis

Cost-benefit analysis

1. Cost-minimization analysis (CMA)

Assumptions in CMA

- The emphasis is on keeping costs as low as possible.
- Only costs are evaluated.
- Clinical outcomes are the same.
- Example: guidelines for thrombolytic therapy; streptokinase vs. TPA

2. Cost-consequences analysis (CCA)

Assumptions in CCA

- Consequences of two or more alternatives are measured as well as the costs, but costs and consequences are listed separately.
- Example: comparison of early discharge of low-birth weight infants whose care was managed by advanced practice nurses compared with traditional physician care

3. Cost-effectiveness analysis (CEA)

Assumptions in CEA

- Outcomes are measured in the same units between alternatives, such as dollars per life-year gained or cases avoided.
- Example: evaluation of pain management interventions for patients with chronic arthritis

4. Cost-utility analysis (CUA)

Assumptions in CUA

- CUA is a special type of cost effectiveness analysis that includes measures for quantity and quality of life.
- Individual preferences for different health outcomes are sought and included.
- CUA is a difficult comparison; the goal is to compare $/QALY (quality adjusted life years).
- Example: comparison of cost of diabetic teaching in groups vs. individual teaching to QALY

5. Cost-benefit analysis (CBA)

Assumptions in CBA

- Outcomes are measured according to some monetary unit.
- A single dollar figure, representing costs minus benefits, is calculated.
- Example: is the cost of a pain management clinic covered by revenue generated? Cost $500, Revenue $750 = 50 % ROI

EVALUATION: MULTIPLE MEASURES

Template of Measures

	Quality	Productivity	Cost
Patient	Clinical outcome Satisfaction with care	Length of stay Length of procedure Time to treatment	Cost of service Charge per case
Employee	Competence/credentials/certifications Level of education Satisfaction with work	Hours per unit of service Skill mix % Turnover Registry staff % Overtime %	Wages and benefits
Organization	Reputation in the community Licensure status Accreditations	FTE/AOB	Net income margin Departmental margins

Evaluation of Pain Management Specialist (CNS) program

	Quality	Productivity	Cost
Patient	Increased satisfaction 5% specific to pain relief. Pain relief improved from 3 to 2 on 10-point pain scale.	Length of stay decreased 0.5 day for 2 DRGs.	Charge per case decreased 10%.
Employee	Pain specialist and direct caregiver satisfaction increased 4 percentage points.	No change in turnover.	Increase cost of $50/day/patient on pain protocol (CNS).
Organization	Availability of pain management clinic improved community reputation. No deficiencies in recent licensure review specific to pain management.	No change.	Margin for 2 DRGs increased 10%.

EVALUATION:
MEASURING STAFF EFFECTIVENESS

Did the amount and level of skill provide the desired patient care outcomes?

☐ The evidence-based approach to evaluation of adequacy has been advanced with the introduction of the JCAHO Staffing Effectiveness standard (2002). The goal of this standard is to correlate actual staffing of a unit to patient outcomes. Screening indicators must include indicators sensitive to staffing effectiveness from the clinical and human resource categories. Clinical patient outcomes are affected by multiple variables: variables related to clinical expertise, technology, the physical environment, availability of therapeutics, and human resource levels of staffing.

☐ The BEMC Staffing Effectiveness diagram represents the application of this standard on the basis of the patient care delivery model. The patient care delivery model is the focus of the evaluation. The human resource characteristics of the model—that is the types of caregivers, hours of care, and support services comprising the interdisciplinaryteam—are examined in relationship to clinical outcomes. The clinical outcomes examined include patient satisfaction, caregiver satisfaction, patient falls, medication errors, and nosocomial infections.

Dashboards & Scorecards

Dashboards and scorecards have become useful to leaders in managing the plethora of data specific to organizational performance. The scorecard model provides a framework in which to measure and trend the most critical variables in one's area of responsibility. This framework can be used effectively in monitoring staffing effectiveness.

Note:

Single metrics seldom provide information to adequately evaluate the effectiveness of work processes.

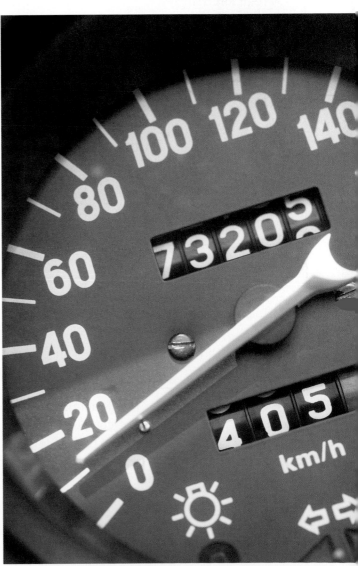

STAFFING EFFECTIVENESS: SCORE CARD

Evaluation of resources and their effect on outcomes is an essential attribute of cultures supportive of professional accountability. In this analysis, the human resource indicators reflect the inputs that produced the clinical outcomes on the right side of the table.

Human Resource Indicators		Clinical Indicators	
Hours of care: % registered nurses	850 hours/62% RN	Number of patient codes	8
Hours of care: respiratory therapy	125 hours/2% RT	Patient falls with injury	2
Hours of care: social worker	50 hours/0.5% of patient hours	Medication omission	30
Hours of support: advanced practice nurses	150 hours/10% APN	Medications late (>60 minutes)	55
% Core staff	80%	Surgical site infections	0
% Registry staff	20%	Patient satsifaction with skill of nurses	88th percentile
Admission support	55% admissions completed prior to unit	Employee satisfaction	75th percentile

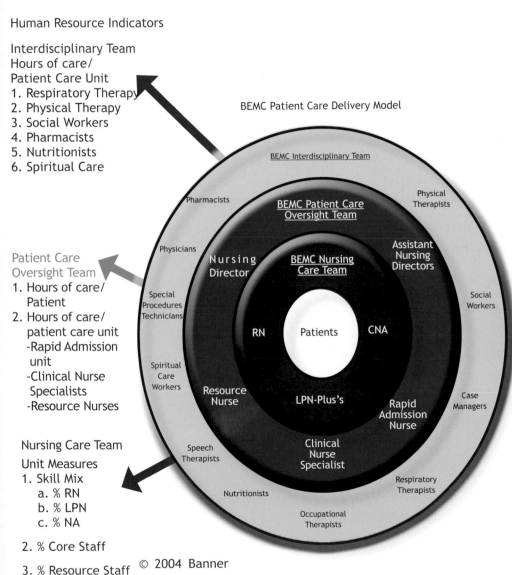

BEMC Staffing Efectiveness 2005:
Measuring the Impact of the BEMC
Patient Care Delivery Model

Human Resource Indicators

Interdisciplinary Team
Hours of care/
Patient Care Unit
1. Respiratory Therapy
2. Physical Therapy
3. Social Workers
4. Pharmacists
5. Nutritionists
6. Spiritual Care

Patient Care
Oversight Team
1. Hours of care/
   Patient
2. Hours of care/
   patient care unit
   -Rapid Admission
   unit
   -Clinical Nurse
   Specialists
   -Resource Nurses

Nursing Care Team

Unit Measures
1. Skill Mix
   a. % RN
   b. % LPN
   c. % NA

2. % Core Staff

3. % Resource Staff   © 2004 Banner

BEMC Patient Care Delivery Model

BEMC Interdisciplinary Team

Pharmacists

Physicians

Special
Procedures
Technicians

Spiritual
Care
Workers

Speech
Therapists

Nutritionists

BEMC Patient Care
Oversight Team

Nursing
Director

BEMC Nursing
Care Team

Assistant
Nursing
Directors

Physical
Therapists

RN   Patients   CNA

Resource
Nurse

LPN-Plus's

Rapid
Admission
Nurse

Clinical
Nurse
Specialist

Social
Workers

Case
Managers

Respiratory
Therapists

Occupational
Therapists

Clinical Indicators

BEMC Quality Measures
1. Patient Satisfaction
   Press Ganey:
   a. (D-3) promptness
   in responding to call
   button
   b. (D-4) amount of at-
   tention paid to special
   needs
   c. (D-6) skill of the
   nurses
   d. (J-2) How well
   ICU/CCU nurses helped
   you understand your
   treatment, tests, and
   condition
   e. (J-3) ICU nurses'
   sensitivity and responsiveness to your pain.
   f (L-3) How well your
   pain was controlled
Press Ganey Items
2. Patient Codes
3. Patient Falls with
   Injury
4. Medication Errors
5. Nosocomial infection
   -Central line infections
   (aggregate)
   -Ventilator associated
   pneumonia (ICU)
   -Surgical site infections
   (aggregate)
   -UTI (unit)
6. Restraint use

References

Buerhaus, P. (1998). Milton Weinstein's insights on the development, use, and methodological problems in cost-effectiveness analysis. *Image: Journal of Nursing Scholarship*, 30(3), 223-227.

Hardy, R.E. ,& Schwartz, R. (1996). *The self-defeating organization: How smart companies can stop outsmarting themselves*. Reading, MA: Addison-Wesley.

JCAHO facts about staffing effectiveness standards. Retrieved May 15, 2005 www.jcaho org.com.

Kramer, M., & Schmalenberg, C. (2002). Staff nurses identify essentials of magnetism. In M. McClure, & A S. Hinshaw (Eds.), *Magnet hospitals revisited: Attraction and retention of professional nurses*. Washington DC: American Nurses Publishing.

Porter-O'Grady, T. (1996). Multidisciplinary shared governance: The next step. *Seminars for Nurse Managers*, 4, 43-48.

Porter-O'Grady, T., & Malloch, K. (2003). *Quantum leadership: A textbook of new leadership*. Sudbury, MA: Jones and Bartlett.

Schein, E. (1991). *Organizational culture and leadership*. San Francisco: Jossey-Bass.

Weick, K. & Sutcliffe, K. (2001). *Managing the unexpected: Assuring high performance in an age of complexity*. San Francisco: Jossey-Bass.

Suggested Readings

Brill, N. (1976). *Teamwork: Working together in the human services*. Toronto, Ontario, Canada: Lippincott.

Hall, L. M. (Ed.). (2005). *Quality work environment and patient safety*. Sudbury, MA: Jones and Bartlett.

Holden, R. J. (1991). Responsibility and autonomous nursing practice. *Journal of Advanced Nursing*, 16, 398-403.

Krairiksh, M. & Anthony, M. K. (2001). Benefits and outcomes of staff nurses' participation in decision making. *JONA*, 31(1), 16-23.

Longest, B. B. Jr. (1974). Relationships between coordination, efficiency, and quality of care in general hospitals. *Hospital Administration*, 19, 65-86.

MacDonald, C. (2002). Nurse autonomy as relational. *Nursing Ethics*, 9, 194-201.

Wade, G.H.M.R. (1999). Professional nursing autonomy: Concept analysis and application to nursing education. *Journal of Advanced Nursing*, 30, 310-318.

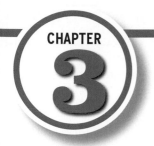

CHAPTER 3

STAFF LEADERSHIP

Retention begins with the recognition of the essential leadership qualities within each professional, regardless on one's formal role designation.

In this section the essential competencies of contemporary caregivers necessary to facilitate satisfaction with the work of health care, managing the workload, and personal retention strategies are discussed.

EVERY CAREGIVER IS A LEADER

As technology increases communication effectiveness and efficiency, the relationship between staff and leaders changes. More information is available to more individuals simultaneously, decreasing the need for much formal communication. The autonomous model of decision making is officially rendered ineffective. The good news is that every caregiver is now able and expected to participate in decision making, and the essence of personal leadership is now a determinant of improved point-of-service care. Leader behaviors are required of every professional regardless of official position in the organization. Assessment, planning, organizing, implementing, and evaluating are present in every role, from the boardroom to the beside.

> *Note:*
>
> **There is no greater disruption than a team member who is unhappy, adversarial, and barely competent to do the work of patient care.**

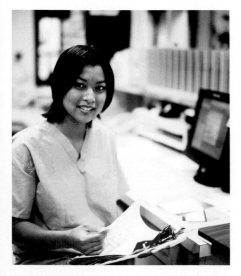

In the health care setting it is easy to focus on the technical, clinical work of the caregiver rather than leader behaviors. Yet the ability of the staff caregiver to assess, plan, organize, implement, and evaluate patient care is the core of the professional health care worker. Thus the organizational structure and supporting processes must ensure that the health care worker is clinically competent and enabled to provide care with the complex health care organization.

The six leadership competencies identified by Longest (1998) are essential to the role of all professional health care workers. The table on the following page identifies specific behaviors for each of the categories. Each professional is accountable to develop expertise that embodies all six competencies.

Leadership Competencies (Longest, 1998)	Staff Nurse Performance Competencies
CONCEPTUAL Knowledge and skill to envision one's place in the larger society	1. Understands the vision of nursing 2. Uses problem-solving skills to meet the complex needs of patients 3. Appreciates ambiguity 4. Articulates nursing's contribution within the larger organization 5. Formulates creative ideas and new solutions 6. Understands the organizational culture
TECHNICAL The direct work performed in one's domain	1. Demonstrates knowledge of health care service enough to support it with necessary resources and to ensure an acceptable level of quality 2. Uses problem-solving skills 3. Educates the patient and family 4. Responds to and/or facilitates change in patient care processes
INTERPERSONAL Human interactions and relations through which one leads other people in pursuit of common objectives	1. Uses effective communication skills 2. Builds collaborative relationships 3. Displays self-confidence 4. Values diversity: holds multiple perspectives 5. Acts as a patient advocate 6. Builds partnerships with the community
COMMERCIAL Economic exchanges between buyers and sellers in which value is created	1. Uses resources effectively 2. Markets nursing practice 3. Uses appropriate technology
POLITICAL The dual capacity to accurately assess the effect of public policies on the performance of one's domains of responsibility and the ability to influence public policymaking at state and federal levels	1. Has knowledge of relevant health care regulation, legislation, and certification 2. Identifies policy changes needed to improve patient care efficiencies and outcomes 3. Recommends possible solutions to regulatory and legislative concerns
GOVERNANCE Establishment and enactment of a clear vision for the organization	1. Articulates the organization's desired environment for practice 2. Articulates a vision for nursing practice 3. Responds to and/or facilitates change 4. Demonstrates continual learning 5. Uses appropriate technology

STAFF LEVEL LEADER COMPETENCE

Leadership requires that the professional be more than a technician with good communication skills. Expertise in the professional role requires knowledge of the vision and mission of the specific professional role as it fits within society and the existing organizational culture. Knowledge and understanding of the commercial value of the professional is an expectation that can no longer be set aside by the bedside caregiver. The cost of each caregiver and the relative effect on the patient's health status is a requirement for responsible use of health care resources. No one is better suited to assess the effectiveness of patient care processes and to make recommendations for change when these processes are no longer effective or compromise patient safety.

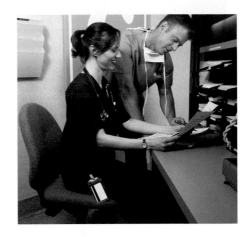

Competent professionals not only know their work and are able to integrate complex competencies seamlessly, they also know those characteristics of the workplace that support a satisfying experience and those that are frustrating and demoralizing. It is important NOT to develop a list of standard satisfiers, but rather to discover myriad preferences, motivations, and values of the workforce that can be personalized to each nurse. Attempting to eliminate variation or forcing widely disparate groups into one standardized group creates discontent and frustration before the work of nursing ever begins.

The following characteristics and behaviors reflect professional practice:

- *Nurse-directed care:* satisfied nurses are able to participate on practice councils, make recommendations specific to the patient care delivery model, and address staff issues.

- *Recognition:* sincere and timely feedback is received from leaders and is specific to the quality of patient care.

- *Valued:* leaders see the nurse as an essential member of the team. Nurses are able to access leaders easily. Leaders seek input from caregivers regularly.

- *Celebrated:* humor is used appropriately to reduce stress and promote creative thinking.

- *Flexibility:* nurses are able to self-schedule and to negotiate for time off within the defined needs of the patient population.

- *Continuing education opportunities:* sessions are available at least monthly both within the organization and externally to broaden nurse knowledge.

NURSE SATISFIERS

• Minimize the requests to work overtime or for changing schedules.

• Involve in creating activities that include family members.

• Encourage self-scheduling.

• Request participation on performance improvement teams specific to clinical area.

• Request participation on teams to evaluate new equipment and replace outdated equipment.

• Ensure that ongoing educational opportunities are available.

• Create reward options that include attendance at conferences or seminars.

• Ensure the availability of housekeeping and messenger services; include teams to address support service issues.

• Request feedback on communication effectiveness and recommendations to improve current methods.

• Ensure that personal safety is a priority and regular feedback is solicited on perceptions of personal safety.

• Provide secure locker space for personal belongings; provide security escorts after dark.

• Include on teams to review and improve the physical space for patient care specific to patient lifting, adequacy of patient care workspace, and nurse workstations.

Greene (2005) has identified nurse dissatisfiers on the basis of age and values of nurses. This information is best used to address issues of greater interest to each group. This is not to say that the issues are not important to both groups, rather certain issues are of greater priority to each group and can assist leaders in addressing the issues for the overall good of the workforce.

SOURCES OF DISSATISFACTION

Nurses Younger Than Age 32
• Work/personal life balance

• Organization not focused on patient needs

• Outdated medical equipment

• Insufficient development opportunities

Nurses Older Than Age 32
• Ancillary and support services

• Teamwork and coworkers

• Lack of information sharing

• Security services

• Physical plant

EVALUATING THE EXPERIENCE: CHECKING IN WITH COLLEAGUES

Traditional unit meetings focus on communication of new policies and projects as well as discussion of areas of poor performance—much of which is one-way communication and could be accomplished in memos. Amore satisfying and empowering process is needed. Focusing on a process of checking in with colleagues about their experiences offers a new approach to communication, valuing the experience of nurses and thus determining how to modify the work when indicated. The stories and satisfaction of nurses are best found in the narrative description of their experiences of being a nurse.

To create full engagement to the work of health care, the following topics are useful in beginning the dialog about the experiences of care, especially those memorable moments, times of stress, and times of opportunity that can now be discussed in a specific context. Such storytelling validates the value of the experiences and reinforces the therapeutic richness of health care.

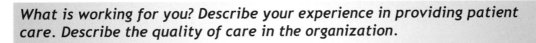

What is working for you? Describe your experience in providing patient care. Describe the quality of care in the organization.

Rationale for this question: 57% of nurses leave their first position within 2 years because of concerns about patient acuity and patient safety. Learning about experiences provides opportunities to address issues and affirm positive behaviors.

1

How are you supported by your colleagues and your supervisors?

Rationale: 22% of nurses leave their first position due to lack of support and guidance and too much responsibility

2

What are the activities you have engaged in to increase your knowledge in providing patient care?

Rationale: Support for advancement is a key satisfier for nurses. Learning about the activities that support professional development provides an opportunity to reinforce positive behaviors.

Describe the level of patient safety in the organization.

Rationale: Often times, nurses do not believe the environment of the organization is supportive of patient safety. Validation of the state of patient safety is essential in creating optimal nurse engagement.

Are you able to manage your stress appropriate to the expectations of your job? What's not working? What ethical dilemmas have you been facing?

Rationale: The vast majority of new graduates believe that the working environment is stressful. Discussion of stress levels provides opportunities to assist colleagues in developing better coping strategies.

Please comment or make suggestions to improve your work experience.

Rationale: No set of questions can ever hope to cover or address all issues. Asking an open-ended question allows team members to ask the unaskable!

MANAGING THE WORK OF HEALTH CARE

Health care workload is the basic challenge for all caregivers. Leaders routinely manage the multiple variables that are involved in getting the right caregiver with the right patient at the right time. Knowing what the patients' needs (patient classification) is a significant part of the picture, along with the availability of competent caregivers (core scheduling) and the availability of caregivers at the time (staffing) they are needed by patients. Every professional is aware of staff issues and is confronted with different challenges everyshift or day worked.

Workload Management

The Ultimate Goal:
Getting the Right Caregiver
with the Right Patient
at the Right Time!

Workload management is an integral component of hospital operations. Because nursing constitutes the majority of the workforce in a hospital, nurse leaders in particular are faced with the increasing demand to ensure efficient and effective service delivery. For years nurse leaders have relied on their experience, intuition, judgment, and traditions to create and justify their caregiver staffing plans. However, given the amount of clinical and financial data that are now available, the focus has shifted to managing the data to guide effective decision making, specifically evidence-based staffing. The challenge for nursing continues to escalate as the health care industry struggles with patient safety, demands for staffing ratio legislation, and increased collective bargaining units.

Workload management includes (see next page) the processes of establishing a core schedule of staff hours and skill mix, adjusting that core schedule on the basis of patient needs identified in a valid and reliable system, adjusting the hours and skill mix again on the basis of available staff, and finally managing the differences between what is needed and what is available. This is no small task and must be done everytime there is a change in caregivers—a new shift, a new day or a new case.

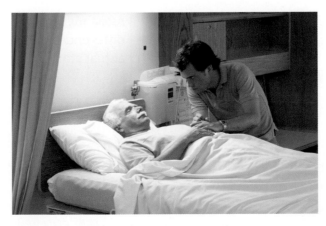

Workload Management

Workload management includes five distinct processes with specific characteristics, processes, and goals.

Caveat: Continuing to attempt to amalgamate patient classification, scheduling, staffing, retention, and recruitment into one process serves only to decrease system validity and frustrate workers with additional unproductive tasks.

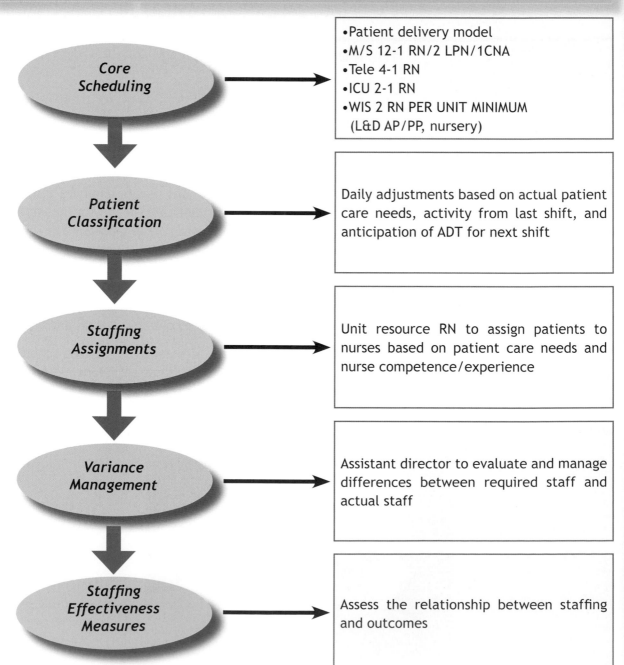

Core Scheduling
- Patient delivery model
- M/S 12-1 RN/2 LPN/1CNA
- Tele 4-1 RN
- ICU 2-1 RN
- WIS 2 RN PER UNIT MINIMUM
  (L&D AP/PP, nursery)

Patient Classification

Daily adjustments based on actual patient care needs, activity from last shift, and anticipation of ADT for next shift

Staffing Assignments

Unit resource RN to assign patients to nurses based on patient care needs and nurse competence/experience

Variance Management

Assistant director to evaluate and manage differences between required staff and actual staff

Staffing Effectiveness Measures

Assess the relationship between staffing and outcomes

STAFFING REGULATIONS: HELP OR HINDRANCE?

Patients and the public are concerned about their ability to get quality health care as a result of insufficient staffing. As health care resources become scarcer, patients are finding it increasingly difficult to gain access to services. At the same time, patients and the public are concerned about the rising cost of health care.

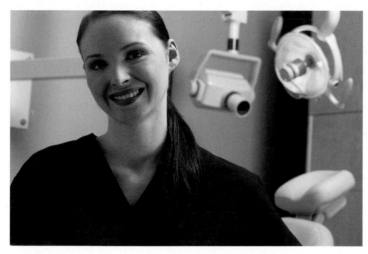

Legislators have responded by studying the issues and enacting laws to prevent harm to patients and support safe staffing. Numerous regulations and accreditation standards have been created to address the need for adequate staffing. Although the health care industry has yet to create adequate systems to manage the cyclical staffing shortages and ensure patient safety, the need still exists.

Rather than work to create more legislation and more accreditation standards, leaders are challenged to develop new and innovative solutions for the work of health care that incorporate the value produced, resources available, and the associated costs. To be sure, the issue of safe staffing is a complex problem that affects all members of society. Solutions will not be forthcoming by simply mandating more staffing.

Staffing Regulations and Recommendations
- Centers for Medicare and Medicaid Services (CMS)
- Joint Commission on Accreditation of Healthcare Organizations (JCAHO)
- State regulations
- American Nurses Association (ANA)

Four major groups provide guidelines or statutes specific to patient care staffing, as outlined in the box above. The next two pages provide summarized ANA Principles of Staffing. JCAHO staffing effectiveness standards are available through the organization (*www.jcano.com*).

CENTERS FOR MEDICARE AND MEDICAID SERVICES

Medicare Conditions of Participation
482.23(b) Standard: Staffing and Delivery of Care

The nursing service must have adequate numbers of licensed registered nurses, licensed practical (vocational) nurses, and other personnel to provide nursing care to all patients as needed. There must be supervisory and staff personnel for each department or nursing unit to ensure, when needed, the immediate availability of a registered nurse for bedside care of any patient.

Interpretive guidelines include the following:

- There must be written staffing schedules that correlate to the number and acuity of patients.

- There must be supervision of personnel performance and nursing care for each department or nursing unit.

- To determine if there are adequate numbers of nurses to provide nursing care to all patients as needed, take into consideration:

  —Physical layout and size of the hospital.

  —Number of patients.

  —Intensity of illness and nursing needs.

  —Availability of nurses' aides and orderlies and other resources for nurses.

  Source: *www.cms.gov*

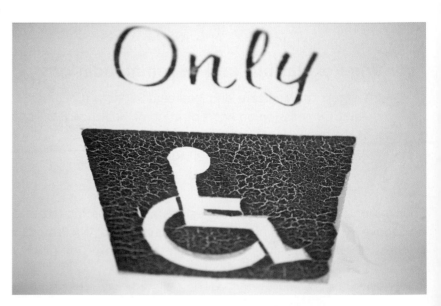

ANA PRINCIPLES OF STAFFING

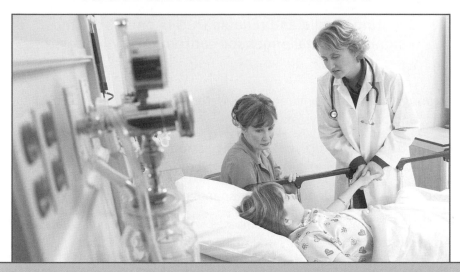

- Appropriate staffing levels for a patient care unit reflect analysis of individual and aggregate patient needs.

- Retire or seriously question the usefulness of the concept of nursing hours per patient day (NHPPD).

- Unit functions are necessary to support delivery of quality care.

- Specific needs of various patient populations should determine appropriate clinical competencies required of the nurse practicing in that area.

- Registered nurses must have nursing management support and representation at both the operational and the executive levels.

- Clinical support from experienced registered nurses should be readily available to those registered nurses with less proficiency.

- Organizational policies should reflect a climate that values registered nurses and other employees as strategic assets.

- Organizational policies should recognize the many needs of patients and nursing staff.

- All institutions should have documented competencies for all nursing staff, including agency or supplemental traveling registry nurses for those activities they have been authorized to perform.

From American Nurses Association. (1999). *Principles of nurse staffing*. Washington, DC: American Nurses Publishing.

Patient Classificaton Systems (PCSs)

Creating a valid and reliable PCS is one of the most significant challenges for contemporary leaders.

Definitions

- *Workload management:* the comprehensive system that includes patient classification, scheduling, staffing, and budgeting systems

- *Patient classification:* the process of grouping patients into homogeneous, mutually exclusive groups to determine their dependency on caregivers.

- *Acuity:* the level of need or dependency of an individual patient

- *Scheduling:* the long-range plan that combines your organization's goals, legislation, regulation, and accreditation requirements and planned patient demand

- *Staffing:* the real-time adjustment of the schedule based on census, acuity, and the mix of available resources

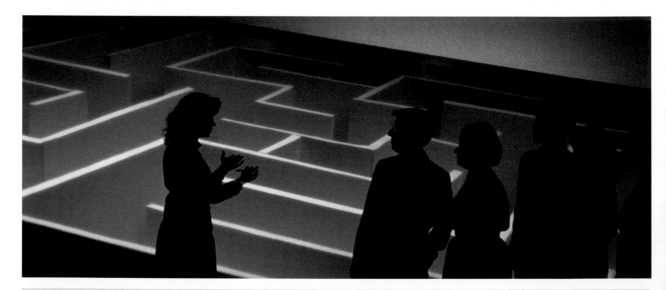

Ratio Staffing Is NOT Enough!

Staffing ratios or staffing grids based on budget hours or state regulations offer only the beginning step in safe staffing. Fixed staffing numbers (ratios) cannot be considered as remedies to improve quality patient care (Bolton et al., 2001). Patient-nurse ratios identify the minimum staffing levels whereas patient classification systems define the amount of staff needed for a particular situation. Ratio-staffing levels are data derived from a valid and reliable patient classification system and from knowing the range of patient care needs. Ratio data are best used in the aggregate for budgeting and scheduling, not for day-to-day staffing.

WHY WE NEED A PCS

☐ To understand the relationship between patient care needs, interventions, desired outcomes, and the skill level of caregivers as a prerequisite to determine the appropriate type and number of caregivers and support staff needed to provide safe and effective patient care

☐ To define the amount of staff needed for a particular situation

☐ To create a valid and reliable system that defines and defends the work of professionals, increase visibility of the role of professional health care practice, protect patients from complications, and decrease the vulnerability of professional caregiver staff to budget cuts

The challenge to create valid and reliable systems for staffing may indeed seem to be an uphill and impossible challenge. As the pressure continues to escalate in the health care industry for systems that ensure patient safety and address staff shortages, demands for ratio legislation, and increased bargaining units, nurse leaders must respond with more effective and data drive systems. In response to the increasing complexity and challenges, some leaders are considering the elimination of PCSs in light of the inadequacies of system validity and reliability.

Indeed, many patient classification systems lack validity and reliability, but nurse leaders may be expecting more than is possible from the system. At best, the PCS can provide an accurate record of care provided; predictions of staffing needs for the next shift are limited by the stability of the patient population. The degree of validity of one's current system in the organization, whether it is a purchased system or developed internally, can be assessed using the checklist discussed on pages 367-370.

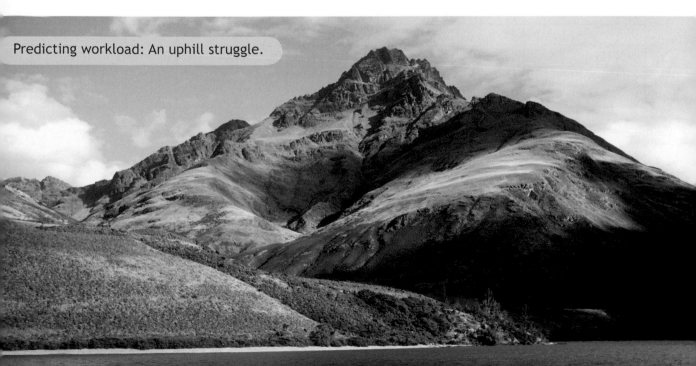

Predicting workload: An uphill struggle.

VARIANCE MANAGEMENT

Perhaps one of the most often missed processes in workload management is the identification of and management of the variance between needed staff and actual staff hours. Managing the difference between actual hours of staff and required hours of care requires analysis of individual caregiver variances as well as total variance hours. The following screen shot of a variance analysis data form displays the actual, required, and variances. Once a significant variance is determined, variance actions are implemented and documented. These data provide valuable trend information for nurse leaders as they continually work to create effective workload management systems.

> ## Note:
>
> **Expecting caregivers to "do one's best" in an impossible situation fuels the flames of caregiver dissatisfaction, resulting ultimately in premature exit from the workforce.**

Variance Management: 016100 Evening Shift 02-10-2004

	Actual Hours	Required Hours	A-R Var Hours	%	Budget Hours	R-B Var Hours	%	A-B Var Hours	%
RN	24	29	-5	-16	24	5	19	0	0
LPNN	16	28	-12	-43	8	20	251	8	50
Licensed Total	40	57	-17	-29	32	25	77	8	20
NA	40	16	24	155	16		-2	24	60
TECH	0	0	0		0	0	0	0	
Unlicensed Total	40	16	24	155	16		-2	24	60
INDIRECT	0	0	0		0	0	0	0	
Total Evening Shift	80	72	⑧	11	48	24	51	32	40

> NEG Called in additional help.
> NEG Used staff overtime.
> NEG Used resource nurse.
> NEG Reassessed for overestimation.
> NEG Redefined nonessential tasks.
> NEG Found missing or errors in scores.
> POS Floated staff to another unit.
> POS Cancelled staff.
> POS Cancelled registry.
> POS Sent staff home early.

Variance Management Actions

Examination of the required staff needed for care and the actual staff is a routine activity of nurse leaders. What is not routine is the systematic documentation of the difference between required and actual hours and the interventions to address and mediate the variance or gap. NOTE: Both positive and negative variances need to be addressed and documented.

Examples of interventions to address the variance or gap between needs and actual staffing include:

- Postponing admissions.
- Calling additional staff.
- Floating existing staff to the unit in need.
- Reevaluating patient acuity ratings.
- Postponing nonemergent patient care.
- Sending staff home early.

Staffing Scheduling and Patient Classification: Magnetism Checklist

Evaluation of staffing, scheduling, and patient classification systems considers the infrastructure, the processes, and the outcomes of the integrated workload management system.

Three areas are included in the checklist:

- infrastructure
- process
- evaluation

Leaders will find the checklist on pages 368-369 helpful in reviewing their existing systems and identifying areas for improvement.

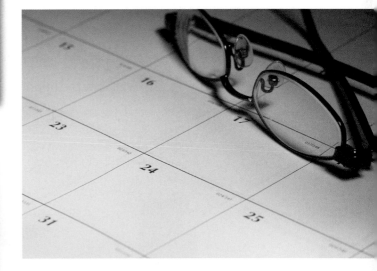

Assessment: Infrastructure for Excellence

1. There is a clearly defined patient care delivery system that includes support for nursing participation in decision making at the point-of¬service, expectation for professionalism, and shared decision making.

2. A valid and reliable system to determine patient care needs drives the staffing process. Specific consideration is given to:

    - Number of patients.

    - Acuity of patients.

    - Length of stay/intensity factor.

    - Unit geography.

    - Skills and experience of caregivers.

    - Appropriate skill mix.

3. Scheduling/staffing systems are developed collaboratively by leaders, managers, and direct caregivers.

4. Consideration for unit functions that support the delivery of patient care is included in staffing hours (indirect time).

5. Staff clinical competencies are identified for differing patient populations.

6. Expert resources are available to support less experienced staff.

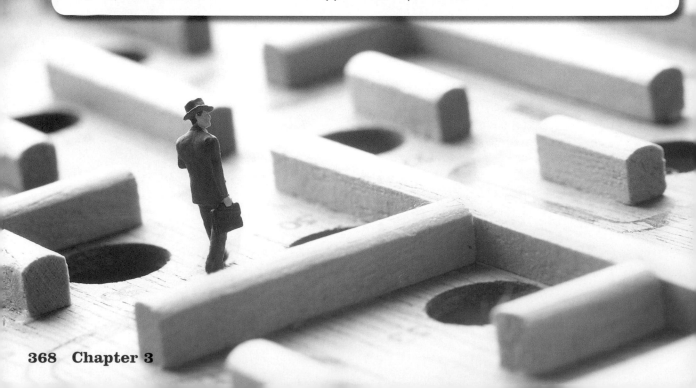

Assessment: Process Excellence

1. Collaborative scheduling is the norm. Historical trend data, patient care needs and staff preferences (in that order) serve as the basis for scheduling. Note: Patient care needs are always the first priority.

2. Mandatory overtime is not used.

3. The fatigue factor is recognized; long stretches of 12-hour shifts are not considered safe practice. Nurses do not work more than three l2-hour shifts in a row.

4. Leaders and staff work together to manage variances (staff shortages) between available staff and patient care needs.

5. Experienced clinical experts are available to assist less experienced staff in organizing and providing patient care.

Assessment: Evaluation Excellence

1. Multiple indicators are used to evaluate staffing effectiveness. Indicators include patient outcomes, staff satisfaction, and organizational cost. Performance indicators do not focus solely on hours per patient day (HPPD).

2. Analysis includes individual patient care as well as aggregate analysis. Ranges as well as averages are evaluated.

3. Analysis includes both census averages and outliers (ranges).

4. Indicators sensitive to nursing scheduling and staffing are examined at least monthly. These include but are not limited to:

   • Patient satisfaction with response to call lights.

   • Patient increased knowledge of clinical condition.

   • Patient and family's increased ability to manage their own care.

   • Absence of adverse outcomes, e.g., dermal ulcers, nosocomial pneumonia, patient falls, and medication errors.

Assessing Your
Patient Classification System

- Is there an adequate representation of the work of nursing or interventions for the specific unit? Are the majority of nurse interventions included in the system?

- Are patients correctly distributed across classes and job categories? Is there a bell curve of distribution of the lowest- to highest-need patients?

- Is standardized language used throughout the tool? Are the definitions consistent from one clinical area to another?

- How accurate is the calculation of hours of care and skill mix for each patient or shift? Does the system estimate total hours of care for each patient and the skill mix for each intervention?

- Is administrative caregiver time distinct from direct caregiver time? Is there time allocated for unit support activities—activities that cannot be attributed to a specific patient such as shift report, counting supplies and medications?

- Are variances calculated and addressed each shift?

- Is the system simple to use? Can the nurse learn the system in less than 1 hour?

- Is minimal time required to rate a patient? Can the nurse rate each patient in less than 1 minute?

- Is inter-rater reliability specific to ratings and documentation greater than 85% for all units? Note: Accurate data are essential and nonnegotiable. System users must rate patients accurately and consistently.

- Is the system computerized? Are the downtime policies and practices effective and efficient?

- Is there evidence of direct caregiver involvement in the development and ongoing evaluation of the system?

- Is there a policy specific to patient classification? Are there references and rationale for the work processes?

- Is the system evaluated annually by caregivers?

PERSONAL RETENTION: MANAGING YOUR PROFESSIONAL REPUTATION

Before you look to others to improve your work life,
look first to yourself!

If you are not fully committed to the work of patient care and the organization in which the work is occurring, it is difficult if not impossible to influence others to remain in their positions, and your reputation as a professional is at risk. Examine the message you are sending about your work and how it influences others. Consider the retention questions on the following page.

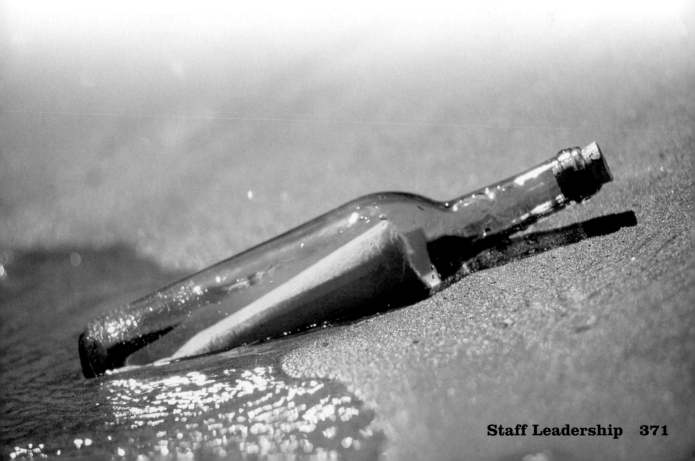

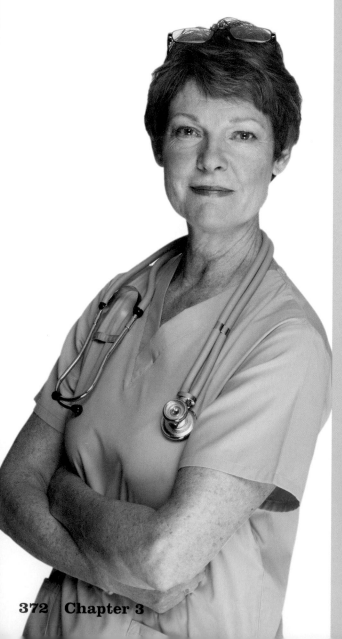

Can you continue to commit to the clinical and emotional challenges of death and dying? Of adults, geriatric patients, infants?

Can you continue to commit to the work of a clinical setting—pediatric, adult, geriatric, trauma, etc.—that ranges from the mundane activities of daily living to the complexities of drug titration and patient resuscitation?

Can you continue to commit to working with patients who are resistant, challenging, and at times abusive?

Can you continue to commit to working to impro the work environment for nursing?

Can you continue to commit to the ongoing mentoring of new colleagues?

Can you continue to commit to lifelong professional development?

Can you continue to commit to involvement in pr fessional nursing organizations?

Can you continue to commit to being a great colleague and team member? Can you commit to addressing colleague (including physician) behavior that is inappropriate in a timely and professional manner?

Can you continue to commit to endless changes i technical systems and electronic documentation modules?

References

American Nurses Association. (1999). *Principles of nurse staffing*. Washington, DC: American Nurses Publishing.

Bolton, L. B., Jones, D., Aydin, C. E., Donaldson, N., Brown, D. S., Lowe, M. et al. (2001). A response to California's mandated nursing ratios. *Journal of Nursing Scholarship*, 33(2), 179-184.

Greene, J. (2005, March). What nurses want: Different generations different expectations. *Hospitals and Health Networks*, 34-42.

Longest, B. B. (1998). Managerial competence at senior levels of integrated delivery systems. *Journal of Healthcare Management*, 43(2), 115-135.

Suggested Readings

Bethune, G. , Sherrod, D., & Youngblood, L. (2005). Tips to retain a happy, healthy staff. *Nursing Management*, 36(4), 4-29.

Bolton, L. B., Jones, D., Aydin, C. E., Donaldson, N., Brown, D. S., Lowe, M. et al. (2001). A response to California's mandated nursing ratios. *Journal of Nursing Scholarship*, 33(2), 179-184.

Bowles, C., & Cabndeal, L. (2005). First job experience of recent RN graduates. *JONA*, 35(3), 130-137.

Ibarra, H., & Lineback, K. (2005). What's your story? *Harvard Business Review,* 83(1), 65-71.

Malloch, K., & Krueger, J. (2005). Patient classification systems (Chapter 19). In J. Dunham-Taylor, J.Z. Pinczuk (Eds.), *Health care financial management for nurse managers: Merging the heart with the dollar*. Sudbury, MA: Jones and Bartlett.

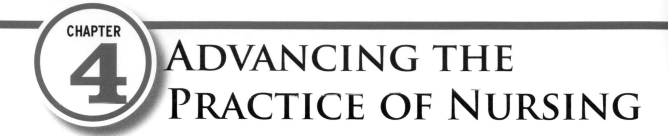

CHAPTER 4 ADVANCING THE PRACTICE OF NURSING

Challenging of the status quo requires vision, courage, and persistence.

Advancing the practice of nursing requires a complex balance of stability to support the completion of current work AND an eye on the future to continually ask "Is this the best way to provide patient care?" There is no checklist or strategy that can simplify the work of managing the balance of getting the work done and being open to new technology, new processes, and the elimination of current work that is no longer valued.

Excellent leaders recognize that this work is filled with risk taking, the essence of thriving in vulnerable situations, celebrating successes when they occur, and gracefully changing course when necessary. In this section, strategies to work toward the balance of accomplishing work and moving into the future are discussed, specifically, the importance of challenging the status quo, removing barriers to the future, the mandate for an evidence-based mindset, and another iteration of the clinical ladder.

Moving to the Future...Leadership Challenges

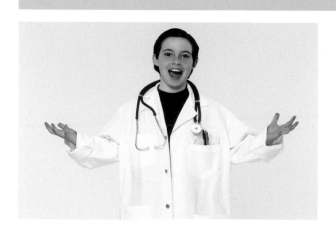

- Workforces are fragile.
- We must work on retention with a new generation of "movers."
- We don't know everything.
- We can't control others.
- It is very risky out there!

REMOVING BARRIERS TO THE FUTURE

Most nurses believe they are providing patient care that is contemporary and evidence based. Few nurses believe their work is outdated or lacking supportive rationale and evidence. Yet for most nurses, evidence-based practice is not the norm, and this can become the greatest barrier to a better future. Not knowing that current practice should be challenged is a barrier that can be removed with education and a new mindset to continually challenge the status quo. It is the role of the leader, steeped in the value of excellence, to continually challenge the status quo and instill the courage in others to become comfortable and competent to continually seek the best nursing practices—practices that are based on evidence!

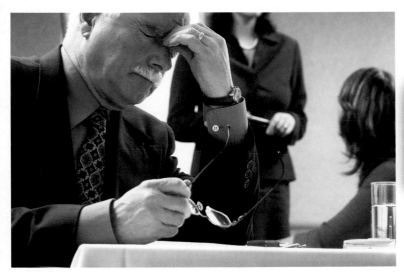

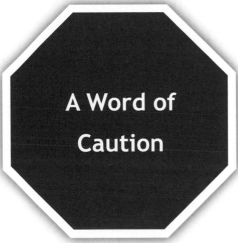

A Word of Caution

Change for Improvement—With EVIDENCE!

Change is a natural and important fact of organizational life. Changing structure, processes, and policies for the right reason or on the basis of evidence is a mark of leadership excellence. Knowing what to change, when to make changes, and how to fully engage the team requires knowledge and sensitivity to the current work and an eye toward the future. Courage to challenge the status quo and decision making based on evidence, a commitment to transforming the health care experience, new reward structures, and sensitivity to the varying characteristics of each nurse are but a few of the considerations necessary to advance the practice and profession of nursing.

The work of removing barriers is a lifelong journey—as one barrier is removed, often new barriers are identified. Examples of behaviors, some overt and some subconscious, that create barriers to progress are identified in the table on the following page.

Barriers to a Better Future

☐ *Out of Balance*
- Boundaries are unclear or nonexistent between obligations to employer and time away—always at work! Ever-present email.
- Overstimulation.

☐ *Abuse of Power*
- Mandatory overtime is acceptable .
- Intolerance toward diversity.
- Underdeveloped middle management skills

☐ *Inequitable Compensation*
- Performance is based on employee longevity rather than contributions to the mission of the organization.

☐ *Impersonal Downsizing*
- Employees are viewed as expendable nuisances. Respectful disengagement is not the norm.
- The cost of doing business.
- It's about the bottom line—it's not personal!

☐ *Integrity at Will*
- Filling vacancies based on personal relationship; holding vacancies when applicants are not likable.
- Age discrimination—too young or too old
- Religious discrimination (members of my church are more trusted)
- Different thinking styles—he takes too long to make a decision.
- Sarbanes Oxley violation—a little inappropriate behavior won't matter!

☐ *Failure to Manage the Careerist*
- Employees are retired on the job and tolerated.
- High-maintenance employees are tolerated.
- Entitlement is encouraged.
- Clear and evolving job expectations are not identified.

☐ *Tolerance of Antisocial Behavior*
- Sexual harassment
- Dishonesty
- Gossip
- Stealing supplies

☐ *Bureaucratic Structures*
- Filtered decision making
- Permission is required to provide patient care
- Restricted communication
- Overcontrol—tell me everything!

☐ *Toxic Mentoring*
- Continuing practices that worked in the past but are not suited for the future
- Is the wise elder really wise?

EVIDENCE-BASED PRACTICE

The integration of the best research evidence
with clinical expertise and patient values (Sackett et al., 2000)

Removing barriers to allow caregivers to be open to better solutions is the first step in becoming an organization known for its excellence because the work is based on evidence. The next step is developing knowledge and competence in the use of evidence.

The formalization of evidence-based practice occurred in England and Canada in the 1980s with the goal of using the best evidence so health care could be delivered in a cost-effective way using the best research. In the United States, the Agency for Healthcare Research and Quality has been the leader in generating evidence-based standards for health care providers (*www.ahrq.gov*).

Previously, the emphasis had been on research utilization—a more structured way of using research findings. This approach looks at research outcomes in a selected area of practice, reviews the literature, and bases practice changes on qualitative and quantitative research findings. Evidence-based practice uses the broader patient preferences, expert opinion, and data on the costs of care.

Evidence-based practice and research utilization require caregivers to learn to search for and analyze the evidence. Making decisions with good information is the goal for all health care professionals, yet consistent evidence-based decision making does not occur routinely in health care.

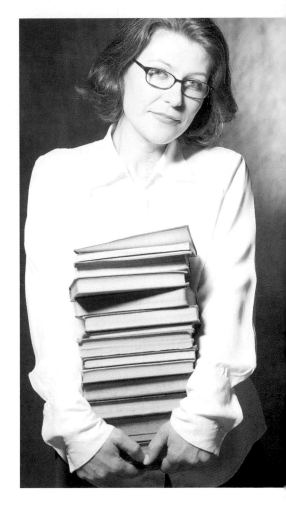

> Evidence-based practice is a way of thinking that requires discipline and experience to continually challenge practices and ask, "Is there evidence and support for this work?"

LEADING WITH EVIDENCE...

Evidence-Based Practice

The term EBP is probably derived from the definition of evidence-based medicine, which is "the conscientious, explicit and judicious use of current best evidence in making decisions about the care of individual patients." The practice of evidence-based medicine means integrating individual clinical expertise with the best available external clinical evidence from systematic research (Sackett, 2000, p. 2).

The Leader as Transformer

Contemporary leaders must shift from traditional leadership based on education, experience, and tradition to an evidence-based approach in which the available evidence, experience, expertise, and values of the organization direct the work. Interestingly, leaders have recognized research, experience, and personal values as important. The difference with the evidence-based approach is that the linkages among the three—research, expertise, and value—must be inexorably linked. Failure to make these connections can only result in less than optimal work processes, misuse of resources, and poor outcomes.

The journey to evidence-based perspective can begin simply with a reflection on the negative events occurring in the current patient care experience, such as patient falls or medication errors. These experiences can serve as the beginning issues for discussion in which the leader uses an evidence-based approach, thus becoming the springboard for the transition to a more effective model, to transforming health care into a service that is healing, therapeutic, evidence based, safe, patient centered, and affordable.

Creating evidence based practices is not about fine-tuning current practices; rather it is about reviewing research evidence, integrating leadership expertise in the revision of patient care delivery processes, considering the physical environment, and modifying the organizational culture and norms to support a new way of thinking (Institute for Healthcare Improvement, 2004).

Transformation Leadership	*Transformational Leader Competencies*
The ability to envision, energize, and stimulate a change process that coalesces communities, patients, and professionals around new models of health care and wellness	Achievement oriented Analytical thinker Community oriented Information seeking Innovative thinker Strategic orientation Source: National Center for Healthcare Leadership, 2004

LEADING WITH EVIDENCE: THREE KEY CONCEPTS

Three key concepts of evidence-based practice—research evidence, expertise, and values—can be translated into the work of leadership. These applications provide clarity of purpose and direction for evidence-based leadership as defined by DeGroot (2005).

Evidence-Based Leadership

A transformational relationship involving organizational stewardship, decision making, and vision translation through reasoned application of empirical evidence from management, leadership and patient care research (DeGroot, 2005).

1 *Best Research Evidence*

Common sources of evidence include the systematic literature review, meta-analysis, integrative review, and exhaustive integrative reviews. Systematic review is a type of inquiry that summarizes all of the evidence related to a specific research issue. Meta-analysis involves a systematic review that uses statistical methods for combining results of individual studies. An integrative review summarizes the findings of research on a particular topic and draws conclusions from the body of the literature. An exhaustive integrative review may meet the same standard as primary research in regard to clarity, rigor, and replication. The validity of each of these reviews can be assessed by asking the following questions: (a) Is the clinical question well focused? (b) Are the criteria for including articles in the review appropriate? (c) How likely is it that relevant studies were missed? (d) Are the results similar from study to study? (Sanares & Hiliker, 2005)

Clinical Research

Refers to clinically relevant research, often from the basic health and medical sciences, but especially from patient-centered clinical research. Scientific findings, an external source of evidence, are considered to be the most credible, clinically relevant, systematically derived and empirically based information available.

Leadership Research

Refers to relevant research specific to organizational structure, team building, culture, measurement, and strategic planning, often from the humanities, anthropology, and management sciences. Scientific findings, an external source of evidence, are considered to be the credible, relevant, systematically derived and empirically based information available.

2 | *Expertise*

Clinical expertise means the ability to use clinical skills and experience to rapidly identify each patient's unique health state and diagnosis, individual risks and benefits of potential interventions, and personal values and expectations. Clinical expertise is an internal source of evidence derived from clinical training and classroom or other formal methods of didactic education, systematic observations and analyses of previous clinical encounters, and the ability to weigh these sources in light of the individual patient situation. Clinician experience includes knowledge of biological principles, access to benchmarking data, knowledge of local, national, or international standards of practice, quality improvement data, and cost information. Also, the clinician incorporates psychosocial principles of care and the assessment of a patient's individual concerns and needs.

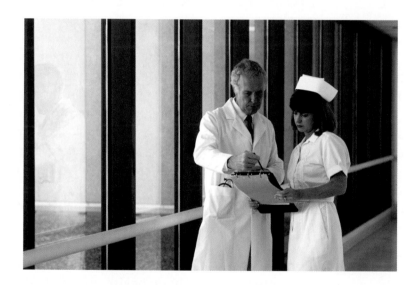

Leadership expertise means the ability to use leadership skills and experience to rapidly identify each of the skills and abilities of employees, the unique characteristics of the organization, available resources, cultural norms, and the emotional intelligence expressions that provide service and direction for the work being led. Leadership expertise is an internal source of evidence derived from leadership training and classroom or other formal methods of didactic education, systematic observations, and analyses of previous manager and leader roles, and the ability to assess the situation and synthesize all of the variables of the situation into productive and effective work. Leadership experience includes knowledge of management principles, access to benchmarking data, knowledge of local, national, or international standards of practice, quality improvement data, and cost information.

3 $\quad$ Values

Patient values refer to the unique preferences, concerns, and expectations that each patient brings to a clinical encounter and that must be integrated into clinical decisions if they are to serve the patient. Patient preference is an internal source of evidence and requires the intentional solicitation by health care professionals of their patient's treatment-related wishes, which are influenced by the patient's values, beliefs, culture, and previous or family experiences. By incorporating these into patient care and evidence-based guidelines, the patient's autonomy and ability to participate in treatment related decision making are protected.

Leadership values refer to the unique preferences, concerns, and expectations identified by organization specific to healing, employees, patient care delivery, productivity, and financing. Further values are expressed in the order of importance of the identified values. Leadership values are internal to both the individual and the organization. The solicitation of individual values and internalization to the existing organizational values require constant attention and validation. The collective values of the organization may be quite different from individual value, which produces dysfunction if not recognized and addressed. Individual values must be identified prior to hiring and deemed consistent with the organization in an open and honest dialog. Congruence of values supports the employee's ability to be a viable member of the team and participate in the organization's work effectively.

It is not a secret to caregivers who remember these protocols that new evidence has emerged, been accepted, and changed the way patient care is provided. These changes occur over and over again. The challenge is to be appropriate and timely in choosing the best evidence.

REMEMBER WHEN...?

- Sippy diets were the standard treatment for gastric ulcers?
- Sandbags were used to stabilize the head after cataract surgery and the patient remained on strict bed rest for 7 days in the hospital?
- Back pain was treated with pelvic traction and complete bed rest for 10 days?
- Taking of blood pressure was restricted to physicians?
- Milk and magnesia paste was standard treatment for pressure ulcers?

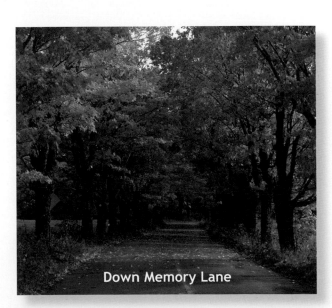

Down Memory Lane

Advancing the Practice of Nursing   381

RATIONALE FOR EVIDENCE-BASED THINKING

The rationale for using evidence is clear—it's the right thing to do for better health care. Choosing not to practice based on evidence is unethical.

Closing the Gap among Tradition, Intuition, and Value

In addition to the obvious logical reason to use evidence for decision making, other reasons exist for the transition:

- Focusing on the work of health care can only assist researchers and expert practitioners to give structure and substance to the invisible work of caregivers—the work of assessing, monitoring, caring, coordinating provider work, and preparing for events not readily evident to others. This work has long been referred to as the soft stuff of health care rather than as being part of the essential interventions necessary to ensure positive patient outcomes.

- There is an urgent need to determine the value or cost-effectiveness of the work of caregivers. This emphasis expands the focus to both process and outcomes of work. For example, using an evidence-based analysis of the admission of a patient can no longer be considered the completion of the assessment form. The quality and appropriateness of the information collected in the assessment becomes the vital information.

- The demand for resources is overwhelming, particularly in the area of patient safety. The need to be judicious in the use of resources has never been greater as the cost of health care continues to rise rapidly.

- Unnecessary variations in practice persist and continue to affect the health care system negatively

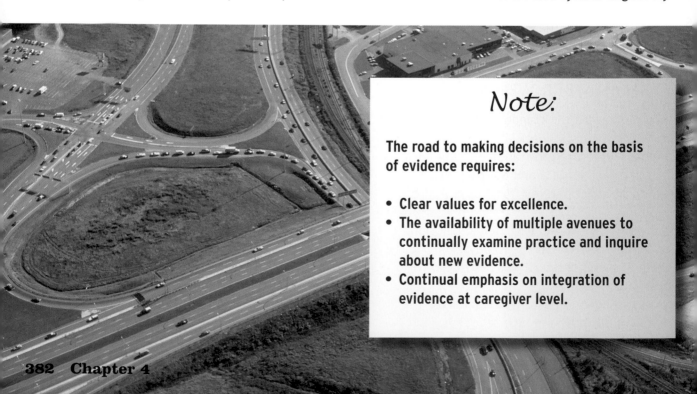

Note:

The road to making decisions on the basis of evidence requires:

- **Clear values for excellence.**
- **The availability of multiple avenues to continually examine practice and inquire about new evidence.**
- **Continual emphasis on integration of evidence at caregiver level.**

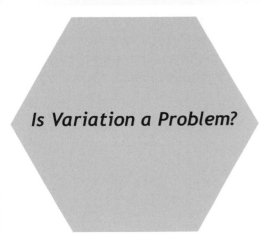

Is Variation a Problem?

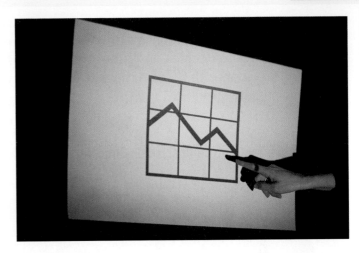

In most cases, variation is problematic because of different interpretations, applications, and evaluation of work processes. The delicate and dynamic challenge to balance variation and standardization is forever present. Expert clinicians must determine the principles that should be standardized and when to vary in applying those principles. Consider counseling a colleague in private as the standard way to do business, but when safety is threatened, the intervention may be done in the presence of hundreds. The greater good prevails—along with good sense!

Wennberg, the principal investigator and series editor of the Dartmouth Atlas, has documented significant geographic variations in medical practice since the early 1970s. According to Wennberg (2004) Medicare patients with similar chronic conditions receive strikingly different care, even among hospitals identified as "best" for geriatric care. The studies show that the frequency of physician visits, the number of diagnostic tests, and rate of hospital and intensive care unit (ICU) stays vary markedly. The studies show that a higher intensity of care and higher level of spending are not associated with better quality or longer survival times even in the most renowned teaching hospitals.

Comparison of Provider Services
for Cancer, CHF, and COPD (Risk Adjusted)

	Lowest	Highest	% Variation
Days in the hospital	8.5	32.3	25
Days in ICU	0.6	13.4	45
Physician visits	13	99	37

Data from Wennberg, J.E., Fisher, E.S., Stukel,T A & Sharp, S.M. (2004). Use of Medicare claims data to monitor provider-specific performance among patients with severe chronic illness [web exclusive]. *Health Affairs: The policy journal of the health sphere.* Retrieved November 21, 2005, from *http://content.healthaffairsorg/cgi/reprintinlthaff.var5v1.*

Variation documented by Wennberg and colleagues (2004) is difficult to explain or justify. The same analysis of caregiver variation is also needed to identify which standards of care represent best practices and best outcomes. In light of the variations in provider practices, the work of caregivers must vary in response to the variations of length of time in the facility, in the ICU, and in assisting the physician during rounds.

Based on the Table of Comparisons, Consider the Following Questions:

The hours of care required for patient care similar conditions has an effect on the number and skill mix of nurses needed. If the variations are standardized, would the skill mix of licensed and unlicensed nurses change in order to achieve the same outcomes?

What are the hours of care variations for ICU care for these three conditions? If there is a 45% variation in ICU days, could standardization of practices—assuming the same outcomes—positively affect the nursing shortgage?

If the number of physician visits varies by 37%, assuming that new orders are written each visit, could standardization of practices result in fewer medication errors, less time for treatments, more time for patient teaching, or entirely different outcome?

EBP RESOURCES

Numerous resources for evidence emerge everyday. The following represent a small sampling of readily available resources. The highest level of evidence continues to be the relevant randomized control trials (ROT). However, the humanistic nature of the health care experience requires qualitative, experiential evidence as well as the quantitative evidence of the gold standard RCT.

Cochrane Library
www.cochrane.org

Central: Cochrane Central Register of Controlled Trials Contains details of published articles taken from bibliographic databases and other published and unpublished sources

HTA: Health Technology Assessment Database Contains details of ongoing projects and complete publications from health assessment organizations

DARE: Database of Abstracts of Reviews of Effects

CMR: Cochrane Methodology Register A bibliography of publications that report on methods used in the conduct of controlled trials

EED: Economic Evaluation Database Contains structured abstracts of articles describing economic evaluations of health care interventions; papers compare the costs and the outcomes of alternatives

BARRIERS TO EVIDENCE-BASED PRACTICE

Needed Evidence

There are many areas in which there is a need for evidence to both support long-held practices and the emerging technology and physical environment configurations. Examples of areas of need include:

☐ What is the minimal nurse-to-patient hours and skill mix for safe and effective staffing in medical-surgical units?

☐ What is the clinical efficacy for patient safety interventions? Given the research supporting the elimination of side rails, why are they still so prevalent?

☐ What is the effect of centralized vs. decentralized nurses' stations on nurse satisfaction, accuracy of documentation, and number of codes?

☐ What are the indicators of the optimal physical environment that result in optimal patient outcomes?

☐ Why is hand washing still done less than 40% of the time when research identifies clean hands as the single most important factor in reducing the spread of dangerous germs in health care settings?

– Not seen as important to nurses
– Lack of time/work overload
– Reluctance to ask questions
– Information overload
– Lack of role models/ mentors for evidence-based practice
– Limited accessibility to research findings
– Anticipated outcomes of using research
– Organizational support to use research/time
– Support from others to use research
– Lack of authority to change practice
– Lack of collaboration/physician buy-in

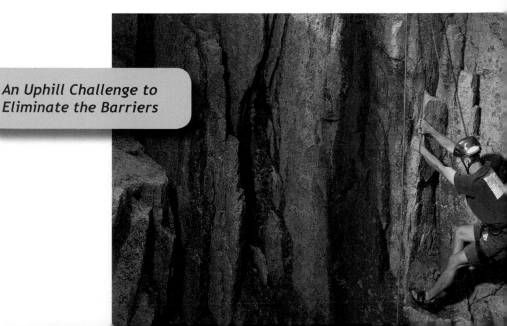

An Uphill Challenge to Eliminate the Barriers

STRATEGIES TO INCREASE EBP

Multiple strategies are needed to transform the mindset of the caregivers from a traditionalist to an evidence-based practitioner. Leaders are encouraged to use the following strategies to assist others in the transformation.

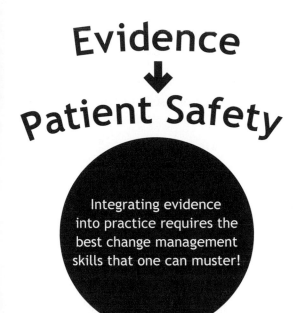

Evidence
↓
Patient Safety

Integrating evidence into practice requires the best change management skills that one can muster!

Think in systems. Everything is connected! Be sure to examine issues within the context of both the local unit and the whole system.

Reinforce learning with access to resources. Currently access to resources is inconsistent.

- ☐ 95% of facilities provide textbooks on units.
- ☐ 66% provide nursing journals.
- ☐ <20% provide nursing research journals.
- ☐ 60% Internet/online resources are in nurse manager offices.
- ☐ 35% Internet/online resources are in patient care units.

Not only encourage but also require staff to challenge policies and make changes when appropriate

Rethink Journal Clubs for Staff

The journal club is rich with ideas, discussion, and stimulates new thinking—the reality is that few survive for any length of time because participants' needs change. Staff no longer need to learn how to review and discuss complex topics—that was met in the first three meetings. The needs are now person-specific to their work and no journal club can meet the needs of all staff.

ESP: LEADERSHIP CASE STUDY

Identifying the appropriate number of individuals that one can supervise is an issue for leaders. Using the evidence-based practice approach, one can begin to address this age-old issue. Several responses are included, others are left to be determined as more information is identified. This situation is like many leadership challenges, the solution is not readily available. More questions are identified and further discussion is needed.

1. **Identify an issue**
   Leaders are unsure of the right number of employees that one manager can supervise effectively.

2. **Develop the question**
   What is the optimal span of control? What are the measures of effectiveness?

3. **Search for evidence**
   Search literature for information specific to the number of individuals supervised. A range of 5-10 individuals were identified with differing levels of education, expected job functions, availability of clinical experts, and budget allocations. No studies examining spans of control greater than 10 individuals were found. Span of control for greater than 10 is common in practice.

4. **Evaluate the evidence**
   The evidence is not conclusive as to the appropriate number of employees that one should supervise. New questions emerge: What are the variables of number of employees supervised, job role expectations, and the resulting patient outcomes, caregiver outcomes and costs to the organization of the present span of control? Based on this analysis, which set of variables results in optimal outcomes for patients, caregivers, and the organization?

5. **Make recommendations**
   Collect information for each unit and summary data for the department(s) specific to number supervised, education level of managers and staff, number of evaluations'manager, number of support roles, patient falls, medication errors, nosocomial pneumonia, number of codes, caregiver satisfaction, hours per patient day, and cost of care per patient.

6. **Determine feasibility for implementation**
   Data collection is feasible.

7. **Develop implementation plan**
   Data collection template should be created and distributed for submission within 1 month.

8. **Implement change**
   To be determined when information is available. Reorganization of responsibilities or new programs may be selected to implement the planned change in span of control.

9. **Evaluate results**
   Evaluate the outcomes when the number is identified and implemented. Outcome measures should address the presenting issue. These data will also provide new evidence for spans of control greater than 10 and should be submitted for publication.

TRANSFORMATION REQUIRES COURAGE

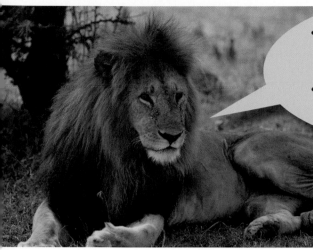

- What stops you from stepping up to a challenge?

- When was the last time you felt courageous? Courageous AND successful?

Identifying the barriers to a better future is the first step for the leader to assist others in opening the organizational culture to be more receptive to the uncertainties of the future. As always, knowing as much about yourself and your leader behaviors is critical for effective leadership.

Asking yourself and others how you approach work provides important insight into your level of courage and willingness to challenge the status quo—seldom a comfortable position or one that is welcomed by colleagues engaged in fast-paced, complex work.

☐ First, answer these four questions yourself.
☐ Then ask a trusted colleague to respond to the questions based on their observations of your behavior.
☐ Compare the responses.
☐ How similar are the answers?
☐ What new behaviors should you consider to develop your courage?

Note:

Courage often does not emerge until the pain of not doing something exceeds the fear of doing it.

Once you have answered the questions, consider the list of courageous behaviors on the final pages of this section. Are there behaviors at which you are particularly competent? Behaviors that you would like to develop? Select one at a time and work with a colleague to become competent with the new behavior.

Be Courageous!

ASSESS YOUR WILLINGESS TO BE COURAGEOUS

1. Is there evidence that you are able to share your own values and ideas, especially when they are different from the majority?

2. Is there evidence of your strong, persistent, and vocalized commitment to new ideas?

3. Is there evidence of your vigor and vitality when managing a project even when activities are not going as planned?

4. Are you considered by others as honest, forthright, and candid or do you give away integrity with half truths?

5. Is the code of silence your mantra?

6. Share an experience in which you did step up to a challenge.

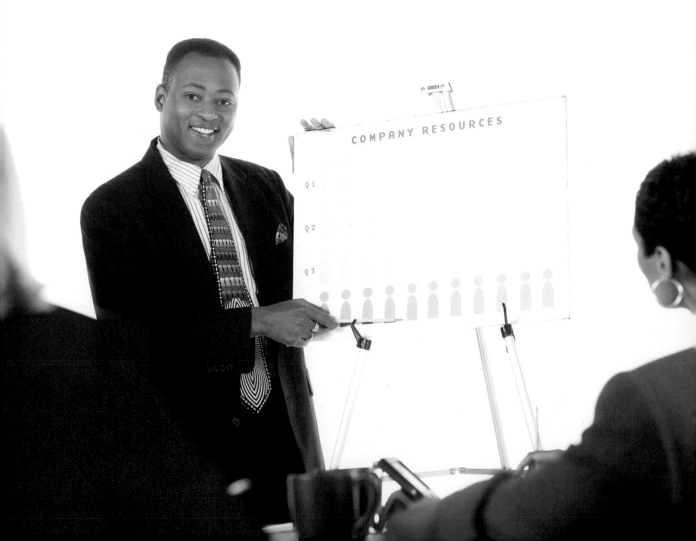

Courageous Behaviors

Different situations require different considerations and behaviors

Remove the dogma brick wall

- Review current policies; support what is working, retire what is not working.
- Motivate others.
- Be enthusiastic.
- Persist without impulsiveness.
- Believe in others.

Minimize professional antagonism

- Bring issues into the open for discussion.
- Expect collaboration as the only way to work.
- Address issues as they arise.
- Remain focused and objective.
- Believe that others care as much as you do!

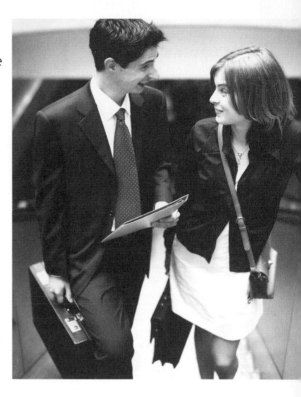

Never stop learning

- Create, defend, and fund a culture supportive of learning.
- Believe that knowledge is necessary for survival.
- Participate enthusiastically.
- Never waver in commitment.
- Believe that others share the same values—ask for validation when you are not certain.

Provide value-based service

- Continually examine services, measures, and systems to ensure value.
- Believe that hope can be restored through value in caring work.
- Be alive and committed!
- Consistently support the belief that value-based service is the only acceptable product of health care.
- Believe that caregivers intuitively know the right path for value.

COURAGEOUS BEHAVIOR
Different situations require different considerations and behaviors

Maintain mental fitness
- Create a culture that supports consistency in recognition.
- Develop a personal commitment to ensuring hardiness and resilience as essential characteristics.
- Continually strive for personal mental fitness.
- Establish a program of self-examination and renewal.
- Recognize that no individual is an island and each person needs relationships, support, and feedback to function.

Use time wisely
- Recognize that everyone can improve their use of time.
- Focus on the importance of balancing one's energy rather than efficiency.
- Share the spirit of the reality that there will always be a shortage of time and excesses of desires—a never-ending struggle to close the gap! THIS IS LIFE!
- Stay focused and be aware of personal performance.
- Support others less successful in time balance, knowing there are opportunities to improve for all.

Balance career and job emphasis
- Create compensation systems that recognize a multiplicity of values.
- Pursue change with enthusiasm.
- Be vigilant and persistent.
- Stay focused and committed among resistance.
- Believe that others are interested in new approaches as well.

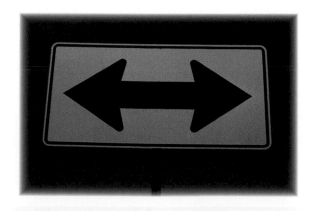

ONE MORE TIME! IS THERE EVIDENCE FOR CLINICAL LADDERS?

Advancing the practice requires not only evidence for decision making and the courage to make the needed decisions but also programs that reinforce and validate those behaviors. Recognition of excellence in the performance of caregiver work has been a long-standing challenge. Often, clinical ladders are like patient classification systems—you can't live with them, but something tells you that you need them! The right kind of recognition for direct caregivers should be credible, measurable, and linked to patient outcomes. Traditional recognition programs for caregivers that are easy to administer, measure, and manage have been based on attendance and committee participation. More contemporary clinical ladder systems are emerging that simply, but effectively, recognize caregiver expertise based on credentials, the ability to plan, coordinate, deliver and evaluate complex patient care. In addition, these ladders assess the coaching and mentoring of less experienced nurses.

The goals of a contemporary clinical ladder program include:
- Rewarding competent caregivers for contributions to patient and nurse outcomes.
- Achieving a higher standard of care and patient outcomes for organization.
- Ensuring that the values of clinical excellence and lifelong learning are integrated into organizational programs.

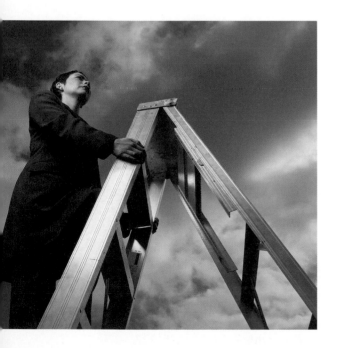

Challenges of a clinical ladder program include:

- Ensuring that the program is credible to key stakeholders across the organization, from staff nurses to senior leadership.
- Ensuring staff nurse involvement in the development and maintenance of the program.
- Developing and sustaining a program that is credible but not overly complex in order for participants to demonstrate their competence.
- Ensuring that the expenses of the program are actually an investment in the outcomes of patients and in the staff members.
- Sustaining an annual evaluation process to ensure program validity and appropriateness for the current environment.

References

DeGroot, H. A (2005). Evidence-based leadership: Nursing's new mandate. *Nurse Leader*, 3(2), 37-41.

Institute for Healthcare Improvement. (2004). Innovation series 2004: Transforming care at the bedside. Cambridge, MA Author. Retrieved November 21, 2005, from www.ihi.org/IHI/Topics/MedicalSurgicalCarefTransformingCare.

Sacket, D. L., Straus, S. E., Richardson, W. S., Rosenberg, W., & Haynes, R. B. (2000). *Evidence-based medicine: How to practice and teach EBM*. London: Churchill Livingstone.

Sanares, D., & Hiliker, D. (2005). A framework for nursing clinical inquiry: Pathway toward evidence-based nursing practice. In K. Malloch, & T. Porter-O'Grady (Eds.), *An introduction to evidence-based practice in nursing and healthcare*. Sudbury, MA Jones and Bartlett.

Wennberg, J. E., Fisher, E. S., Stukel, T. A, & Sharp, S. M. (2004, October 7). Use of Medicare claims data to monitor provider specific performance among patients with severe chronic illness [web exclusive]. Health Affairs: The policy journal of the health sphere. Retrieved November 21, 2005, from http://content.healthaffairs.org/cgi/reprint/hlthaff.var.5v1.

Suggested Readings

Green, J. (2005). What nurses want: Different generations, different expectations. *Hospitals & Health Networks*, 79(3), 34-42.

Hinds, P. S., Gattuso, J. S., Barnwell, E., Cofer,M., & Kellum, L. (2003). Translating psychosocial research findings into practice guidelines. *JONA*, 33(7/3), 397-403.

Malloch, K., & Porter-O'Grady, T. (2005). *Quantum leader. Applications for the new world of work*. Sudbury, MA Jones and Bartlett.

National Center for Healthcare Leadership. (2004). NCHL health leadership competency model (version 2.0). Chicago: Author. Retrieved November 22, 2005, from vvvvvv.nchl.orginsidocumelits/NewVenn.ppt.

Pravikoff, D. S., Pierce, S., & Tanner, A., (2003). Nursing resources: Are nurses ready for evidence-based practice? *AJN*, 103(5), 95-96.

Swan, B.A., Lang, N. M., & McGinley, A M. (2004). Access to quality health care: links between evidence, nursing language, and informatics. *Nursing Economic$*, 22(6), 325-327.

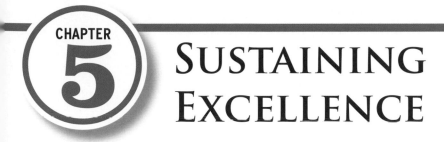

CHAPTER 5

SUSTAINING EXCELLENCE

Excellence begins with the individual!

The organizational structure must be dynamic to sustain a high level of functionality. As mentioned in Unit 5, Chapter 1, changing the fundamental elements of one's organizational structure when there is evidence that a change would improve functionality is the only rational reason to modify the span of control, decision-making expectations, level of authority, or role-essential responsibilities. Before one modifies an organization's structure, it is important to know also about the passion of employees, their commitment to the work of the organization, the level of teamwork that is occurring, and the diverseness of the team. If any of these behaviors are less than optimal, structure changes that redefine the work of defined roles and the accountabilities of employees may be indicated. Knowing where the structure is weak provides leaders with direction and focus in making structure modifications and most important, when and how to sustain the infrastructure that has been able to support excellence.

> **First, create your own story or self-portrait.**
>
> **Second, celebrate your accomplishments.**
>
> **Third, flaunt it—tell the world!**

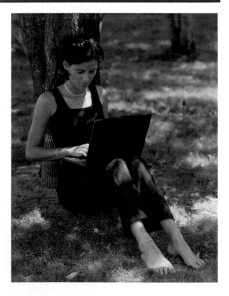

If these behaviors are overwhelmingly successful, leaders need to ensure continuing stability of the structure until there is a need to modify roles or reporting relationships. Changing roles and reporting structures seldom improve passion, energy, commitment to health care, or teamwork. The essence of the work begins with the individual.

In this section, more focused and personal processes are presented as the ultimate factors in sustaining the level of excellence created by the foundational organizational structure. The process of managing one's own reputation through personal assessment, creation of stories, and reflections on teamwork is discussed. A discussion of diversity—internal and external—is shared to celebrate the realities of differences as well as to recognize the limitations of too much diversity. The right mix of diversity, often illusive and indeterminate, is an important ingredient is sustaining excellence—excellence that is always improving.

THE STORY:
SHARING THE EXPERIENCES OF CAREGIVERS

Recognize the Best in Yourself

Talking about the experiences of nursing is the first step in creating a story that recognizes your strengths and realities of nursing.

Focus on the Positive

Feedback that focuses on identification of shortcomings can lead otherwise talented managers to over invest in fixing perceived weaknesses, thus preventing one from moving from good performance to outstanding performance. The intent is not to ignore or deny shortcomings, but to provide feedback that taps into one's strengths and contributions and serves as an inspiration to others.

Note:

You have more to gain by developing your gifts and leveraging your natural skills than by trying to repair your weaknesses.

CREATE YOUR STORY

The stories told by caregivers can either entice and engage interested individuals or give them reason to never consider the health care profession. By telling stories about the richness of the work of caregivers, a highly respected individual can lead others to explore and eventually commit to the health are profession.

Telling stories of overwork, long hours, and disrespectful colleagues gives potential health care workers every good reason to NOT pursue health care and good reason to wonder about your personal sanity in remaining in a profession with so little satisfaction.

The Elements of a Story

More than 2300 years ago, Aristotle defined the classic story structure used to reflect how the human mind wants to organize reality. The key elements of a story include:

- *A protagonist the listener cares about*: This is you or the patient and something that is occurring; a new event or insight that reflects a point of no return. There is a break from the past. If all goes well in the story, the tension is resolved and a new chapter is started.

- *A catalyst compelling the protagonist to take action*: This could be an experience with a patient, a coworker, or a family member. "I discovered that I am good at...; this gives me real pleasure...." Include personal and professional impetus.

- *Trials and tribulations*: How to get there—obstacles and challenges to overcome

- *A turning point*: It felt better.

- *A resolution*: Here I am!

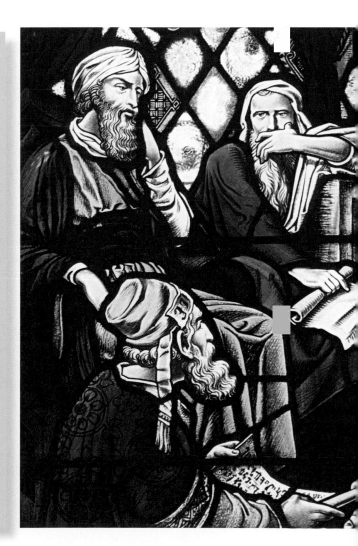

As You Create Your Story, Consider the Following:

☐   *Think about what you want others to know about you and about your career as a health care worker. If you love your work and feel fulfilled, your stories become a source of satisfaction and the best recruitment tool there is.*

☐   *If you are not fully committed to patient care and to the organization in which you work, it is difficult to stay committed to the work and influence your colleagues in a positive way.*

☐   *Your story is your resume in full, living color!*

☐   *Take the time to examine your story and be sure that you are sending the message that you want about your work as a caregiver.*

☐   *Reflect the Forces of Magnetism: the image of nursing, involvement in decision making, quality care, consultation and support from advanced practice nurses, and the role of the nurse-teacher in your work life.*

☐   *Health care stories are rich with experiences and lessons to compel new journeys. If you have a story in which you experienced an ah-ha moment or learned something that remains with you, share it with others.*

☐   *The kinds of stories one tells provide insight into how well one copes with change. Identify what challenges you and how you respond. Remember, not all stories are fairy tales with a great ending. Some stories may be unfinished and thus allow others the opportunity to reflect and complete the story themselves.*

☐   *A little humor is always healthy. Never belittle others—laugh at yourself and what you learn from living. Others will understand and in many cases empathize with you.*

A Nurse Healer's Story: Music as Therapy

This heartwarming story of professional practice was identified in the course of routine conversation. A colleague invited Debbie to create the story and share it with others.

Debbie, a nurse at hospital in the Southwest, shared this story about a recent patient care experience in which she received great satisfaction and a sense of accomplishment from her care, her colleagues, and the patient. Mary, a retired concert violinist, was a patient in severe pain and dying from cancer, a diagnosis and fate she had come to accept. Debbie, her nurse, recognized Mary's pain, 8 on a scale of 1 to 10, and offered her pain medication. Mary declined due to religious beliefs of the value of suffering and the need to endure the condition. Debbie also recognized that Mary had been actively dying for several days, but the pain seemed to be holding her back. Debbie was feeling inadequate and wanted to administer morphine because she knew it would relieve Mary's pain. Mary again declined. Debbie remembered that Mary was a concert violinist and loved symphony music. Debbie and her team secured a headset and a CD with symphony music, offered the headset to Mary, and watched her begin to relax, then fall asleep listening to her favorite music. A few hours later, into the next shift, Mary died peacefully. The nurse who followed Debbie and cared for Mary as she died called Debbie to let her know that Mary had died peacefully.

The lesson is in learning to understand the values and needs of the patient, recognizing the therapeutic value of music, and making it available for the patient. The traditional administration of medication was within Debbie's scope of intervention, but a violation of the patient's values and wishes. Debbie was able to gain an understanding of the patient's needs and synthesize her knowledge of pain management with the personal preferences of the patient. The lesson is also about how nurses care for each other. Calling Debbie following Mary's peaceful death was an act of caring for one's colleagues; an action not required in any plan of care but one of utmost importance and validation of the value of Debbie's nursing work. This is a most healing story—a story that many nurses can understand and employ. Thank you, Debbie, for sharing your experience.

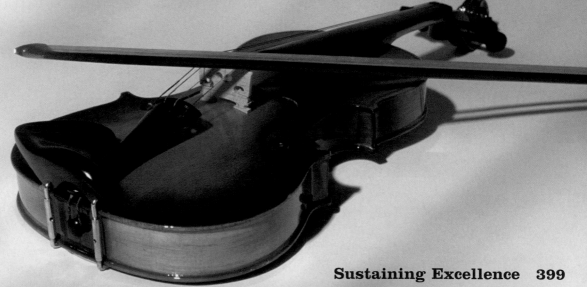

MENTORING FOR BALANCE: MANAGING PASSION

The specific role of the mentor varies widely depending on the skills of both the mentor and the mentee. Learning the techniques of leadership and the processes of building effective relationships, and the processes of decision making, experiencing the actual work of leaders, and modeling overall professional demeanor are the foci of many positive mentoring relationships. What is often overlooked is the need for skilled leaders to share their expertise in creating balance in the emerging leader's work life: balance not only between hours of work and home, but within one's daily work. Emerging leaders are often highly enthusiastic and energized to accomplish great things in a very short hart period of time. Internal, personal pressure to be the best is significant and must be channeled to ensure that emerging leaders do not become stressed, burned out, and disenfranchised.

More Work to Manage... Results in Attention Deficit!

The transition from the industrial age to the information age has resulted in increased organization complexity and additional work expectations. This complexity is further complicated by the fact that in spite of the creation of new and more efficient systems and tools, little work has been given up. In spite of the availability of complex electronic data management and storage systems, printing copies of electronic documents has become the norm. The need to be an efficient multitasker has become the topic at management development workshops. Yet leaders and caregivers are stretched to the limit of their capacity, and a variation of the well-known attention deficit disorder—attention deficit trait—emerges.

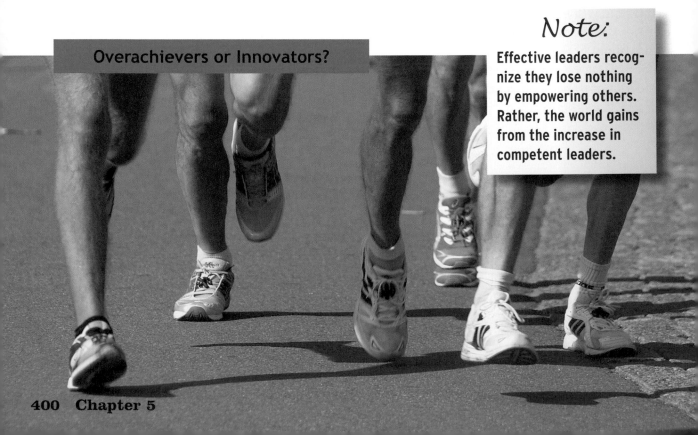

Overachievers or Innovators?

Note: Effective leaders recognize they lose nothing by empowering others. Rather, the world gains from the increase in competent leaders.

Hallowell (2005) has noted that brain overload occurs; employees are easily distracted, internally frenzied, and unusually impatient. Employees have difficulty staying organized, setting priorities, and managing time. Otherwise talented leaders are subtly, but strongly undermined by the overload of input data. To be sure, the problem is not simply poor time management, it is about an environment gone wild with data coming at leaders relentlessly and from all directions. Most leaders lack the capacity to attend fully or thoroughly to anything. Feelings of low level panic and guilt are commonplace.

This phenomenon labeled attention deficit trait (ADT) by Hallowell (2005) has positive and negative outcomes much like the well-known attention deficit disorder (ADD). Leaders are challenged to not only reflect on their own personal behaviors but also strategize with emerging leaders in helping them set limits and manage the never-ending work of health care.

ATTENTION DEFICIT DISORDER: LEADERSHIP BEHAVIORS

At best, individuals with ADD are gifted with rare talents, are creative and original, display ingenuity, improvise well under pressure, have the ability to field multiple inputs simultaneously, and can be strong leaders during times of change. They tend to rebound quickly after setbacks and bring fresh energy to the next project.

As the human brain is asked to process dizzying amounts of data; its ability to solve problems flexibly and creatively declines and the number of mistakes increases.

ADD is the response to the hyperkinetic environment of today's world and is considered by some as essential to function in the contemporary culture. The quest for speed in data transfer with cell phones, personal digital assistants, and video conferencing drives the frenzied activity with little possibility of any slow-down.

At worst, individuals tend to procrastinate, miss deadlines, struggle with disorganization and tardiness, are forgetful, and drift away mentally in the middle of a conversation. Results are inconsistent.

REVERSING DISENFRANCHISEMENT

Overachievers or Innovators?

Too often, passionate, energetic professionals become overachievers destined to become underperformers. Innovative ideas are conceptualized but seldom brought to fruition. The lack of focus and systematic planning can quickly result in frustration, discouragement, and ultimately disenfranchisement. Good ideas are not transitioned to better practices. Bright, competent professionals are burned out quickly when support and coaching to recognize, prioritize, and manage new ideas is absent.

What's wrong with this picture?

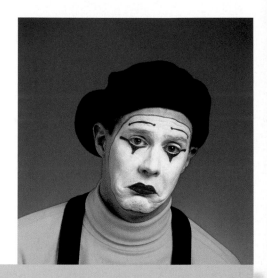

- Caregivers—energetic and enthusiastic, are filled with ideas that are often met with rejection or statements like, "This is how we do it here; you'll learn."

- Overusing the competent nurse for every committee, every function, and every extra shift!

Strategies to Manage the Frenzy

Innovative ideas come from multiple sources; actual experiences, reading, conferences, and recommendations from others. A structure and systematic process to encourage the evaluation of new ideas is needed in each organization.

- It is impossible to eliminate the activities in one's environment, but it IS possible to control and filter the activities.

- Assess your environment for the level of frenzy. Is multitasking an expectation? To what degree?

- Work to segment projects into manageable sections; recognize limitations—easier said than done in this environment; negotiate.

- Focused activities result in better outcomes with fewer feelings of incompleteness.

- Working on multiple overlapping projects often results in second-rate thinking.

- Are leaders in your organization required to manage multiple projects simultaneously? When are they effective? When are they overwhelmed?

SUSTAINING PASSION FOR PATIENT CARE

The heart of the nurse is a very critical element necessary for excellence in health care. In times of overwork, stress, conflict, or loss, the heart of the healer often becomes broken or at best demoralized and sad and disconnected from the tough work of caring. Caregivers come to the health care field with passion, commitment, and the belief that all other health care workers are equally motivated and passionate. When the passion is dampened, there is a need to look both inward and outward. As discussed in Unit 4, Chapter 3, personal commitment is essential; however, the culture of the organization may also require improvement to reverse this disenfranchisement of caregivers.

According to Peter Block (2004), noted bestselling author, the current crisis may be not about the work of the caregiver, but how to create fulfillment in the work.

Empowering caregivers to control their work is an important first step in regaining the once felt fulfillment in healing work. Self-scheduling, eliminating mandatory overtime, and evidence-based patient care assignments are important strategies to attain the goal of fulfillment. Allowing caregivers to control their work and to have a say in their assignments allows them to provide the care needed and to experience the essence of being a healer.

Facilitating Fulfillment
Improve the capacity of caregivers to set limits and boundaries for themselves.

Lack of Fulfillment Indicators

- *Feelings of abandonment*
- *Staffing shortages*
- *Excessive regulations*
- *Reduced reimbursement*
- *Overwhelming legal constraints*

- *Loss of control*
- *Devaluation/disrespect*
- *Overextension*
- *Fragmentation and frustration*

TEAMWORK

The quality of health care depends on how well team members communicate, coordinate care, and negotiate their interdependencies in practice to achieve a cohesive treatment plan for patients. Working in groups requires knowledge, commitment, excellent communication skills, respect, and the ability to share and trust in others. As leaders work to sustain the highest level of excellence and respond to the changing conditions in the environment, the need for effective teamwork has never been greater. There is little room for personal agendas, private negotiations, and reluctance to collaborate; the work is now!

Teamwork is defined as that work which is done by a group of people who possess individual expertise, who are responsible for making individual decisions, who hold a common purpose and who meet together to communicate, share and consolidate knowledge from which plans are made, future decisions are influenced and actions determined (Brill, 1976, p.10).

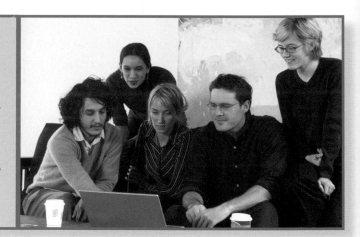

Collaboration and coordination of work are essential characteristics of successful teams. Work that reflects the highest level of coordination cannot be realized unless there is attention to the coordination of work processes; conversely, partially developed work by selected members of the team cannot be realized even with the best coordination of work plan.

Collaboration: the interaction between nurses and physicians with trust, respect, and joint contributions of knowledge, skills, and value to accomplish the goal of quality patient care (Krairiksh & Anthony, 2001, p. 17).

Coordination: the process of assembling and synchronizing differentiated activities so that they function effectively in the attainment of the organization's objectives (Longest, 1974, p. 65).

Group cohesion can mediate the frustrations of high workloads, lack of recognition, and low morale. Team members who work together effectively on a regular basis are able to achieve better outcomes and are more productive.

BUILDING TEAM STRENGTH: ONE CODE AT A TIME

Every practicing nurse knows the phenomena of good codes and bad codes. These scenarios serve to describe how the work of effective teams does indeed occur. Effective teams, or work groups dedicated to excellence are like good codes all the time. Team members know the work to be done, trust the skills of team members, manage the uncertainties of activities to come, and regularly compliment the work of others. Further, when the team is not working well together, members recognize the activities as team dynamics that need to be adjusted rather than personal failings.

The Good Code

Nurses describe a good code as an emergency situation in which a team of qualified staff comes together to assess, treat, and stabilize the condition of a patient who has experienced a cessation or near cessation of vital functioning. In a good code someone assumes charge of the code. There is the right number of participants, each one competent to perform the necessary actions in a timely manner. Supplies are available and in the right location; equipment is available and functioning. There is very little noise-often no one is speaking, just acting, and a staff member is with the family supporting them during the code. The patient may not survive, but in all cases the team members feel they did their best.

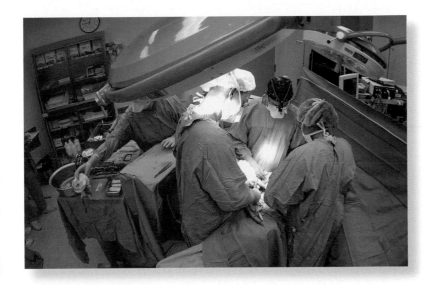

The Bad Code

Nurses describe a bad code as an emergency situation in which the team has been called to intervene on behalf of a patient whose life functioning has ceased. Multiple people run down hallways to reach the patient room, some qualified, and some not qualified. No one and everyone is in charge, equipment and supplies are missing, and participants throw items and scream obscenities at each other. The family is alone and crying uncontrollably. The patient may or may not survive. In all bad codes, team members are demoralized and frustrated by the lack of professionalism and control of a difficult situation.

Diversity: Internal and External

External

Each nurse is an individual with unique personal and professional needs, desires, and aspirations. Different generations value different incentives and support. Multiple retention strategies that provide choices to nurses are necessary. Diversity abounds among nurses in age differences, culture, religion, education, and income. The box below describes the differing external generational characteristics.

Internal

In addition, the internal diversity of an organization is significant. Differences exist in unit cultures from one unit to the next; the emergency department is quite different from the critical care unit and different from the oncology unit. Each unit has its own culture and personality. The values, beliefs, motivations, and how the work is approached in the differing areas add value to the work. The image shown on the following pages describes multiple internal characteristics that come together in the formation of the team.

Four Distinct Generations of Nurses in the Workforce

Matures, born 1922-1943: These nurses believe in hard work, paying dues, conformity and long-term commitment to one employer.

Baby Boomers, born 1944-1960: These nurses tend to define themselves through their jobs and equate work with self-worth. They like to change things and are willing to work long hours.

Generation X, born 1961-1980: These nurses were latchkey children, which has made them independent. They seek connection with managers on an equal footing and are highly comfortable with technology.

Generation Y, born 1981-2000: These nurses are technologically, savvy, optimistic, and street smart. They expect diversity and crave structure.

From Greene, J. (2005, March). What nurses want: Different generations different expectations. *Hospital & Health Networks*, 34-42.

The Culture of Caregivers

The culture of caregivers includes myriad differing attributes in all combinations from shift to shift, unit to unit, and from facility to facility. The interconnections between the attributes is as complex and varied as one could imagine. Knowing who we are is the first step in learning to honor the diversity among health care workers and not minimize the differences but to value and integrate the best of every caregiver to create the most positive experience of care.

Assessment of the differing attributes within the workforce should serve as the foundation for succession planning. Who do we have currently and with what skills and attributes? Does the organization need more caregivers who speak Spanish? More male caregivers, Native Americans, baccalaureate nurses, bilingual pharmacists? Even more important, does the organization need more critical thinkers, more technical staff, more planners, more technologically savvy caregivers? The list is long to be sure, but important in creating a succession plan for the future. Succession planning is more than finding a replacement for one's position, it is about planning for the next generation of work.

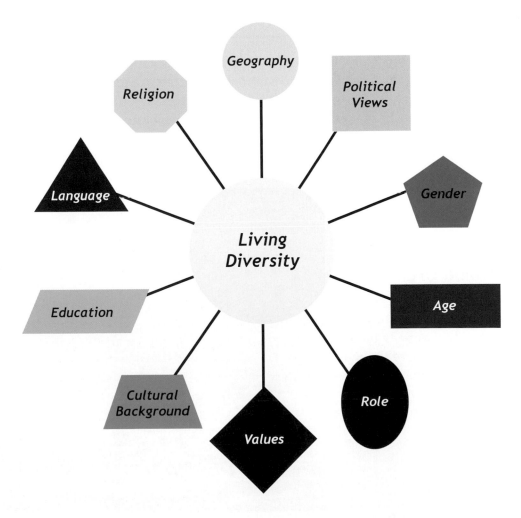

SUCCESSION PLANNING:
A PERSONAL, TRANSFORMATIONAL EXPERIENCE

Moving to the future requires the assurance someone will be able to do the work not only of today, but also the work of tomorrow. The role of the leader is paradoxically to eliminate the work of today when it is no longer needed and transform the role of the worker to one that is suitable to the newly defined work.

Leaders should continually focus on eliminating their leadership work as they know it today and create roles more suited to the knowledge and technological advances of the future. Yet so much of the work is about sustaining the present with less time to envision and adjust for the future.

Succession planning for managerial positions is practiced in less than 20% of organizations. Very little, if any, succession planning is done at the caregiver level—the most vital point of service in health care! As organizations struggle with recruitment and retention, an obvious source of retention is career planning for and with each caregiver.

Although the annual performance review is an optimal time for this discussion, the diverse members of the workforce require more than annual discussions of their future and role in the organization. Creating a succession planning team on each unit recognizes the untapped potential in the unit, the need to consider new ideas, and a willingness to confront the future in a proactive manner. This is not to minimize succession planning for key leadership roles—the message is that the leader must also embrace succession planning at the point-of-service in order to facilitate leadership evolution.

A Finely Tuned Orchestra!

The health care team functions at its best when there is a clear understanding of what the work is today and recognition that the team will face the needs of tomorrow with enthusiasm and the knowledge that all are in this work together.

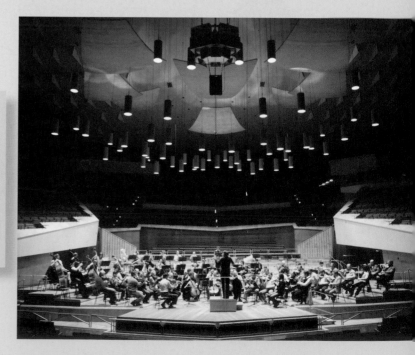

SUSTAINING CULTURE WITH AN EYE ON THE FUTURE

Much has been written about the electronic medical record and its potential benefits. Even more is being written and implemented specific to evidence-based architecture. Health care leaders, faced with new and uncertain processes, technology, genomic therapy, and physical space innovations, will be in the best position to create the best solutions for implementing new work and work processes. Leaders engaged in this future work will transform the health care experience from multiple perspectives.

The integration of facility design and technology into clinical processes must improve the quality and efficiency of patient safety, clinical outcomes, and caregiver satisfaction. In this section, information specific to the transformation of the workplace technology and architecture is presented.

Note:

The environment in which computerized and noncomputerized systems continue to exist is by nature less productive than either in isolation. The paradox of the transition from the age of paper and manual processes to the age of technology is that the initial inefficiency is inescapable. Until the transition has reached a critical tipping point of processes, productivity gains will be intermittent and limited. To halt all efforts in the name of productivity would be shortsighted and have serious quality and efficiency of patient negative long-term results. Working to manipulate current productivity system to extract value from processes in transition is frustrating and nonproductive.

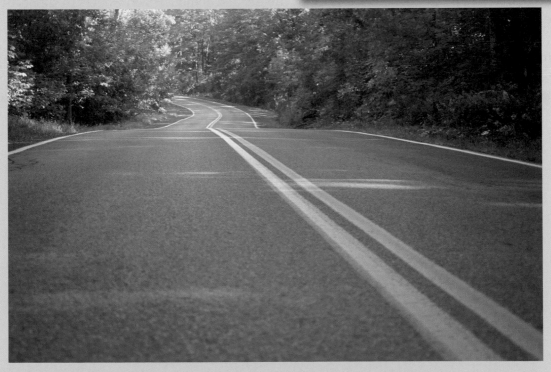

TECHNOLOGY CONSIDERATIONS

Fully wired environments create real-time data documentation and accessibility to multiple clinicians; availability of standardized care protocols for treatment and consistent documentation; and increased patient satisfaction with fewer requests for the same information.

Technology Innovations

Communication:
- Wireless personal phones for all caregivers, personal digital assistants, and multifunction email-phone-schedule-calendar products

Information Management:
- Decision support systems for schedules, cost-revenue management, clinical data processes and outcomes analysis; bar-coding documentation

Clinical Monitoring Systems:
- Physiologic monitoring of body functions

Virtual/Distance Health Care:
- Telemedicine for diagnosis and treatment

Clinical Documentation Systems:
- Electronic health record of all patient care, diagnostic results, treatments, medications, and outcomes. Multiple device strategies such as tablets and computers on wheels to support real-time documentation.

Interface Technology:
- Integration of appropriate systems

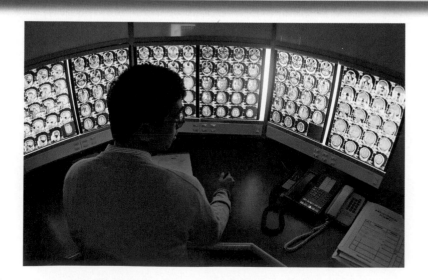

PHYSICAL ENVIRONMENT CONSIDERATIONS

More than 650 studies specific to evidence for designs in health care facilities have identified several characteristics that indeed will affect patient healing. The box to the right includes a representation of the most significant recommendations.

Physical Environment Innovations

- Private rooms
- Patient rooms with views of nature
- Enclosed medication administration rooms
- Decentralized and centralized workstations
- Multiple hand washing dispensers located based on human factors research
- Multipurpose interventional suites for surgery, catheterization labs, endoscopy, and interventional radiology
- Admission units for all patients except critical care
- Family space in all patient rooms
- Healing modalities of music, water features, and gardens
- Attractive space for staff lounges
- Separated greeter and unit clerk space

EXPECTED OUTCOMES

As leaders examine new technology and new architecture, they need to consider the composite health care environment. None of the changes can be done in isolation; there is an effect on the nurse, the patient, and the available physical space to accommodate the new equipment.

Leaders must examine each and every new option from the perspective of the mission and values of the organization and the ever-present question, "Will this change sustain or improve our level of excellence and at what cost?" What is the evidence for making this change?

The following list is a sampling of outcomes that are anticipated as a result of the ongoing projects dedicated to creating futuristic facilities, optimal technology and a culture of healing that positively impacts, patients, caregivers, the organization and the community.

1. Reduce staff stress and fatigue

2. Decrease patient falls

3. Decrease preventable adverse medication errors

4. Decrease nosocomail infections

5. Increase physician satisfaction

6. Improve accuracy and timeliness of documentation

7. Increase compliance with best practice protocols

8. Decrease employee back injuries

9. Decrease the need for medications

10. Decrease turnover

11. Increase fulfillment level of caregivers

12. Decrease turnaround time from order to treatment

New Communication Technology for Improved Management of Patient Care Events

Consider the situation in which a sentinel event occurs on a patient unit. With available wireless communication technology and the fully wired electronic medical record, multiple individuals can communicate, collaborate, and develop a real-time plan of action-all remotely, if needed. The action plan to correct the situation can be communicated to all caregiver's voice communication followed by an email notification-this is real-time performance improvement! What is the effect on the organization? On existing committee? On turnaround time? On patient care outcomes?

References

Block, P. (2004). Creating healthy conditions for service: A time to heal. *Reflections of Nursing Leadership*, 29(4), 20-22.

Brill, N. (1976). *Teamwork: Working together in the human services*. Toronto, Ontario, Canada: Lippincott.

Greene, J. (2005, March). What nurses want: Different generations different expectations. *Hospitals & Health Networks*, 34-42.

Hallowell, E. M. (2005). Overloaded circuits: Why smart people underperform. *Harvard Business Review*, 83(1), 55-62.

Krairiksh, M., & Anthony, M. K. (2001). Benefits and outcomes of staff nurse participation in decision making. *JONA*, 18(5), 16-33.

Longest, B. B. Jr. (1974). Relationships between coordination, efficiency, and quality of care in general hospitals. *Hospital Administration*, 19, 65-86.

Suggested Readings

Dolan, T. C. (2005). Increasing succession planning. *Healthcare Executive*, 20(3), 6.

The Center for Health Design: The Pebble Project. Concord, CA: Author (www.healthdesign.org/research/pebble).

Watson, C. A. (2005). Integration of technology and facility design: Implications for nursing administration. *JONA*, 35(5), 217-219.

Ulrich, R., Quan, X., Zimring, C., Josepy, A., & Choudhary, R. (2004). *The role of the physical environment in the hospital of the 21st century: A once-in-a-lifetime opportunity*. Concord, CA: Center for Health Design.

UNIT 5: SEARCHING FOR EXCELLENCE: RECRUITING THE BEST

1. ASSESSING THE WORKPLACE

2. MARKET REALITIES OF RECRUITING

3. SELLING YOUR ORGANIZATION

4. INTERVIEWING FOR EXCELLENCE

5. SOCIALIZING NEW EMPLOYEES

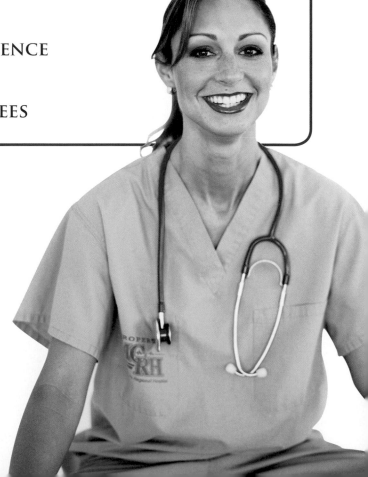

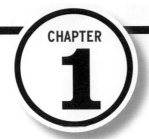

CHAPTER

1

ASSESSING THE WORKPLACE

No workplace remains stagnant. Regular and focused assessments are important processes in ensuring that the appropriate caregivers with the appropriate skills are available to do the contemporary work of nursing.

Recruiting is about more than merely finding warm bodies to fill vacant positions. In times of scarcity, the desire for goods is paramount—goods that get the job done often without regard to quality. If one desperately needs transportation, any vehicle will suffice—a bicycle, a van, an SUV, a limousine, a brand-new vehicle or one 10 years old. So, too, with the health care field; the significant shortage of numbers of health care workers has resulted in recruitment that is often focused on filling positions with employees that do not always have the essential skills and abilities needed for the work of health care that supports organizational goals and values.

The age-old practice of hiring the first available individual with less than adequate abilities to fill open positions serves to foster dissatisfaction and turnover rather than create a sustainable, highly functioning team. The goal of recruitment is to identify potential employees who will thrive in the organization and be reluctant to leave the organization because of their high level of satisfaction, and select employees who will be protective of the team's integrity. Ultimately, all employees will be able to experience the joy of health care and thrive in a workplace they truly love.

Some recruited individuals do not have values and beliefs congruent with the organization's mission and goals. Individuals with skills for basic care are placed in oncology units or those with average communication skills are placed in complex work environments such as the emergency department or critical care. People are needed with not only expertise in technical services and equipment management but also in building relationships based on therapeutic communication.

In this section, the following planning processes to support recruitment are presented:

1. Describing the characteristics of the organization and specific department

2. Developing a waiting list as the ultimate goal of recruiters

3. Creating a white paper for recruitment that can be used by internal and external audiences to better understand the work and outcomes of the organization

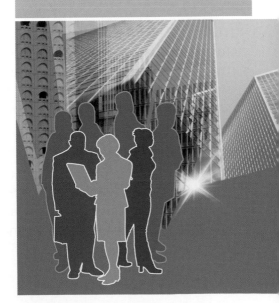

Assessing the Workplace 417

STEP 1.

DEVELOP AN OVERVIEW OF YOUR ORGANIZATION

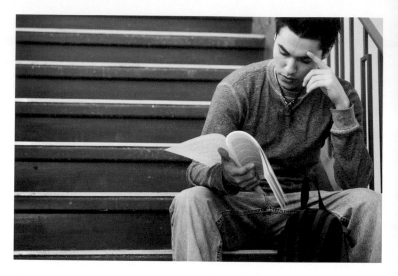

Workplace Desirability

Why would anyone want to work at your organization? Is it the location, the pay scale, benefits, reputation for quality care, research commitment, affiliation with an educational institute, or something else? Potential employees are drawn to organizations for a wide variety of reasons that are often not identified prior to hiring. As organizations seek to stabilize their workforce, knowing the characteristics of the organization can be helpful in identifying and selecting the right employees. This information creates the foundation for the white paper of your particular work setting.

The competition among employers for competent caregivers is intense and relentless. Each employer uses multiple strategies (not all of which are evidence based) to attract new employees. Some recruitment strategies, such as the sign-on bonus, provide a short-term approach but a long-term negative effect on morale.

The complexity and cost of workload management require that leaders recruit on the basis of evidence for efficient and effective use or resources. To market one's workplace, a clear understanding of the workplace is needed: What is the organization selling? What is the work to be done? What is the culture in which the work occurs: How is the work recognized and valued?

The challenges inherent in the health care marketplace with the short supply and excess demand for health care workers are further intensified with turnover of competent practitioners. Knowing that one of every three nurses has reported dissatisfaction with acute care employment calls for significant and meaningful action to stabilize the health care workforce. This begins with filling vacant positions with individuals that fit the work and the culture of the organization.

To begin this process, leaders must identify the specific information that is important to attract and ultimately retain employees. This includes the level of quality of patient care, the level of safety for patients and employees, expected professional behaviors, work processes, teamwork, and technology resources. Each of these affects potential employees in different ways, but are all important in ensuring that the organization is a quality setting for health care. Interested employees want to know what to expect from an organization—the culture, the work, and the accountabilities for each employee.

To attract employees who will fit an organization's needs, the workplace must be desirable, meet the needs of potential employees, and embrace and engage them with a spirit of vitality and concern. In this next section, an overview of each of the six key areas—patient care, safety, professionalism, patient care delivery model, teamwork, and technology (see figure below)—is presented as the basis to assess the workplace and identify those areas of strength that can be used to facilitate recruitment efforts.

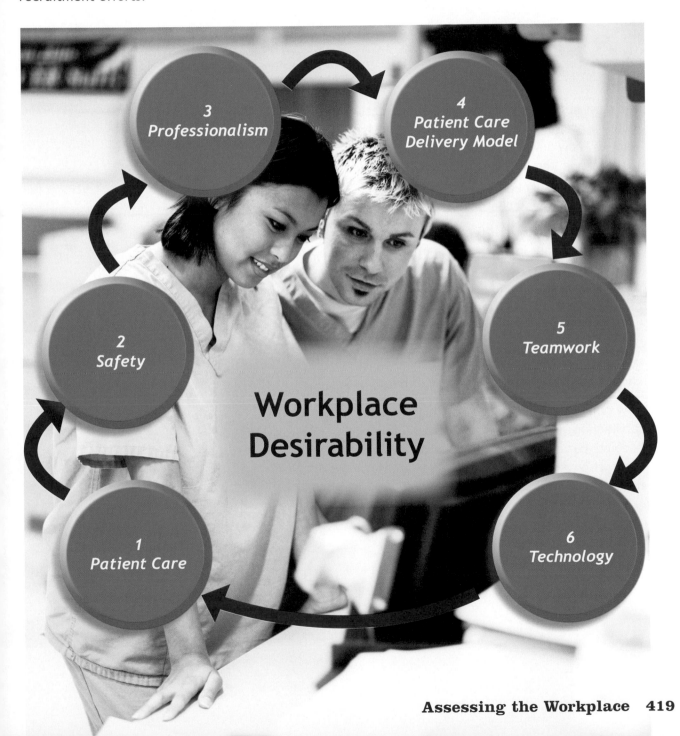

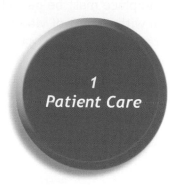

1
Patient Care

The most important variable of workplace desirability is patient care. Prospective employees want to know how the organization cares for its patients and the outcomes of that care. The emphasis on quality patient care is a reflection of the organization's commitment to excellence.

Patient satisfaction is affected by many variables, some more important than others. Most organizations are aware of their levels of patient satisfaction and readily identify areas of strength and opportunity. This information can be leveraged in recruiting employees to be sure that the organization's goals are advanced; potential employees can enhance current success and address areas of need.

New employees who can support high levels of satisfaction and help improve areas of need become partners in supporting high levels of satisfaction and addressing those areas of need.

Patient and Family Expectations

The following list includes expectations from patients and their families:

- Clinical improvement/relief of symptoms (competent caregivers)
- Absence of adverse outcomes (a safe environment)
- Time with members of the health care team (adequate staffing)
- Information and inclusion in plan of care (communication)
- Consideration and respect for privacy, values, preferences, needs, and family enhance current success and address
- Friendly staff
- Timely response to requests (adequate staffing)
- Comfortable setting/relief of pain
- Clean, quiet environment
- Information/instructions for discharge

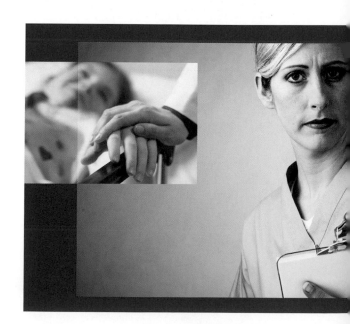

THE SECOND VARIABLE OF WORKPLACE DESIRABILITY IS SAFETY

Selling your organization should include a clear understanding of its commitment to patient and employee safety and demonstration of supportive practices. Specifically, there should be evidence of coordination of work processes—the seamless flow of services, information, and technology that emphasizes flawless execution of processes. This evidence is reflected in the outcomes of patient care, namely, medication errors, patient falls, number of emergency codes (failure to rescue), and nosocomial infections.

Although much attention has been given to patient safety in the past 5 years, there is still a great need for more aggressive improvements. Providers, organizations and policymakers are embroiled in efforts to improve the understanding of errors and creation of incentives that will generate changes in culture, systems, training, and technology to improve safety. More work is needed in securing patient and employee safety.

Recruitment Information

There are many approaches to consider in reducing medical errors. Policymakers, health care professionals, and the public all have ideas but are not in total agreement as to which approaches are the best. Examples of recommendations include the following:

1. Developing systems to avoid medical errors

2. Increasing number of hospital nurses

3. Providing single-bed rooms

4. Ensuring adequate lighting

5. Installing enclosed medication preparation rooms

6. Limiting certain high-risk procedures to high-volume centers

7. Using only physicians trained in intensive care medicine in intensive care units

8. Increasing the use of computerized ordering systems

9. Converting to electronic medical records

10. Requiring public reporting of medical errors

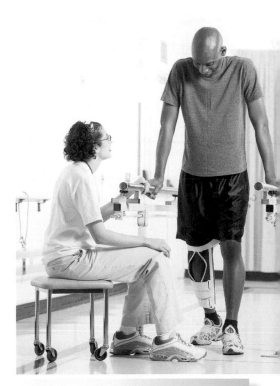

Note:

The most significant design feature to reduce nosocomial infections, reduce medical errors, greatly lessen noise, improve patient confidentiality and privacy, increase social support by families, and increase patient satisfaction with health care is the single-bed room (Ulrich et al., 2004).

EMPLOYEE SAFETY

Health care ranks as the second highest industry for occupational injury and illness in the country. Back injuries, needlesticks, workplace violence, and exposure to respiratory agents are among the leading incidents affecting worker safety.

Characteristics of a Safe Environment

- Protocols for safe staffing

- Availability of physician intensivists

- Unit-based pharmacists

- Read-back verbal orders practice

- Standardized abbreviations and dose designation

- Clearly executed advance directives

- Pressure ulcer evaluation on admission

- DVT evaluation upon admission

- Prophylactic beta-blockers for at-risk surgical patients

- Effective methods of preventing central venous catheter-associated bloodstream infections

- Commitment to handwashing/decontamination

- Medication preparation rooms clean, orderly, well lit, and free of clutter, distraction and noise

- No-lift environment

- Equipment to support no-lifting

- Protection from patient violence

- Evidence-based architecture

Safety Checklist

✓ Is there a safety and health committee?

✓ Is the membership multidisciplinary?

✓ Do staff members participate on the committee?

✓ Is there equipment to assist with patient lifting and prevent caregiver injury?

✓ Does the facility use safer needle and sharps devices and needleless systems?

✓ Is there a program for fit testing respiratory masks?

✓ What precautions are in place to address latex allergies?

✓ What systems are in place for emergency preparedness such as bioterrorism, mass casualties, and natural disasters?

✓ Is there open discussion of errors?

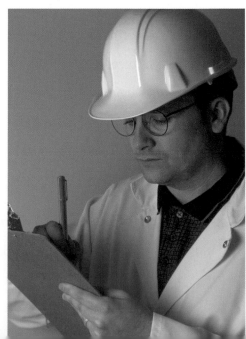

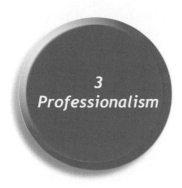

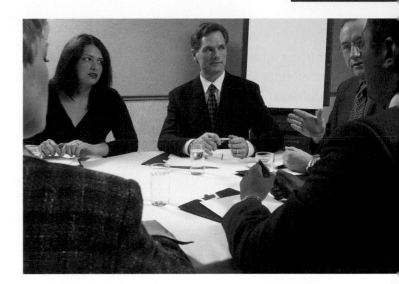

3
Professionalism

The third variable of workplace desirability to include in recruitment discussions is professionalism. Most leaders believe their organization supports professionalism through management style, policies, models of care, and role expectations. They support professional behaviors and in turn act as professionals themselves.

Every member of the organization is a recruiter and an exemplar of the value and excellence of the organization. Although not always in the "recruiting" frame of mind, each employee reflects attitudes, values, and respect for the work and the organization in which they work. Leaders are challenged to ensure that the appropriate images and messages about the organization are given by employees in their daily work. Many individuals have been influenced by the caring, competent work of nurses in the emergency department, the delivery room, and nearly every other area of patient, family, and caregiver interaction.

UNPROFESSIONAL BEHAVIORS

The following behaviors are considered unprofessional and undermine efforts to achieve high levels of professionalism:

1. Communicates subversively; seldom addresses concerns to the right person
2. Communicates with sarcasm
3. Fails to take accountability for actions: seldom admits to making a mistake
4. Fails to follow rules
5. Manipulates others and misrepresents the real issue
6. Rationalizes aberrant behaviors
7. Threatens others
8. Criticizes the organization to others
9. Resists self-assessment of behaviors and their effect on others
10. Rarely apologizes for inappropriate behaviors

PROFESSIONAL BEHAVIORS

Recruiting information should include specific information as to how the organization defines professionalism and the behaviors expected of employees. The expressions of professionalism can be seen in many positive and negative or unprofessional behaviors. The following five behaviors reflect high levels of professionalism and should be expected of all employees:

1. **Emotional competence:** All employees should be able to sense their setting and moderate actions appropriately. Such behaviors reflect the professionalism and maturity essential for health care workers. The ability to be able to motivate oneself and persist in the face of frustrations; to control impulses and delay gratification; to regulate one's moods and keep distress from swamping the ability to think; and to empathize and to hope is the expectation of health care workers.

2. **Membership in a professional organization** is evidence of commitment to one's discipline. Individuals who support and contribute to the standards of one's discipline are able to assess compliance with expected behaviors and make recommendations for changes when the practice is outdated. Leadership behavior implies that one is involved in shaping the standards of the discipline. New employees need to understand the expectations of the employer regarding professional organizations, and employers must understand the individual's commitment.

3. **Leading and following:** Professional behaviors include the art of followership. Not everyone can be in charge; someone needs to lead and others need to follow to get the work done. Individuals can be leaders and followers depending on the specific situation and expertise needed. Knowing when to lead and when to follow requires self-management, effective communication, teamwork, and engagement to the work of the organization. An understanding of the expectations of leading and following within the context of shared leadership is essential. Whereas this discussion is often confusing, both the employer and potential employee need to be clear that in organizations dedicated to excellence, shared decision making is the norm; however, in some situations such as compliance to regulations, there can be no discussion about the regulation and followership is the appropriate behavior. Too much control over decision making reflects an autocratic approach.

4. **Accountability for personal development:** An important professional behavior is ensuring continuing competence, owning ongoing development, and implementing new behaviors when appropriate. Most organizations support professional development for employees; however, the recruitment concern in selecting new employees is to identify the past practices of the individual in continuing personal development. Is continuing education evident through the work experiences as well as personal responsibility for development? The real question for employers is "Does the prospective employee expect the organization to provide 100% of lifelong learning experiences and funding or is it a joint accountability?"

5. **Ethical behavior:** Both the employer and potential employee need to be clear about how difficult patient care situations are addressed. If caregivers believe that their primary obligation to the patient is compromised, an ethical dilemma is present. When there is a lack of congruency between individual patient needs and the demands of the organization, caregivers become disenfranchised and dissatisfied with their work and turnover may result.

Being able to work in an organization in which difficult patient care problems are discussed and decided so the primary obligation to the patient is honored is essential for caregiver satisfaction and retention. Caregivers are empowered, trusted, and included in the decision-making processes of ethical dilemmas.

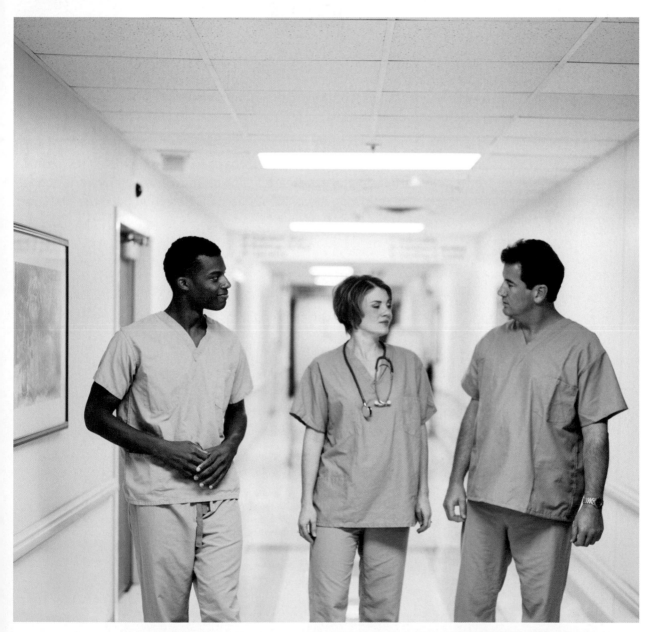

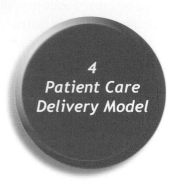

4
*Patient Care
Delivery Model*

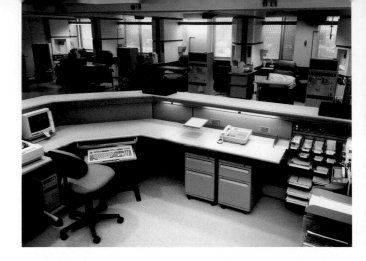

The fourth variable of workplace desirability is the patient care delivery model. The work of the organization requires complex processes and structures to ensure that the desired level of excellence is supported. The way in which the work of the organization is viewed, valued, supported, and evaluated reflects the culture of the organization.

Perhaps the most important issue is the individual's daily work assignment—what is expected each day? Employers want to know how prospective employees approach work, and employees want to know how they will be treated. Potential employees clearly want to know how the work is accomplished and their role in the work. The following areas should be considered by both the employer and potential employee.

Delivery model:
- Is there a team approach or is work expected to be done by the individual—primary care versus team nursing?
- What is the core staffing plan?
- What is the percentage of licensed, credentialed, skilled, unlicensed, and support staff?
- What is the percentage of external staff?

Decision making:

- Is the role of each professional valued as an autonomous professional with accountability for interprofessional collaboration?
- Is permission required from certain individuals on a routine basis to accomplish work? From physicians, nurses, or LPNs?

Assignments:

- Who makes the assignment?
- Does the employee have input into the assignment process?
- Is work overload addressed? Or are employees expected to "do their best" when there is additional work, without additional assistance?
- Are the assignments adjusted during the shift? If yes, how and when does this happen? If no, why does this happen?

Span of control:

- How many individuals report to the supervisor?
- How often does communication occur between the supervisor and the staff person?

Levels of education:

- What is the percentage of employees with a high school education, college education, and graduate education?
- Is there support for continuing education?

Shift lengths/schedules/overtime:

- Who makes the schedule?
- How are requests managed?
- Are shift lengths variable?
- Is overtime expected?

Evaluation: satisfaction, turnover:

- What is the level of satisfaction for the employees in the department?
- How frequently is staff feedback requested?
- What is the turnover percentage for the past year, the past 6 months?
- How do external staff (registry, travelers) describe the work environment?

Expectations:

- Are the target levels of performance identified for patient care?
- Are target levels of performance identified for employee satisfaction?
- Are target levels of performance for turnover identified?
- Are there standards for communication? Email etiquette? Response/turnaround time, etc.?

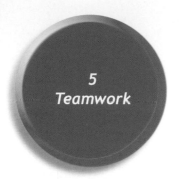

5
Teamwork

The Best Recruiting Strategy: A Fully Engaged Caregiver

How many times have you heard someone tell the story of a positive experience about the care of a loved one? Indeed, the best recruitment tool is a caregiver who is engaged and loving the work of the healer and shares that dedication by living the role of the healer.

The fifth variable of workplace desirability is teamwork. Health care recruiters are challenged to discover the "real" person—how the potential employee functions as an individual and as a team member. Unfortunately, minimal information is gained in the interview due to the artificial nature of the process, yet this information is vital to be sure that the prospective employee is competent to support collaborative practice.

In spite of the fact that patients and professionals benefit from collaboration, team members often experience strained and adversarial relationships. Expertise in collaborative practice and interdisciplinary approaches to patient care has been developed primarily through individual education and experiences in the practice setting. More recently, formalized training has been included in medical schools to promote interprofessional acceptance and respect of team members as a means to create more productive alliances. Effective collaboration decreases the cost of health care and benefits both the patient and team members. Misunderstandings are clarified, effective dialog occurs to develop the optimal plan, and an atmosphere of openness allows for further discussions without fear of criticism and rejection.

Learning to work with others is a cooperative venture for physicians, nurses, therapists and support staff that is based on shared authority and responsibility, open communication, and shared decision making as the means to provide optimal clinical service and patient empowerment.

Collaboration is a complex process that requires ongoing self-development, team development, and work in basic communication skills. The prospective employee needs to know how collaboration is valued by the organization, specifically how the members of the department interact and what the expectations are for successful employment.

ATTITUDES FOR EXCELLENT TEAMWORK

Effective collaboration and teamwork require constant attention and affirmation of appropriate behaviors and eliminating or at least minimizing the barriers to collaboration.

> Team members are viewed as collaborators and colleagues.

> Team members are not viewed as assistants to each other.

> Interprofessional collaboration requires mutual goal setting and satisfying work relationships.

> Healthy, effective relationships require attention and nurturing; validation and regular feedback as to the effectiveness of teamwork are essential.

> All team members are expected to identify issues and recommend changes that will improve communication, relationships, and patient care outcomes.

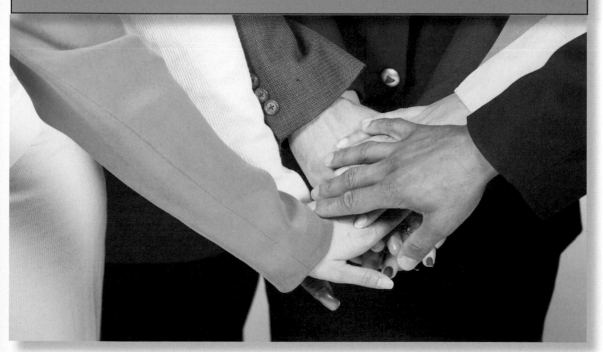

Barriers to teamwork and effective collaboration are both subtle and overt. The following list identifies cultural, educational, economic, and communication styles that can create barriers.

BARRIERS TO TEAM COLLABORATION

- Differing education levels: highly educated to illiterate

- Differing cultural/ethnic values and beliefs

- Social status: established in the community, financial level

- Sex role stereotypes: male, female, preferences

- Language: polished, high-level vocabulary, slang

- Professional elitism

- Role ambiguity

- Independent decision making: elitist, non-team players

- Acting spontaneously

- Withholding information—partial sharing of information

- Scapegoating; looking for someone to blame

- Disruptive team members—side conversations, joking, coming late to meetings

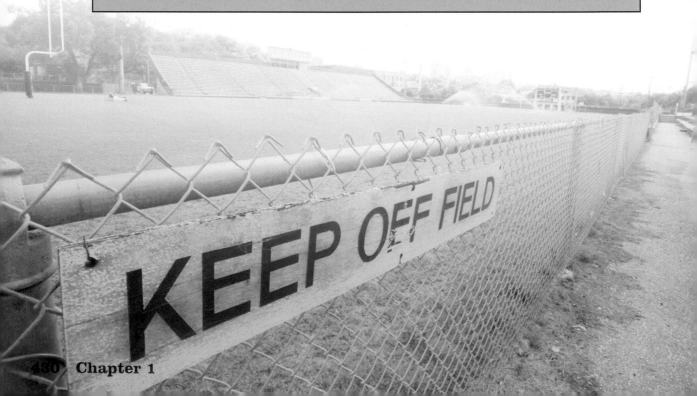

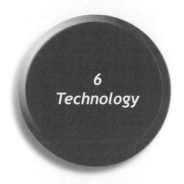

**6
Technology**

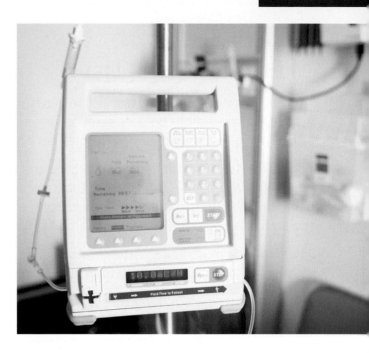

The sixth variable of workplace desirability is technology. There is no escaping technology in health care—automated phone systems, talking elevators, computerized billing systems, bar-coded employee badges, electronic documentation, and integrated-computerized infusion pumps that record doses administered and vital signs simultaneously. The integration of technology into the humanistic work of caregivers requires mastery of the work of healing and the competency in the use of technology as a means to an end. Although the effect of an increasingly hi-tech environment of the work of caregivers continues to become increasingly visible, the real effect on the work of caregivers has yet to be realized. The goal is to recognize technology as merely a means to an end and not the end in itself.

Recruiters are challenged to determine both the prospective employee's level of comfort with technology and the attitude and engagement in the process of continuing introductions of new devices and processes. Most applicants proclaim their support and strong interest in technology generically. Others claim they are not good with technology or they are not a "computer person."

Be specific in where the organization is in the technology transformation, what support is provided to assist employees in the development of expertise, and the accountabilities of employees specific to technology.

Technology Levels
- Keyboard skills
- Software program knowledge
- Hardware knowledge
- Device knowledge: handhelds, computer on wheels (COW)
- Troubleshooting systems
- Downtime procedure knowledge

In general, all technology is evolving, and the challenge is to determine how comfortable and flexible each individual is with the processes of moving to new devices and systems. Is it an adventure that is embraced or is it an overwhelming interference that impedes workflow? Both types of individuals are present in organizations. How the leaders guide these processes is significant in maximizing use of each piece of technology.

STEP 2.

CREATE A WAITING LIST

The notion to create a waiting list in times of shortage may seen unrealistic, yet revolutionary visions are needed. To be successful an organization has to stand several levels above the crowd. Although that effort is daunting, it must not be considered impossible.

Now is the time to challenge and change the mental models about the workforce. Leaders must create new approaches that support the transformation of traditional recruitment practices to those based on belief in the ability of the system to change, the power of one, the strength of teams, and the ethical accountability to create a better health care experience.

To begin, one must first create new expectations and work to make the vision a reality—create a waiting list for the opportunity to be a health care worker!

People want to work in the presence of excellence. The best hospitals and health care organizations have less trouble getting the required resources. They have become the beacons of hope for health care workers. They have proven by their results that they are the best places to work— employees are valued, are able to do the work for which they are prepared, feel like a member of the team, and are compensated fairly. Besides being excellent workplaces, top-performing organizations consistently and methodically integrate all recruitment work as a reflection of the mission of the organization. Fragmented, faddish, and short sighted activities are seldom, if ever, used by high-performing organizations.

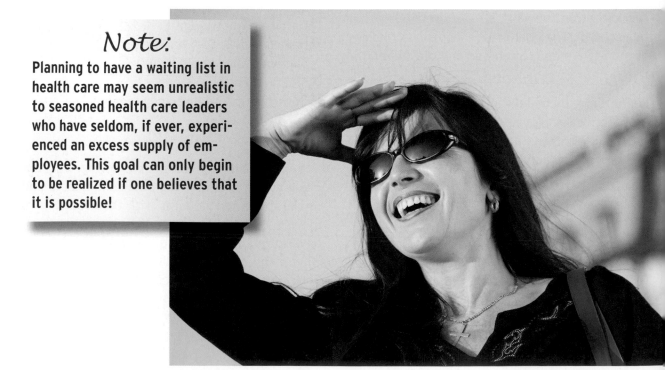

Note:

Planning to have a waiting list in health care may seem unrealistic to seasoned health care leaders who have seldom, if ever, experienced an excess supply of employees. This goal can only begin to be realized if one believes that it is possible!

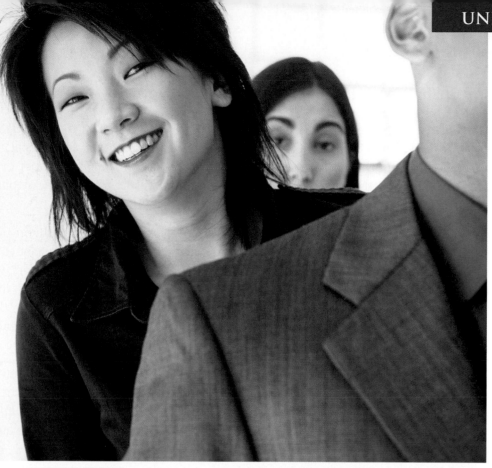

Key Steps in Creating a Waiting List

☐ *Identify why the organization or unit is the best and only place to work.*

☐ *Create a white paper for each department in the organization that describes the workplace culture, goals, and accomplishments.*

☐ *Define a waiting list—applicants with completed paperwork, tentative acceptance of a position.*

☐ *Create target goals for the waiting list, for example, a minimum of two acceptable candidates for each position.*

☐ *Create processes to stay in touch with those on the waiting list, for example, institute monthly personal communication with each individual on the waiting list.*

☐ *Encourage temporary employment for interested staff to work in a temporary on-call position to learn more about the organization.*

STEP 3.
CREATE A WHITE PAPER

Prospective employees need to know as much as possible about the organization before making a commitment. Unfortunately, the traditional interview is often brief, formal, and an unnatural setting to learn about the critical issues of the organization. The white paper offers a vehicle to summarize the characteristics, expectations, and outcomes of the specific department as well as the organization.

A white paper typically argues a specific position or solution to a problem. Although white papers take their roots in governmental policy, they have become a common tool to introduce technology innovations and products. A typical search engine query on "white paper" will return millions of results, many focused on technology-related issues. As a recruitment tool, the white paper argues for the organization of interest and provides specific information to assist the employer and prospective employee in making an evidence-based employment decision. Health care white papers can serve as a recruiting document and template for interviewing interested candidates.

Most white papers give important and substantive information; however, the information is only the tip of the iceberg. Educated and knowledgeable individuals appreciate the information and are appreciative of the organization's willingness to share essential information and take time to explain the issues encountered by the organization. Interested individuals are more able to make intelligent decisions about the organization.

> **The white paper is a clear, concise overview of the organization and the work of the department.**

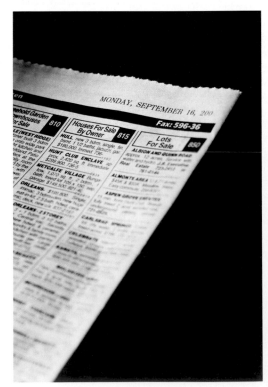

Note:
For two centuries, the British government has published its official policy statements between white covers. Somewhere along the line, "white paper" became shorthand for "official report." Today, any short treatise intended to educate customers is called a white paper.

WHAT'S IMPORTANT IN A WHITE PAPER?

Clarity

Readers of white papers are usually individuals looking for information about a specific topic. They appreciate clear explanations, charts, and diagrams. They won't read material that is dense with jargon.

Actionable Intelligence

A good white paper doesn't just explain; it provides context. Most readers aren't fascinated by broad descriptions and lofty goals. They want to understand how these issues are relevant to them.

Balance

The white paper is more than a sales pitch. It brings the interested individual to the level of understanding that's needed to understand the issues and situation. It lays out the information in a balanced way, and explains the positive and negative attributes of the issue.

THE HEALTH CARE WHITE PAPER: AN EXAMPLE

Creating a white paper for potential staff and leaders is the first step. It can serve as the template for interviewing and as an informational tool for current employees.

My Health Care Organization, USA
The White Paper

We need you in our organization! Our organization is looking for individuals willing and able to commit to the best health care service possible. We are working to achieve Magnet accreditation and national recognition as a Top 100 Hospital in the country. We are dedicated to evidence-based practice in a healing environment. Our facility is 5 years old; has all private rooms, which includes family space; and has a moderate amount of technology and computerization.

Patient care: Our unit provides care to medical patients with primary diagnoses of congestive heart failure, pneumonia, and diabetes. More than 50% of our patients are Hispanic and most speak Spanish only. Patient satisfaction is at the 87th percentile; our goal is to be above the 90th percentile by the end of the year.

Other satisfaction scores are:

Nurses' attitudes toward requests	78th percentile
Accommodations and comfort for visitors	92nd percentile
Noise level	88th percentile
Physician concern for patients	91st percentile
Adequacy of pain relief	94th percentile

Clinical outcomes:

Falls	3 per 1000 patient-days
Medication errors	<6 per 1000 patient-days

Safety: All departments have a unit-specific safety committee that has membership on a facility-wide safety committee. In addition to falls and medication errors, emphasis is placed on patient identification with the new bar-coding system, and handwashing to minimize nosocomial infections, which are fewer than three per 1000 patient-days.

The physical environment is very important in our organization. Adequate lighting, enclosed medication preparation rooms, and noise minimization are important. Employee safety is stressed through our no-lift environment, no-carpet environment, and motorized beds. Needlestick injuries were fewer than four last year; four minor back injuries occurred last year with no lost work time.

continued

continued from p. 433

Professionalism: 45% of caregivers are certified in their specialty and 28% belong to their professional organizations.

Staff satisfaction is above average. Several areas of opportunity exist in the relationship between the staff and immediate supervisor. Overall satisfaction is 4.1 on a 5 scale. Other scores include:

My immediate supervisor is a good coach	3.8/5
Change has occurred as a result of the last employee survey	4.1/5
My opinions count in this organization	4.3/5

Patient care delivery model: The team model is used for patient care delivery and assignments. Each caregiver is expected to be autonomous in their own specialty and integrative with the team. No decisions are ever made in isolation. Daily assignments are made by a designated staff member familiar with the patients and the staff providing the care. In general each supervisor is responsible for five to nine employees and meets with each employee at least monthly. The levels of education range include high school, college, and some graduate. Most nurses are associate degree prepared. The skill mix is 65% licensed and 35% nonlicensed; 8% external travelers are used. There is no mandatory overtime. Employees participate in creating work schedules within defined guidelines. Current facility turnover is 9% and unit turnover is 12%.

Teamwork: The team consists of physicians/hospitalists, advanced-practice nurses, registered nurses, licensed practical nurses, nursing assistants, social workers, therapists, and nutritionists. Teamwork is assessed monthly using an electronic survey available to all employees. Latest results are as follows:

My team functions at a high level	4/5
Everyone carries their share of the workload	3.5/5

Technology: Daily documentation is computerized for all caregivers except physicians. Medication administration is also computerized but not completely implemented. Clinical monitoring systems are electronic for vital signs, and cardiac monitoring, and are integrated into the documentation system. The goal of the organization is to be fully computerized and wireless in 3 years.

References

Stelzner, T. (2005). *What is a white paper?* Poway, CA: Stelzner Consulting. Retrieved November 21, 2005, from www.stelznercom/WhitePaper.

Ulrich, R., Quan, X., Zim ring, C., Joseph, A, & Choudhary, R. (2004). The role of the physical environment in the hospital of the 21st century: A once-in-a-lifetime opportunity. Concord, CA *Center for Health Design*, Robert Wood Johnson.

Suggested Readings

Berney, B., Needleman, J., & Kovner, C. (2005). Factors influencing the use of registered nurse overtime in hospitals, 1995-2000. *Journal of Nursing Scholarship*, 37(2), 165-172.

Hojat, M., Fields, S. K., Veloski, J. J., Griffiths, M., Cohen, M. J. M., & Plumb, J. D. (1999). Psychometric properties of an attitude scale measuring physician-nurse collaboration. *Evaluation & the Health Professions*, 22(2), 208-220.

Lindeke, L. L., & Sieckert, A M. (2005). Nurse-physician workplace collaboration. *Online Journal of Issues in Nursing* 10(1).

Wachter, R. M. (2004). The end of the beginning: Patient safety five years after "to err is human." *Health Affairs*, 23(2), W4-534-545.

CHAPTER 2

MARKET REALITIES OF RECRUITING

The challenge to match demand for health care services to the supply of resources is ever present for all leaders in all organizations.

The supply of competent health care workers fluctuates cyclically based on market conditions, changing job roles, social initiatives, financial resources, and competing job fields. Due to the very nature of the changing environment, each cycle is different from the last. Decreasing the gap between demand for health care services and the supply of resources to meet the needs of the community remains the primary goal of health care leaders.

In this section, the complexities of the health care marketplace are examined. Given that providers comprise the greatest portion of health care expenditures, knowledge of the marketplace is essential. Basic principles of economic theory, demand, supply, and price along with strategies to mediate the gap among demand, supply, and price are presented to assist leaders in making the best decisions possible in their challenge of providing safe staffing for quality patient care.

The gold standard of economics resource allocation in a perfectly competitive market has five characteristics:

1. There are many buyers and sellers with no single economic agent influencing the exchange of goods among market participants.
2. There is a standardized product.
3. There are no barriers to movement of firms into or out the market.
4. There is perfect information about market conditions that is available to all market participants.
5. There is a fully defined system of property rights in which ownership of all products and productive resources is assigned.

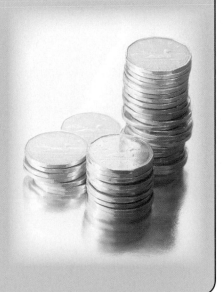

An understanding of the economic perspective on decision making is essential to understand in the current health care marketplace. In general, the economic system seeks to address the following:

1. What goods and services shall be produced?
2. How will services be provided?
3. For whom are the services provided?

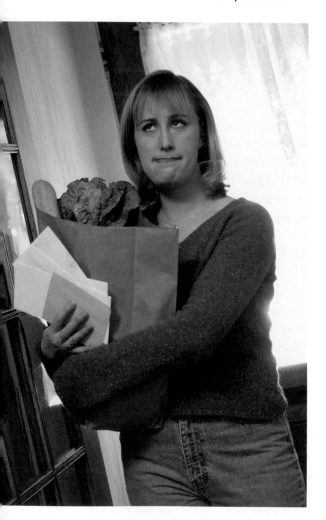

ECONOMICS: FIVE KEY CONCEPTS

1. **Economics**
   The social science that studies the production, distribution, and consumption of goods and services; how consumers, firms, governmental bodies, and other organizations make choices to overcome the problems of scarcity.

2. **Demand**
   The amount of services or product that consumes are willing and able to buy at a specific price.

3. **Supply**
   The quantity of a service or product that providers are willing and able to sell at a particular price.

4. **Scarcity**
   Scarcity exists when there are not enough resources to satisfy all demands.

5. **Unanticipated consequences**
   An interesting but sometimes confusing concept is that of "unanticipated consequences." Sometimes supply and demand get out of balance and cause additional problems. If demand goes astray, consumers may choose to stockpile the goods in anticipation of a shortage. As a result, the demand increases to unnecessary levels, causing producers to increase production—an unanticipated consequence. If this stockpiling did not occur, the rate of production of the goods would have met the demand. Similar scenarios can be instructive for those in the marketplace—perceived demand-supply imbalances must be analyzed carefully before taking action.

ECONOMIC PRINCIPLES AND HEALTH CARE

The market for health care services is considered an imperfect market because:

1. Health care is a heterogeneous product because the patient can experience a range of outcomes.

2. Patients who are insured have third-party payers covering their direct medical expenses.

3. A market price is lacking; there is no feedback mechanism that reflects the value of the resources used in health care.

4. Hospital patient costs are different for patients (consumers), providers (suppliers), insurance companies (third-party payers), and society.

5. The economic effects of pain and suffering are of concern to the patient and society, but may notbe relevant to a purely economic analysis of costs from the perspective of health care providers or third-party payers.

6. The range of productive inputs available to a health care leader and the outputs produced is significant.

In spite of the fact that many health care leaders attempt to apply the gold standard of economics to the health care marketplace, the reality is that there is very little congruence with these standards and the health care marketplace. Health care resources are allocated quite differently; there are limited economic agents (insurers, regulators, and payers), who strongly influence the exchange of health care services, products and services are personalized to each patient, numerous restrictions to competition exist through regulations and licensure, information diffusion is limited, and health care organizations are owned by both the community and the stockholders.

The complexity of health care services and products does not easily translate to discrete items that can be pulled off the shelf in a store, placed in a shopping cart, and paid for at the register. The result of health care services or products cannot be guaranteed; the outcome depends on many interrelated factors that are often beyond the control of the provider or the consumer-patient. Recruiting caregivers in this system requires that leaders possess knowledge of and sensitivity to the dynamic conditions of health care economics. Key players in the system are identified in five categories; consumers, providers, payers, suppliers, and regulators.

Health Care Key Players

Consumers: Those who use or intend to use the services of health care.

Providers: Those who provide and support health care services—physicians, nurses, pharmacists, therapists, technicians, and support personnel.

Payers: Those who pay for the services—patients, employers, federal and state programs, and commercial insurance plans.

Suppliers: Those who provide the technology, products for patient care, and pharmaceuticals.

Regulators: Policymakers who create and uphold standards for health care from a statutory, credentialing, or accrediting perspective.

DEMAND INFLUENCES

1. The community needs for health care services vary based on age-groups in the population.
   - Adult
   - Children
   - Elderly
   - Disabled
   - Mentally impaired
   - Medical, surgical, oncology, women and infants, rehabilitation

2. The source of funding for health care or who traditionally pays for health care. Three major sources of funding include:
   - Public
   - Private
   - Commercial

3. The location of services also influences demand. Access to care is a significant influence on the demand. Also, transportation to and from service providers is a significant influence. Major categories of service location include:
   - Urban
   - Suburban
   - Rural
   - Home health
   - Schools

4. Consumer knowledge/values/preferences. Consumer beliefs about health and the expectations about services directly affect the amount and specific services to be provided.

5. The levels of income from poverty to affluence affect demand for and location of service.

6. Available technology.
   - Computerized medical record
   - Clinical monitoring systems
   - Clinical information systems
   - Diagnostic equipment
   - Management information systems

7. Regulations/policy mandates. Numerous regulations specific to physical facilities, safety, clinical standards, operations, and staffing affect the level of demand for health care services.

DEMAND ASSESSMENT:
DETERMINING SPECIFIC COMMUNITY NEEDS FOR HEALTH CARE SERVICES

The specific health care needs of each community should be the guiding force in determining the demand for services. Knowing the needs of the community specific to the ages, clinical needs, values, cultures, and location of patients should be matched to the supply side of the health care equation. Each community must examine the need and determine how to create the most appropriate supply characteristics. For example:

1. If the ages of the community include a high birth rate and an increasing population older than 85 years, services must include women and infants, long-term care, and end-of-life.
2. If the community is predominantly Hispanic, health care services must be based on Hispanic values including Spanish-speaking providers.
3. If cancer, obesity, and mental illness are the common disease entities, then oncology, weight management, and mental health services must be available.

National Health Care Needs Categories: National Rankings

1. Cardiovascular
2. All cancers
3. Stroke
4. COPD
5. Accidents
6. Diabetes
7. Pneumonia/influenza
8. Alzheimer's
9. Nephritis
10. Septicemia

From Centers for Disease Control

Demographic Variables: National Population Data 2003

Births:	4,089,950 per year
Deaths:	2,443,387 per year
Average life expectancy:	
Male:	74.8
Female:	80.1
Older than 65:	15% of population

From Centers for Disease Control

Ethnic Groups: National Percentages

92%	White
1.5%	Hispanic
7.1%	African Americans
0.1%	Native Americans
0.5%	Asian/Pacific Islanders

From Bureau of Labor Statistics

SUPPLY INFLUENCES

Multiple factors influence the supply of health care services; providers, clinical expertise, funding, equipment/technology, and combinations of these In addition, variations in each factor necessarily affect other factors. For example, if funding for salaries increases, the supply of providers is affected positively. The following overview of supply influences and facts about the current supply of health care resources demonstrates the complexity and wide-reaching dynamics.

- *Physician*
- *Advanced-practice nurse*
- *Registered nurse*
- *Pharmacists*
- *Respiratory therapists*
- *Social workers*
- *Nutritionists*
- *Rehabilitation therapists*
- *Medical imaging technicians*
- *Licensed practical nurse*
- *Assistive personnel*

- *Cultural*
- *Age groups/generations*

1. *Available providers: specific types and levels of services*

2. *Clinical expertise/skills/competence of providers*

3. *Physical environment: number, types, and location of facilities*

4. *Funding for providers: source of payment for services*

5. *Equipment/technology*

- *Surgical*
- *Medical*
- *Women and infants*
- *Oncology*
- *Rehabilitation*

- *Urban*
- *Suburban*
- *Rural*
- *Home health*
- *Schools*

- *Private*
- *Commercial*
- *Federal/state*

- *Clinical monitoring systems*
- *Management information systems*
- *Clinical management systems*

SUPPLY FACTS: HEALTH CARE WORKERS

FACT

Health care services accounted for almost 20% of all job growth from 1994 to 2005. Employment opportunities in the health services industry are projected to increase 28% through 2012, compared with 16% for all industries combined.

Bureau of Labor Statistics, 2005

FACT

Nursing tops the list of the 10 occupations projected to have the most growth between 2002 and 2012.

Bureau of Labor Statistics, 2005

FACT

There are 2,694,540 licensed registered nurses in the United States.
- 5.4% of RNs are men.
- 9.1% of RNs are younger than the age of 30.
- 38% of male RNs are younger than age 40 compared with 31% of female RNs.

FACT

More than 126,000 registered nurse positions are unfilled in the United States; 400,000 will be needed when the baby boomers reach retirement.

Spratley et al., 2000

FACT

59% of all RNs work in a hospital.
18.2% of all RNs work in community/public health settings.

Note:

Men, particularly older men, probably looking for better employment options and economic security, are entering the nursing profession in greater numbers than ever before.

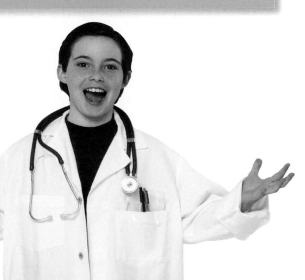

Market Realities of Recruiting   445

FACT

The average age (45) of the registered nurse workforce makes nursing the oldest occupational group in the United States. RNs are retiring faster than the system can replace

FACT

The number of nurses in the United States per capita, 7.9/1000, is below the world median.

FACT

Nurse staffing levels/acute care bed in the United States, 1.4 per acute care bed, are above the world median.

FACT

Each discipline has its unique supply and demand issues, particularly nursing. The new signs of increased entry into the labor market are in younger women in their early 30s, and men. However, there is still a significant shortage of nurses.

FACT

The employment of younger nurses (ages 21-34) grew by nearly 90,000 in 2003. This group is attracted to education programs that take the least amount of time to complete; 75% of the growth of younger RNS are recent graduates of associate degree programs.

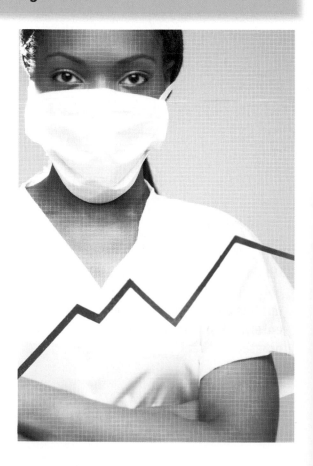

FACT

11% of African American nurses have master's or doctoral degrees compared with 10.4% of white nurses and 8.4% of Hispanic nurses.

FACT

The increase in unemployment in 2003, coupled with the increase in earnings provided a powerful economic incentive to induce RNs, particularly married RNs, to return to the labor market.

FACT

In the recent past, growth in nurse employment was seen from the reentry of older RNs (ages 50-64) into the workforce and the new entry of foreign-born nurses.

FACT

More nurses are satisfied with their jobs; the emphasis on patient care, management recognition for personal lives, satisfaction with salary and benefits, job security, and positive relationships with others and management increased from 21% in 2002 to 34% in 2004.

Buerhaus, et al., 2005

FACT

The growth in employment of RNs ages 35 to 49 decreased in 2003.

FACT

The number of U.S. physicians per capita is below the world median at 2.4/1000.

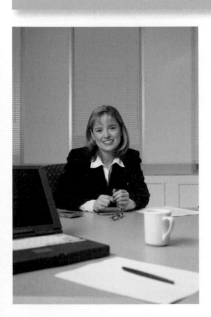

FACT

Between 1992 and 2000, there was a 28% increase in the number of RNs who chose non-nursing jobs because of dissatisfaction with nursing.

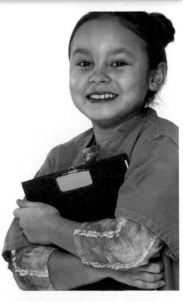

SUPPLY FACTS: SETTINGS AND TECHNOLOGY

There is an explosion of technology and a significant increase in the building of new health care facilities. The information and communications technology with the Internet, new and more sophisticated population databases, and research dissemination have supported the formation and mobilization of alliances with otherwise inaccessible partners. New technology, however, has inherent challenges in managing the confidentiality of information across the Internet and has not reached the disadvantaged groups.

In response to increasing population needs, thousands of hospital construction projects are under way in the United States. In many cases, these efforts have adopted new approaches to design and build patient care areas. Transforming the health care experience to achieve the optimal patient care experience using evidence-based approaches has become the goal for health care organizations involved in both replacement and new building.

Number of hospitals in the United States	5729
Total staffed beds	955,768
Total expenses for all hospitals	$533,853,359

From American Hospital Association (*www.aha.org*)

Note:

The United States is an early adopter of medical technologies. It does not acquire medical technology at high levels once the technology has diffused widely. New technology tends to be adopted in selected areas in limited quantities.

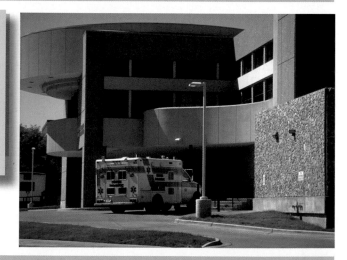

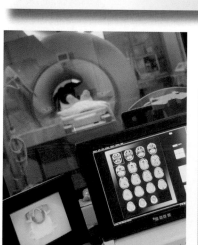

- Resources per capita: The United States has fewer resources per capita—hospital beds, physicians, nurses, MRI and CT scanners—than other countries.
- Hospital beds per capita: The United States is in the bottom world quartile at 2.9 hospital beds per 1000.
- MRI units: The United States is slightly above the world median at 8.2 units per million.
- CT scanners: The United States is below the world median at 12.8 scanners per million.

Price

Supply and demand are fundamentally influenced by price, which is determined and maintained based on complex interrelated market conditions. Several price or cost facts in health care are presented to underscore the multiple variables in the cost of health care.

Health Care Costs: Facts and Figures

For the past 50 years, health care spending has been characterized by unsustainable spending increases that are followed by aggressive cost-containment initiatives. Prices, technology, aging, waste, inefficiency, the legal system, new disease patterns, corporate consolidation, providers, and consumers have all been studied to determine the cause of the spiraling increases in spending.

U.S. Expenditures on Health Care 2002
$1.5 Trillion/Year
14.9% Gross Domestic Product (GDP)

U.S. citizens spent $5440/per capita for health care in 2002, 53% more than any other country.

Cost sharing, rather than reductions in spending is receiving increased attention.

Health Care Funding Sources:
Private 54.1%
Public   45.9%

Believed magic-bullet solutions such as consumer choice, disease management, evidence-based practice, and information technology are of great interest to policymakers but have yet to show evidence of affecting health care spending.

Nursing Wages
The average annual earnings for full-time employed RNs are $46,782.

RN earnings increased in 2003 for a second straight year, but not as much as the increase in 2002.

Data from Anderson et al. (2005).

THE COSTS OF TURNOVER

The costs associated with recruitment and turnover represent significant expenses for the organization. These costs have been estimated and integrated into most organizations' annual financial planning and budgeting processes. Although it is difficult to capture all of the direct and indirect costs of turnover, increasing specificity of these costs are emerging. The following data exemplify the advances in gathering and analyzing these data.

Conservative Estimates of Recruitment/Turnover

1. Direct costs
   $10,800/medical-surgical RN (21% of costs)
   $11,520/specialty RN (18% of costs)
   - Advertising
   - Hiring replacements
     (internal, registry, traveling nurses at 20% above the normal wage and benefit package)
   - Overtime hour for current staff
   - Sign-on bonuses
   - Orientation
   - Initial lower productivity of new hires

2. Indirect cost (79% of costs)
   - $29,200/medical-surgical RN (79% of costs)
   - $47,403/specialty RN (82% of costs)
   - Decreased productivity
   - Decreased quality care
   - Increased burden if responsibility on core staff due to unfamiliarity of external staff with the organization's policies and patients
   - Decreased morale of core staff

$

$

$

$

$

Cost of RN Turnover
Pre-hire costs: *$53,500*
Post-hire costs: *$8,600 to $13,600*
Total: *$62,100 to $67,000*

Data from Jones (2005).

DEMAND, SUPPLY, AND PRICE:
INTERRELATED VARIABLES OF THE MARKETPLACE

The health care marketplace is complex and affected by numerous demand, supply, and cost influences that are often intertwined and difficult to unravel to begin to address the inherent problems in these marketplace factors. An example that is well known to health care leaders is the issue of absenteeism and turnover. What is not well known is how to address the issue. Would turnover decrease if there were more caregivers and less stress? Or would turnover be less if demand were controlled and staffing managed more effectively? The solution lies in continual juggling and readjusting of demand, supply, and price variables.

The rising costs of health care are often explained from the perspective of demand-pull theory or cost-push theory. Demand-pull suggests that increases in health care occur from excess demand and spending on health care with an insufficient supply of goods and services to meet the demand. Cost-push suggests that higher prices result from the rising costs within the business of health care. Efforts to control health care costs are typically regulatory or market based; regulations are enacted to limit spending, or reimbursement policy for certain services might be restricted.

> *Note:*
>
> **The power of the perfectly competitive market is that the perspectives of consumers, producers, and society as a whole converge—this is a goal seldom, if ever, achieved!**

Demand Fact

The demand for health care is increasing in a rapidly aging society with improved health care technology that enables care for those with critical conditions who would have died.

Demand Fact

Approximately 45.8 million people—16% of the population—do not have health insurance.
Bureau of the Census, 2004

Supply Fact: Turnover and Absenteeism

Health care workers have the highest turnover and the second highest rate of absenteeism among employees of so-called extended-hours industries—those that operate beyond a single daily shift, often around the clock. Health care's turnover rate of 19% is higher than transportation (18%) and customer service (17%). Absenteeism in health care averages 14%, just below emergency services (15%).

www.circadian.com

CLOSING THE GAP BETWEEN DEMAND AND SUPPLY

A New Lens!

A Reality of Abundance: Quantum Physics Theory

What we believe is what we get! If one believes there is an unmanageable scarcity of goods rather than an abundance, many supply and demand problems will result. If one believes there is a shortage of pharmacists, one will result; if one believes there are enough pharmacists, there will be enough. The challenge is to change the lens in which supply and demand are perceived.

In the current scarcity reality, this is a radical mental model shift and requires examination. Working to continually mediate demand and supply to achieve the optimal balance becomes the work of leaders that is fundamental rather than work that is directed to alleviate problems of shortages and excesses. It is a continual process of adjusting market realities to achieve the optimal balance for community health.

Health Care Marketplace Assumptions

1. Demand should change as new information, technology, and treatments are discovered.
2. Some treatments and services should be eliminated, some added.
3. Caveat: Evaluation of real changes in demand and supply requires analysis of short- and long-term effects as well as altered work processes resulting from the introduction of new methods to avoid the inclination to document quasi-savings.

> **Key Point**
>
> **Know Your Resources**
>
> *The availability of caregivers seldom matches the need for services perfectly, yet health care must be provided using available resources to thier maximum potential.*

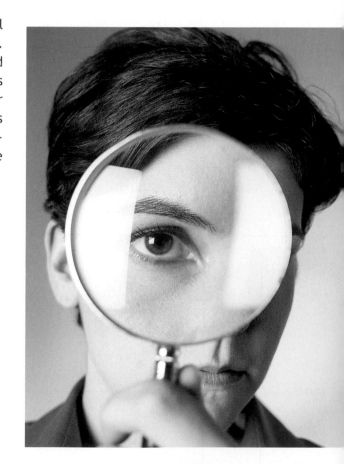

MEDIATING THE DEMAND

Two major areas of opportunity mediate the demand for health care services: establishing the expectation for evidence-based services before payment is approved and implementing new technology to decrease the workload or demand for caregivers.

Historically, most efforts focus on increasing the supply of caregivers, technology, facilities, and pharmaceuticals as the means to decrease the gap between demand and supply. Significant opportunities exist on the demand side of the health care equation. Approaching the gap from this side of the equation is troublesome for many health care workers because of the belief that any decrease in demand will result in loss of employment. There is more than enough health care work to be done; it is the type of work and skills that must be examined and modified to meet contemporary health needs in a technology-enhanced environment. The following are examples of opportunities to decrease the demand for health care services.

Traditional Health Care Marketplace Dynamics

If the demand for pharmacists is suddenly great while the supply is low, an economic problem occurs. The demand is greater than the supply, causing employers to work around the shortage or take action, such as increasing salaries, so more pharmacists will choose to work for the organization. When demand is decreased, salaries level out, and the supply increases. Sometimes the sought-after pharmacists lose their jobs in times of lower demand.

Contemporary Health Care Marketplace Dynamics: Evidence-Based Reimbursement

As the demand for pharmacists increases, with a more contemporary approach, the demand for services is examined to ensure that demands or orders for prescription medications are truly effective, that is, are evidence based and indeed provide value to the consumer (patient). These services would then qualify for reimbursement from payers with established guidelines based on evidence. Challenging the basic request for services is a much different approach than automatically working to meet the demand based on historical practice. The approach is more appropriate than taking action based on the unsubstantiated assumption that all demand for pharmacy service is valid and value producing to consumer outcomes. Finally, this approach integrates both accountability and motivation for evidence-based practice.

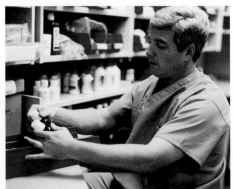

Caveat
Savings, quasi-savings, and downstream savings can result in either net increased costs or savings! Do not assume that short-term improvements provided by technology always result in savings—the changes created may have required unanticipated system changes that are more costly in the long term.

Technology

Adding technology to mediate the demand for services and decrease the need for supplies requires careful planning and evaluation. Whereas technology is typically believed to decrease the need for other resources, the risk of misinterpreting short-term gains as long-term savings is significant. Often, early improvements are realized; however, these savings can be considered as quasi-savings because the changes resulted in unanticipated work increases and overall long-term cost increases. The converse may also be true: improvements in data gathering and documentation may increase costs significantly in the short term through expenditures for computers and decrease expenses in the long term as a result of improved compliance with best practices and decreased litigation expenses.

Computerized documentation is expected to decrease documentation time, time in looking for charts, time in clarifying illegible writing, and throughput time given the ready access of the medical record to all providers. Which positions are affected as a result—clinicians, clerical staff, or both?

Measurement of process savings is challenging due to the multitasking work of caregivers, the initial time required to develop new competence and efficiency with computerized systems, and the substitution of other patient care work to fill the gap created by the increased efficiency.

The reduction in use of paper, cost of copying documents, and storage of forms results in operational savings. Document scanning and equipment to provide timely services replace the traditional management of paper. The analysis of changing demands is best accomplished when there is careful consideration for the initial costs, initial savings, quasi-savings realized, and the downstream changes in supply to meet demands.

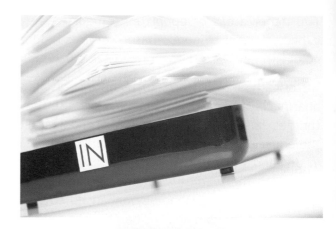

TRADITIONAL PAPERWORK

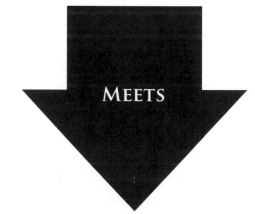

MEETS

NEW TECHNOLOGY

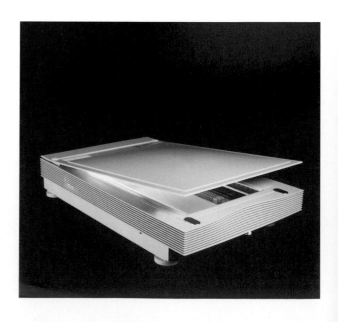

MEDIATE THE SUPPLY

Much attention has been given to the supply side of the health care marketplace. Work to increase access to care, physical facilities, diagnostic equipment, technology, and providers continues to be at the forefront of the local communities and the nation at large. Suggestions that will support supply mediation are discussed from the perspective of the provider and the work environment. Both variables offer significant opportunities to decrease the gap between demand and supply.

1. Begin at the Bedside

IMAGE: The effect of the caregiver is significant. Rather than complaining about working conditions, workload, and pay levels, caregivers can work to address these issues. Recognized and sharing the positive aspects of a health care career is still the least costly, most believable strategy to entice others to join the health care profession. Happy, fulfilled workers are ambassadors for not only their particular profession but also the organization in general. Every act of service becomes a recruitment tool to the patient, family members, visitor, and volunteers. In particular, those individuals considering a second career often choose health care after a positive experience with a kind and compassionate member of the health care team. Further, recruitment into health care often results from a one-to-one discussion with a current, satisfied worker.

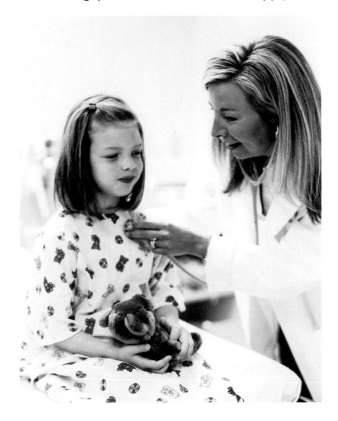

2. Focus on Value/Evidence

To be sure that the work of caregiver results in value to the patient and community, ask yourself and the members of your team:

- How much of what we do really makes a difference?
- How much of this work should be done?
- Is there a better, more cost-saving way to do this work?
- Do we need all of these categories of providers?
- Is the effect of our work sustainable for those we serve?

These questions are certainly reasonable but challenge the very work of caregivers and their security with current work. The real challenge is to eliminate the work that does not affect the patient outcome and create more contemporary, effective work processes that are known to improve outcomes and are aligned with the future.

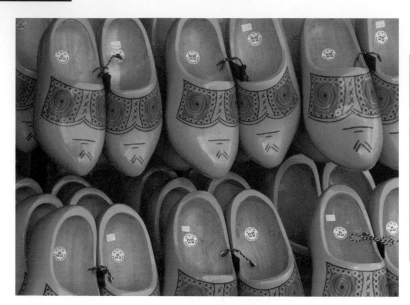

One size fits all when:
- It refers to equity.
- It refers to respect.
- It refers to honesty.

One size does not fit all when:
- Job performance is different.
- Job skills are different.
- Performance is different.

3. Mediate Supply through Human Resource Policies

Health care work is dynamic and always changing and requires new job descriptions and pay scales to accommodate these changes. Yet human resource policies seek to ensure fairness, consistency, and equitable practices, an approach determined to support the greater good of the organization and decrease the risk for discrimination lawsuits. The value of this work cannot be underestimated for many. The difficulty arises when the policies are so rigid and inflexible that adjustments cannot be made to accommodate the wide variations in skills, available technology, values, levels of expertise, and generational differences. Attempting to manage Generation X-ers with baby boomer policies has created numerous challenges in recruitment and retention, and thus the gap between demand and supply is widened.

New models that allow for flexibility in compensation and scheduling are desperately needed in the health care industry. Portability of benefits is also needed for the certain generations who thrive on mobility and skill mastery. Consideration should be given to:

- Statewide benefit plans for health care workers to allow them mobility within the state and uninterrupted coverage for health care and retirement planning.

- Schedule bidding to allow multiple schedule configurations and more weekend flexibility than the traditional every other weekend.

- New job roles for older caregivers that require more intellectual capital than physical strength.

- Expansion of the provision of remote health care services to include nursing, pharmacy, social work, physical therapy, and nutritionists to provide care to great numbers of patients, thereby mediating both the demand and the supply.

4. Improve Supply of Caregivers via Workplace Changes

Much work is needed to increase the supply of caregivers in creating more educational opportunities and articulation between programs to allow continued growth. It is important to note that the work of health care continues to be satisfying; it is the conditions in which caregivers work that create the dissatisfaction. Nurses consistently report that the most enjoyable aspect of their role is helping patients and their families (Lynn & Redman, 2005). The work environment, not the work of caring for patient, is the dissatisfier. Work environment dissatisfiers include:

- Lack of advancement opportunities.

- Verbal abuse on the job.

- Physically demanding work.

- Understaffing.

- Overwhelming paperwork.

The efforts to recognize and value employees in succession planning, implement policies of no tolerance of abuse, equipment that minimizes lifting, management of staffing assignments, and increasing computerization of documentation are all strategies that can positively affect retention, recruitment and ultimately, the overall supply of competent caregivers.

A Final Thought: Recruit to Demand Needs Rather Than Supply!

Wholesale recruiting of any group of health care workers without regard to areas of specific need is destined to further increase the gap in providing needed services to the population. Requesting that any available and interested people fill needs for which they are not suited or worse yet, the demand is not really present, is inappropriate and irresponsible.

For example, continuing to educate and recruit and finance highly specialized staff when the need is primary care serves to increase the gap between the need for primary care and the resources to meet those needs.

Reversing such practices begins with a clear understanding of the marketplace demographics and needs of community members.

References

American Hospital Association. Fast facts on US hospitals from AHA hospital statistics. Retrieved July 16, 2006, at http://www.aha.org/aha/resourcecenter/fastfacts/fast_facts_US_hospitals.html

Anderson, G. F., Hussey, P. S., Frogner, B. K., & Waters, H. R. (2005). Health spending in the United states and the rest of the industrialized world. *Health Affairs*, 24(4), 903-914.

Buerhaus, P. I., Donelan, K., Ulrich, B. T., Kirby, L., Norman, L., & Dittus. R. (2005). Registered nurses' perceptions of nursing *Nursing Economic$*, 23(3), 110-118.

Centers for Disease Control. (2005). Health, United States, 2005. Retrieved July 16, 2006, at http://www.cdc.gov/nchs/data/hus/hus05.pdf#027

Circadian. (2004). Companies with extended hours operations losing major profit gains. Retrieved July 16, 2006, at http://www.circadian.com/media/release-03jul14.

Jones, C. B (2005). The costs of nursing turnover. Part 2: Application of the nursing turnover cost calculation methodology. *JONA*,35(1), 41-49.

Lynn, M R., & Redman, R. W. (2005). Faces of the nursing shortage: Influences on staff nurses' intentions to leave their positions or nursing. *JONA*, 35(5), 264-270.

National Center for Health Statistics. (2005). Fast Facts A to Z. Retrieved July 16, 2006, at http://www.cdc.gov/nchs/fastats/births.htm and http://www.cdc.gov/nchs/fastats/deaths.htm

Spratley, E. (March 2000). *The registered nurse population: Findings from the National Sample Survey of Registered Nurses*. U.S. Department of Health & Human Services, Bureau of Health Professions, Division of Nursing, Health Resources and Services Administration. Retrieved March 15, 2006, at http://nursingworki.orgimemberipracticeffsclemogrpt.cfm

Suggested Readings

American Federation of Teachers. *Empty hallways: The hidden shortage of healthcare workers*. Washington, DC: Author. Retreived November 22, 2005, at www.aft.org/pubs-reports/healthcare/Empty-Hallways.pdf

Buerhaus, P I., Steiger, D. 0., & Auerbach, D. I. (2004). New signs of a strengthening U.S. nurse labor market? *Health Affairs*, 23(2), W4-526-533.

Malloch, K., Davenport, S., Hatler, C., & Milton, D. (2003). Nursing workforce management: Using benchmarking for planning and outcomes monitoring. *JONA*, 33(10), 538-543.

Minority Nurse.com. *Minority nursing statistics*. Chicago: Career Recruitment Media, Inc. Retrieved November 22, 2005, at www.minoritynurse.com/statistics.html.

Pfoutz, S. K., Price, S. A., & Chang, C. F. (2002). Health economics. In D. J. Mason, J. K. Leavitt, & M. W. Chaffee (Eds.). *Policy & politics in nursing and health care* (4th ed.). Philadelphia: Saunders.

Ruggiero, J. S. (2005). Health, work variables, and job satisfaction among nurses. *JONA*, 35(5), 254-263.

CHAPTER 3

SELLING YOUR ORGANIZATION

Selling is not an option—it's necessary for survival!

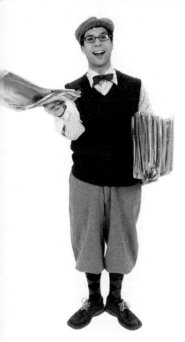

Most health care workers are aware of the historical evolution of healing and its roots as a service for the poor and homeless, but also recognize that in today's society, the work of healing must be compensated. Compensation is a basic expectation of health care workers. Yet the majority of health care workers still struggle with the integration of the hard reality of selling health care services as an integral component of health care processes. In particular, caregivers are reluctant to actively price, sell, and market services to manage pain and suffering. To achieve the desired revenues and compensation from health care services, effective selling of those services to multiple audiences is required. This is necessary so that consumers can make informed decisions about the care they receive, potential employees can select an organization that is congruent with their skills and values, and all stakeholders in the system are compensated for services. In this section, the rationale for selling the health care organization from the perspective of the consumer and the potential caregiver and an overview of the sales cycle are presented within the context of health care services.

Rationale for Health Care Selling

Given that the need for health care services will always be there, one can only wonder why health care organizations actively sell their organizations. Is it really necessary to aggressively sell and market services that most consumers will eventually use? Why would an organization spend time and resources on sales and marketing when resources are already scarce? And when business comes regardless of the sales effort, why spend resources on selling?

The reality is that health care is indeed a business, and more important, not all health care organizations provide the same services or achieve the same outcomes at the same costs. This variation creates significant opportunities for the organization to identify its expertise, describe the exceptional value they are able to provide to consumers, and market and sell those valued services to generate sufficient profits to sustain the organization and fund future operations.

SALES AND THE HEART OF THE HEALER: A REAL CATCH-22

Time to Rethink the Work of Selling in Health Care

Most caregivers are averse to discussing the cost of health care services with patients at the point of service, or for that matter, discussing the costs for caring at all. For the healer it feels like the proverbial catch-22 in which it is illogical to sell health yet the need for personal survival exists. The tradition of treating illness first and then figuring out what the payment will be and if and how it will be paid for has resulted in a marketplace that is significantly out of balance. It is time for all health care professionals to become actively involved in selling their organization using marketplace principles and processes. Selling the specific work of health care organizations further provides clarity to health care professionals specific to the sales encounter, the importance of cultivating relationships, and the incredible complexity of the key stakeholders and their preferences and values. As a result, organizations can expect to improve their processes to ensure that resources are expended logically and rationally.

All Health Care Organizations Are Not Equal

Health Care Organizations Are in Transition

Unsatisfactory cost control and quality levels in healthcare continue to present significant challenges. According to Porter and Teisberg (2004), to address these challenges, efforts are needed to:

1

- Support competition and value.
- Avoid or minimize cost shifting to enhance revenue.
- Avoid large group bargaining when patient costs are actually increased.
- Not restrict choice and access to care at the expense of improved efficiency.
- Not rely on the court system to settle disputes.

Organizations that address some of these issues are:
- Able to identify the value provided for services rendered.
- Able to focus on sharing information about providers, outcomes, treatments, and alternatives.
- Able to provide a simplified billing.
- Able to use a single, transparent pricing system equity to provide services that can be described as better than the norm.

These are examples of the achievements and improvements that health care organizations need to identify, market, and sell to consumers.

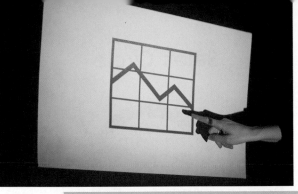

THE FACTS SPEAK!
HEALTH CARE COULD BE BETTER

2 Not All Organizations Provide Comparable Quality

Jha and colleagues (2005) reported high variability in hospital performance in a study of 3558 hospitals. Care of patients with acute myocardial infarction, congestive heart failure, and pneumonia were examined on the basis of 10 quality indicators related to morbidity and mortality; 6 of 10 indicators failed to meet expected standards 10% to 20% of the time, and 4 of 10 indicators failed to meet standards greater than 20% of the time. Further, some organizations excelled in the care of the patient with an acute myocardial infarction and did poorly in the care of patients with pneumonia.

3 Age of Consumerism

Another reason to engage in the selling of the health care organization is the consumer movement, or the age of consumerism. Health care information is readily available to consumers: information specific to quality outcomes, provider competence, levels of adverse outcomes, publication of major safety issues, and provider discipline. There are fewer and fewer secrets in health care.

The age of consumerism and call for safer health care continues to evolve into a world that emphasizes transparency—full disclosure and open sharing of the processes, the challenges, and the outcomes faced by health care organizations.

4 It's an Opportunity!

There is a window of opportunity for health care organizations to sell and benefit from their best practices and outcomes to the public. The opportunity to disclose the organization's achievement of better than average clinical results, high levels of patient and caregiver satisfaction, controlled costs of care, and the efforts taken to address areas that are less than optimal to the community at large have never been greater. Consumers want to know the likelihood that their care will be at least satisfactory and optimally, that the care will be better than expected.

5 The Impact of the Healer

The work of the healer at the bedside, family discussions at home, publications by the organization's members, and professional presentations at local and state are examples of an organization's work. These activities are both informal and formal acts of selling the work of the organization. Each encounter has an effect on someone, from the very positive to the very negative!

The challenge for health care workers is to shift from a mental model in which selling health care organizations is unacceptable to a new mindset in which selling the organization is a formalized and expected behavior that is designed to recognize the accomplishments of the organization, sustain the current customer commitment, attract new customers, and enhance the financial viability of the organization. The following two steps will assist health care workers:

1. Learn the basic sales cycle process.

2. Translate the work of the health care organization into the three phases of the sales process.

Sales Cycle

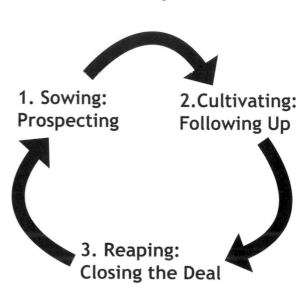

1. Sowing: Prospecting

2. Cultivating: Following Up

3. Reaping: Closing the Deal

EVERY ENCOUNTER IS A SALES PITCH!

DEFINITION: The Sales Cycle

The sales cycle is the sequence of phases that a typical customer goes through when deciding to buy something. As a rule, the sales cycle is described from the customer's perspective. The first phase of the sales cycle may be either the customer's perception of a product, or a perception of a need that the product might satisfy. This is followed by learning more about the product or service and building a relationship to the product or service. Prospective customers research and evaluate the product until the final phase of making the decision to purchase is made.

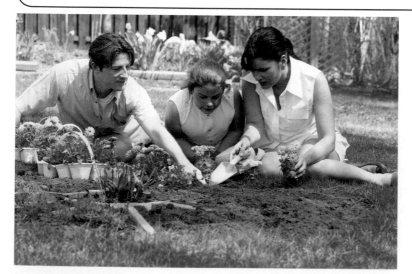

The Law of the Harvest

In order to reap consistent sales, you must regularly sow the right activities to achieve the goals. Sowing the seeds for others to join your organization, following up to solidify the relationship, and finalizing the commitment to the organization require careful planning and execution.

STEP 1. PROSPECTING FOR THE ORGANIZATION

As noted, every encounter between the representatives of an organization and the consumers of health care leaves an impression—sometimes positive and sometimes not so positive. These encounters can be thought of as the first step in the sales cycle, namely, introducing the work of the organization and gaining the interest of consumers.

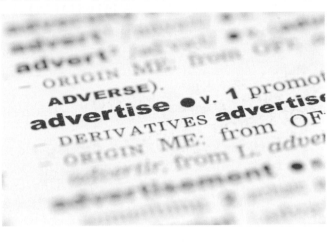

As with any business or service, in order to sustain the work and grow the focus must be on making sure that customers will return. To grow the business, you must do things on a daily basis to keep your name in front of customers. You sow the seed of your message in the minds of as many qualified prospects as possible. For the health care organization, many of these activities of prospecting are already in place. It is important to remember that selling the organization to consumers or potential patients is also about selling the organization to potential employees. The following list of prospecting activities is presented for the organization and the individual to integrate the basic tools of selling in the marketplace.

Organizational Prospecting

> Advertising in newspapers, radio, television, and the Internet

> Sending direct mailers to community members specific to the services that are available, new services added, recent accomplishments, and comments from satisfied patients and employees

> Attending and participating in community events

> Organizing charity events for health care initiatives

> Asking current customers for referrals

> Sponsoring and conducting community focus groups

> Providing educational sessions on mainstream topics such as heart health, diabetes, child care, or nutrition

INDIVIDUAL PROSPECTING

Professional exposure: Provide workshops in areas of expertise.

Network in the community with colleagues from other health care organizations.

Publish: Sharing expertise in local and national venues reflects expertise and commitment to high-quality health care services. Community members value recognized expertise and experience.

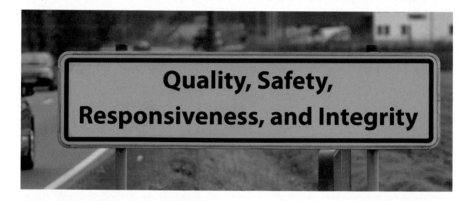

Quality, Safety, Responsiveness, and Integrity

The health care billboard is an example of phase one of the sales cycle, sowing the seeds for community members to be interested in your organization.

The message should appeal to the community at large and be specific to contemporary issues of quality services, safety, responsiveness, and integrity.
The billboard should identify what difference the organization makes, its successes, and its plans.

A True Story: Individual Prospecting

A nurse leader contacted the author of an article in a health care publication to learn more about the topic. The author, located in another state, worked with the nurse leader on the topic, developed a professional relationship, and supported the nurse through her coursework for an advanced degree. When an opening for a nurse leader in the author's hometown became available, the author recommended the nurse leader for the position. The nurse leader interviewed and was selected for the position. The original encounter was not a recruiting effort: the seeds were sown in the relationship and the attractiveness of the organization was shared with the nurse leader, and a goodness-of-fit with the organization emerged as a result.

MORE ON PROSPECTING...

Sowing the seeds for a health care organization requires focused efforts based on the services being sold, the demographics of the community, and target customers.

Products and Services

- Health care services for treatment, prevention of illness, and promotion of health
- Safety
- Goods/equipment/supplies/medications
- Financial stability/sense of security
- Employment for all generations; high satisfaction, skill development
- Health care intellectual capital
- Expert clinicians
- Health for the community
- A reputation for excellence in:
  - ▶ Quality of leadership; describe the leaders
  - ▶ Organizational structure; span of control
  - ▶ Decision making
  - ▶ Models of patient care delivery
  - ▶ Quality of patient care
  - ▶ Quality improvement/management of error

Target Customers

- Patients
- Employees
- Payers
- Educational institutions
- Students
- Community organizations
- Vendors
- Donors
- Policymakers

Customer Demographics

- Age
- Gender
- Income
- Education
- Cultural/ethnic background

SELLING TO GENERATIONS

The complexity of health care and the differing goals of consumers based on generational preferences can serve to enlighten and focus the processes of selling the health care organization. For the first time in decades, there are four separate and distinct generations potentially working together in a stressful and competitive health care workplace. The patient population spans nearly 100 years and more than six generations. Selling to health care consumers cannot be simply standardized into one size fits all. Products and services are based on core values and expectations and then customized to match the more specific needs and values of each generation. The challenge confronting health care organizations is to understand the characteristics and attributes of those it serves and using the groups of generations is a good framework to guide this work. Organizations must create a montage of opportunities and expectations in the environment, expectations that are dedicated and focused on the single goal of value-based, quality health care services for each patient

> **Note:**
>
> Attempting to use values and expectations of one generation for another generation can only result in frustrations and less than satisfactory results.

GENERATIONS: KEY POINTS

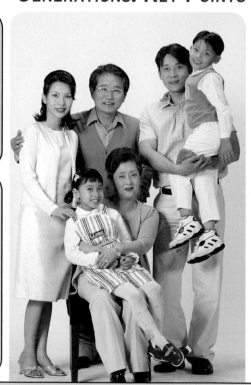

Definition

A generation is an identifiable group that shares birth years, age location, and significant life events at critical developmental stages (Smola & Sutton, 2002, p. 364).

Generational Distinguishing Categories

- Defining events in history
- Childhood experiences
- Economy
- Core values
- Work values

Generation Theory

Each generation is characterized by historical, political, and social events that share the core values, work ethic, and economics movement of its members.

A collective personality of traits provides a reference point specific to each generation.

> *Misunderstandings and differing work ethics create chaos and conflict and negatively affect the quality of work and overall productivity.*

Generalizations about generations serve as reference points from which to comprehend how life experiences affect core values and influence one's work ethic. Generalizations of worker profiles should be avoided given that traits are often overlapping between generations and anecdotal in nature.

SELLING TO THE SILENT GENERATION
OR MATURES (BORN BETWEEN 1925 AND 1945)

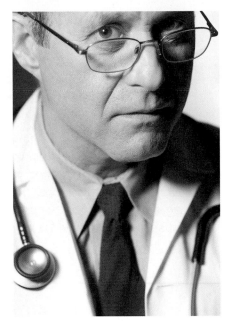

■ Silents are about 95% retired at this point. Soon virtually no Silent will command an industry, a battlefield, anything at all. However, the Silents have continued to exert influence through organizations such as the American Association of Retired Persons (AARP).

■ Approximately 83% of Silent Generation preretirees and 90% of retirees are confident that they have enough money to live comfortably until at least age 85.

■ The Silent Generation spent their working years during an era that was generally more stable for employees, and they are, perhaps, the last generation that will, as a group, have a fairly strong sense of confidence about security in retirement.

■ The majority of those in the Silent Generation have, or anticipate, multiple sources of guaranteed income to carry them through retirement.

■ Silents view leaving an inheritance to someone other than their spouse as relatively unimportant. Less than half of Silent Generation retirees (45%) and preretirees (43%) say that it is important to leave an inheritance to anyone other than their spouse.

1. **Defining events:** the Great Depression, World War II, and the Golden Age of radio

2. **Childhood:** authoritative parenting, overprotective; parents are structured, rigid, and focused on schooling as well as providing clear role models.

3. **Economy:** industrial model, hierarchical workplaces and factories; experienced with economic hardship, they value loyalty, discipline, teamwork, reward for hard work, respect for authority, and seniority-driven entitlement.

4. **Core values:** loyalty, sacrifice, adherence to rules, honor, and resistant to change

5. **Work values:** respect authority, hard work, loyalty, and industrial technology. Given the physical demands of caregiving, they are unlikely to be in direct-care positions, but rather hold senior level leadership positions. Matures require more time, explanation, and assistance with contemporary technology than succeeding generations. Also, they need more detailed reference guides.

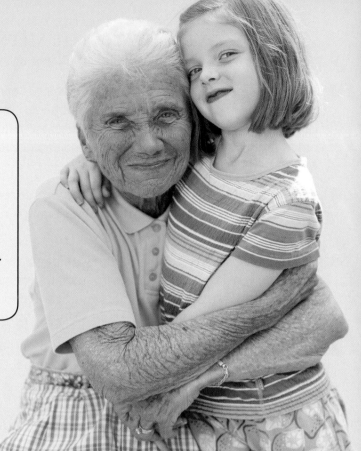

Recommendations for:
patients, employees, payers, educational institutions, students, community organizations, vendors, donors, and policymakers

Although each of these stakeholders represents a different group of expectations and resources, there are strategies that can be focused and helpful in selling the organization.

- Do not expect snap decisions; allow time for consideration of ideas or offers.

- Expect Silents to be loyal to current health care providers and organizations. Recognize Silents for their regular and continuing patronage of the organization.

- Avoid overuse of technology; provide nontechnology options as well as electronic systems to secure services with the Silent generation.

- Encourage more discussion of decisions related to health care services, especially advance directives and HIPAA. Silents tend to not challenge decisions made by others, particularly those with position and experience.

- Anticipate resistance from the Silents due to long-standing loyalty to existing commitments. Request the Silents for changes in practices, products, and standards only when there is good reason.

- Communicate the importance of the organization's strategies and commitment to cost minimization on a regular basis. Inform the Silents that you are working diligently to use their hard-earned dollars wisely.

- Respect the Silents' established protocols and power structures within their consumer groups.

- Provide education and support using experienced, credentialed experts.

SELLING TO THE BABY BOOMER GENERATION
(BORN BETWEEN 1946 AND 1964)

The Baby Boomers are the wealthiest, best-educated and most sophisticated purchasers in today's marketplace. As the baby boomers enter midlife, they face normal emotional and physical transitions, and some unusual financial and employment concerns. The Boomers will face some of the standard chronic health problems and their own mortality. Yet they will strive to control the aging process with beauty products and health treatments more so than former generations. In addition, many baby boomers are facing layoffs as corporations downsize, rather than entering a period of economic certainty, job security, and one's peak earning years. This collective tenuous financial status is compounded by the fact that there is greater uncertainty of the availability and reliability of Social Security. And with many subsidizing their own aging parents, this uncertainty is compounded. As consumers of health care, Baby Boomers play a significant role and influence all stakeholder groups.

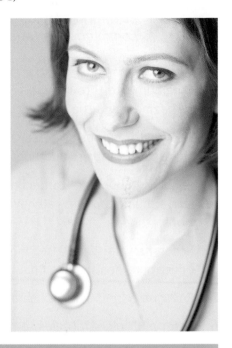

1. **Defining events:** television, man on the moon, civil rights, women's liberation, Watergate, two global wars

2. **Childhood:** doting parents, nuclear family, suburbia, economic prosperity

3. **Economy:** start of the information age. Boomers are distinctly competitive. They are disappointed that technology has not created more efficiency. They are disappointed that robots did not create the promised 20-hour work week.

4. **Core values:** personal gratification, youthfulness, contribution, and involvement are important to Boomers, who are open to improvements. They question the status quo, protest for civil rights, march against war, and demand integrity in leaders. They believe they understand all that is wrong with the world and believe they have the idealism, education, and sheer numbers to change it. Boomers look to external sources for validation of their worth.

5. **Work values:** Boomers challenge or distrust authority. Quality of life and work fulfill personal needs and meaning. Boomers are the dominant generation in the workforce until 2015. They want to be noticed and valued for their contributions through material gain, promotions, titles, corner offices, reserved parking. They tend to be workaholics and are defined by their jobs. Boomers plan to work longer than the traditional retirement age. They are reluctant to hand over the reins of leadership to the next generation and sometimes associate micromanagement with the assurance of quality outcomes.

> *Recommendations for:*
> *patients, employees, payers, educational Institutions, students,*
> *community organizations, vendors donors, and policymakers*

1. Communicate through the television. Boomers prefer TV (75%) followed by radio, newspapers, magazines, and the Internet.

2. Sell youth—exercise, personal appearance, and health promotion. Offer spa-type services that will decrease stress and enhance personal appearance to the Boomers.

3. Encourage Boomers to become involved in two-way mentoring with Generation X and Generation Y members. They all have much to gain from each other, especially from technology innovations.

4. Recognize the expertise and levels of education of the Boomers. Involve them in consumer education, health care financing, and health care reform advisory groups.

5. Recognize their accomplishments publicly; give award certificates, plaques, and so on.

6. Offer multiple strategies to reduce stress.

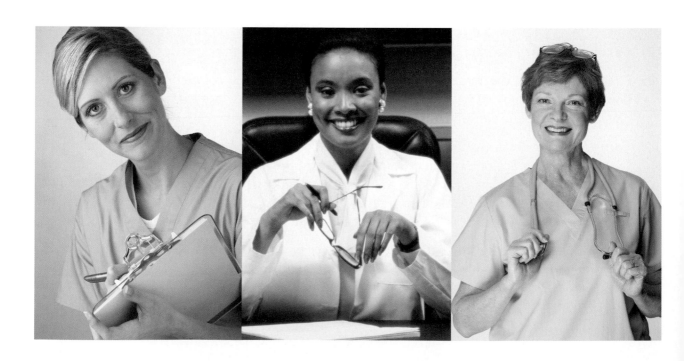

SELLING TO GENERATION X (BORN BETWEEN 1965 AND 1980)

The approach and strategies to sell the health care organization to Generation X should be much different than preceding generations. Their independence and comfort with uncertainty will affect the ability to sow, prospect, and close the sale. Generation X-ers comprise 17% of the population. They have a propensity for technology, skepticism to advertising claims, and attraction to personal style rather than designer price tags. They do, however, respond to high-impact Internet marketing techniques. There are a high number of entrepreneurs in this generation.

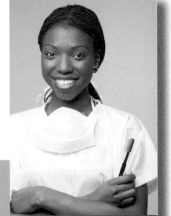

1. **Defining events**: MTV, AIDS, personal computers, *Challenger* space shuttle disaster

2. **Childhood**: latchkey kids, single-parent homes, team-based learn

3. **Economy**: information age, technology driven, and the Internet. This generation believes technology should make things more practical, more efficient, and more functional.

4. **Core values**: balance, self-reliance, diversity, and thinking globally are the values of Generation X. They also tend to have an entitlement mentality and are abrupt and sometimes abrasive in their communication style. A significant difference from the Baby Boomer generation is their focus on balance between work and personal life. They will resist requests to work overtime. They are not intimidated by authority or overly impressed by authority. They have a penchant for pragmatism and street-smarts.

   Additional expressions of their core values include a strong propensity for outcomes rather than process; a greater affinity for information rather than introspection; a desire to know facts over emotions; and an intimate familiarity with ambiguity and flexibility that renders them anxious when faced with fixed, rigidly imposed, or closed-off bottom lines.

5. **Work values**: Generation X-ers tend to ignore authority and look for future opportunities. They move from company to company in search of new skills, contacts, and experiences. They want to be coached and mentored by knowledgeable, confident managers. They resist any approach that smothers or confines their creativity, such as autocratic leadership. It is likely that new generations of graduates will have four or five lateral moves for every promotional move during a working lifetime (Boychuk-Duchscher & Cowin 2004). They do not want to become stagnant in their professional aspirations and accomplishments and have been described as alienated, skeptical, cynical, nonconformist, and individualistic.

   Generation X-ers are well suited for a job market that holds no promise of stability and every assurance of change. They are loyal to a set of principles rather than to an institution. Typically they will seek employability over employment; they are mobile, well educated, and techno-intellectual.

> *Generation X does not like the "hard sell"—it will fall on deaf ears!*

1. In general, members of Generation X make decisions more quickly than previous generations. There is less need to allow time for reflection and consideration for any of the health care stakeholder groups.

    Recommendations for: patients, employees, payers, educational institutions, students, community organizations, vendors donors, and policymakers

2. Generation X responds best when learning from highly qualified, competent resources. Identify and advertise the commitment to evidence-based practices. Share publications of the organization's experts.

3. Generation X members do not like to wait for services—they will leave and seek other resources. Provide as much information and service through electronic media.

4. Generation X patients do not want lengthy explanations of health care issues; they prefer health care information in summaryformat and preferably on the Internet.

5. Create a proactive job mobility program. Identify and support the multiple opportunities for growth and development in the organization but do not be disappointed when the Generation X employee seeks opportunities in another organization.

6. Present the expected outcomes and rationale for expenditures or donations—be clear about what difference will be made in terms of patient care.

7. Include families in organization-sponsored events.

8. Recognize and support the need for worklife—home balance through options for self-scheduling, telecommuting, and flexible hours.

9. Emphasize high reliability organizations (HROs) and the goal of information transparency.

10. Use multimedia selling approaches frequently.

11. Share efforts to achieve and ensure quality outcomes.

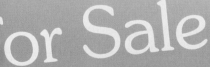

SELLING TO THE NET OR Y GENERATION (BORN BETWEEN 1980 AND 2000)

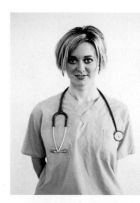

The Y Generation includes approximately 57 million individuals and represents the largest consumer group in the history of the United States. This generation exerts significant influence on many purchasing decisions. They are an interesting mix of ambition and practicality, with a solid underpinning of values. One of their biggest worries is reducing debt; 63% of the college graduates believe they'll have to make some sacrifices to achieve their goals. This is a connected generation. The Internet is their primary source of news: 80% use it frequently as an information source, followed by the radio and television. Boomers and the Y Generations' older siblings see the Internet as something they connect to. But the Y Generation sees the Internet as a way to connect to the world and each other.

1. **Defining events:** violence, Columbine shootings, war in Kosovo, Oklahoma City bombing, Princess Di's death, Clinton impeachment and scandal, OJ trial, fall of Berlin Wall, Mark McGwire/Sammy Sousa homerun contest, Kennedy plane crash

2. **Childhood:** They've been well cared for. Children seem to be valued and cared for most in alternating generations. These folks caught a generational wave in which children are highly valued, and they've benefited from the longest economic boom in history. When they were kids, they got four times the number of toys that their Boomer parents got just 20 years earlier.

3. **Economy:** More affluent, hypereducated, ethnically diverse, and technologically accomplished than any previous generation. Today, nearly 6 in 10 Millennials ages 6 to 17 have their own TV. Teenagers' spendable income is estimated at $60 per week: 22% of the older teens have their own checking account and 42% have a credit card, so they have high expectations.

4. **Core values:** They are notably generous, sociable, practical, and morally civic minded with high self-esteem. They tend to be warm, confident, upbeat, determined, and optimistic. They care deeply about social issues, believe strongly in upholding the individual. They embrace the diversity of their broadened environmental, political, cultural, and socioeconomic communities. Both the Gen X-ers and Y Generation resent previous generations for leaving the world politically disenfranchised, environmentally contaminated, and economically vulnerable; they believe that they will be the redeemers of the 21st century work world. They've got confidence that they'll achieve those expectations too. Some of that is the natural confidence of youth, some comes from growing up in good economic times. According to a Harris Poll of the class of 2001, 88% have established specific goals for the next 5 years, and virtually all (98%) are sure they'll someday get to where they want in life.

5. **Work values:** Members of the Y Generation prefer job mobility within a single company rather than career advancement in the open market. They tend to downplay mathematics, foreign languages, public speaking, selling things or ideas, writing, and editing. The Y Generation tends to thrive working independently, multitasking (instant messaging, cell phones, music), developing personal connections and relationships. Access to technology in the workplace, unit-based Internet access to health research, pathophysiology, and pharmaceutical references are expected.

Recommendations for:
patients, employees, payers,
educational Institutions,
students, community organizations,
vendors, donors, and
policymakers

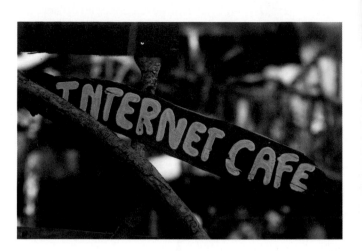

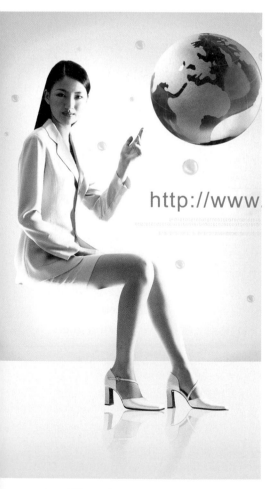

1. Recognize the core values of social consciousness that are different from the previous generation. In general, members of Generation Y are less intense and more socially conscious. They require less formality.

2. Communicate electronically whenever possible. Use the Internet, email, instant messaging, and cell phones.

3. Ask for assistance in achieving organizational transparency from members of the Y Generation using their technology skills.

4. Identify myriad employment opportunities within the health care organization to support stability and diversity.

5. Include members of this generation in discussion of the financial challenges in the funding of health care and in creating new strategies to control costs.

6. Encourage Y Generation members to select a specific area for philanthropy and financial donations.

7. Involve members of the Y Generation in community focus groups to discuss the technology, supplies, equipment, service, treatments, physical setting, and the future of health care services.

Step 2. Cultivating the Relationships

The work of sowing the seeds for sales is typically quite general. In contrast, the focus of phase two, cultivating relationships, becomes more personalized as potential customers are identified. To create meaningful relationships, more specific information must be offered to the prospective customers to assist them in evaluating the organization and to make informed decisions about services that will meet their needs from their set of values, beliefs, and generational perspectives. The organization is always looking for ways to nudge potential customers closer to buying its services and products.

The work of prospecting involves many activities to develop and strengthen relationships as much as possible and give them more reasons to do business with you instead of a competitor. Numerous approaches can be used for this work and include the following:

Share what it is like to be a patient, an employee, or a community member from the perspective of the organization.

Share stories specific to the challenges of the current environment:
- What activities are in place to assess and ensure patient safety?
- How is the stress of the health care workplace managed?
- How are staffing shortages addressed?

Create focused newsletters for specific populations of patients, caregivers, vendors, donors—for example, information for diabetic patients, nurse recruitment opportunities, new opportunities for volunteers and donors.

Tell the story of the positive patient care experience from two perspectives—that of the patient and that of the nurse to provide powerful, clear messages about the organization.

Create focused newsletters to regularly recognize and thank all members of the community for their support of the organization.

Stories

During the prospecting phase, stories from patients, families, employees, payers, vendors and donors are important in describing the character and capabilities of the organization. The art of storytelling is a method of teaching, learning, and informing.

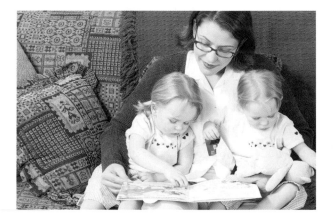

Stories tell much about the organization, the team, and the individual. Motives, character, and capacity to reach goals are often shared through stories. Caregivers have much to share about the work of health care organizations. Stories about how decisions are made, how ethical dilemmas are faced in ensuring patient confidentiality, dealing with grief and disappointment, and all other emotions give life and expression to the challenging work of diagnosis, intervention, and evaluation.

One can share skills and emotions involved in the health care experience to illuminate the knowledge and richness of nursing work that are often taken for granted.

Examples are often able to illustrate:

- The multifaceted nature of caring.

- The complex thinking involved.

- Decision-making challenges that reveal personal and professional wisdom.

Note:

Good Storytellers...
Avoid "telling tales." Stories need to be about accounts that are true and so compelling that others can feel the experience. Telling tales or making up good endings to bad situations misrepresents reality and results in disappointment when the reality is experienced. Avoid stories that demoralize and drive others away.

STEP 3. CLOSE THE DEAL—BEGINNING THE RELATIONSHIP

In health care, closing the deal occurs in many ways. Each stakeholder group makes the decision to use or purchase the services from different perspectives. Patients, employees, payers, educational institutions, community agencies, and donors each have specific needs and expectations. For example, patient selection of a health care facility ranges from choosing a facility in times of crisis based on the nearest location to choosing a facility for elective services based on extensive research and comparisons of quality, cost, and interpersonal relationships. Potential employees may choose the organization due to location, reputation, wages, urgency for employment, and other unknown reasons.

Deal-Closing Activities for Potential Employees

1. *Confirm the new employment agreement in writing or electronically.*

2. *Begin socialization by creating a plan that includes short- and long-term goals of the new employee and the supervisor, specific measures of success, and regular times for assessing progress.*

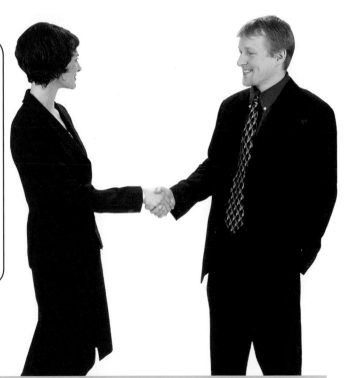

Final Thoughts on Selling the Health Care Organization

1. **Timing is important.**

   - Selling products and services during stressful and grieving times is inappropriate.

2. **Not everyone is a customer.**

   - Individuals with significant criminal histories are not suitable as caregivers.

   - Individuals with unresolved professional discipline are not safe for patient care.

   - Repetitive abusive, combative consumers are inappropriate for the hospital setting.

References

Boychuk-Duchscher, J. E. & Cowin, L. (2004). Multigenerational nurses in the workplace. *JONA*, 34(11), 493-501.

Jha, A, Li, A Oray, J., & Epstein, A M. (2005). Care in U.S. hospitals—The hospital quality alliance program. *New England Journal of Medicine*, 353(3), 265-274.

Porter, M. E., & Teisberg, E. O. (2004). Redefining competition in health care. *Harvard Business Review*, 82(4), 65-76.

Smola, K. W., & Sutton, C. D. (2002). Generational differences: Revisiting generational work values for the new millennium. *Journal of Organizational Behavior*, 23, 363-382.

Suggested Readings

Buchanan, L. (2004). The young and the restful. H*arvard Business Review*, 82(4), 25.

Lancaster, L. C., & Stilman, D. (2002). *When generations collide: Who they are, why they clash, how to solve the generational puzzle at work*. New York: HarperCollins.

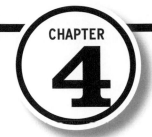
CHAPTER 4

INTERVIEWING FOR EXCELLENCE

There is a need to spend more time with each potential applicant—time and energy dedicated to identifying and selecting the best employees that will optimize the use of resources.

The purpose of an interview is to learn enough about the applicant to be able to determine if that individual is able to meet the identified needs of the organization (Vestal, 2005). Based on this information, the leader is expected to be able to identify and select an individual who will assist the organization in closing the gap between the demand for services and the organization's supply of resources to meet that demand. Historically, interview processes have been only marginally successful given the mediocre levels of engagement of new employees and the turnover in the first year of employment. This is not the result of lack of effort; managers and leaders work tirelessly to interview and hire within the confines of current practices. Significant opportunities exist to improve the process that will support earlier engagement of new employees and decease first-year turnover through more focused, contemporary interview processes.

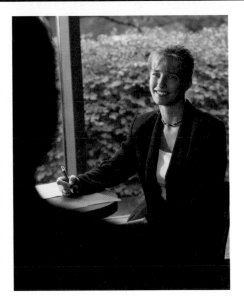

Most leaders are competent in evaluating the required credentials and level of experience of prospective employees; it is determining the level and quality of interpersonal and communication skills that presents the greatest challenge. For this reason, the focus of this section is on creating more effective processes and techniques to discover an applicant's interpersonal skills and communication competence. The topics of discussion include:

- Focused interviewing.
- Evaluating resumes, portfolios, and references.
- Using the white paper as the guiding point for interview questions.
- Examples of interview questions specific to interpersonal skills of collaboration, professionalism, initiative, problem solving, compassion and the 14 Forces of Magnetism.
- Discussion as to how the applicant faces challenges, deals with changing priorities, gives feedback to the right person at the right time, manages disappointment, and adjusts to varying workloads.
- Thoughts on how to reject an applicant with compassion.

TRUE OR FALSE?

Q: Credentials and technical skills will get you hired; however, it is your relationship skills that will sustain your engagement with the organization.

A: True. It is the ability to apply one's credentials and skills into the organization's work that creates a meaningful bond with the team and the organization so that one's expertise can be fully used. If one can't engage in healthy dialog, listen to others, seek alternative solutions when necessary, and act compassionately, the highest credentials and greatest technical skills are useless.

Thoughts on Interviewing

■ Discovering the level of technical competence of the potential employee is typically straightforward and fairly objective. It is the relationship skills that are difficult to unmask in one brief encounter in an artificial setting. Competent interpersonal skills and ability to form meaningful relationships demonstrated by collaboration, professionalism, compassion, problem solving, and initiative are as important as the basic minimum credentials of the applicant.

■ Current interviewing processes are laborious, time consuming, and only partially productive. More effective interviewing processes should be developed that will result in higher employee engagement and lower turnover.

■ A decrease in turnover of 10 clinicians can result in decreased expenses of $670,000 in 1 year! (*Example*: The cost of turnover for 1 RN = $67,000) (Jones, 2005)

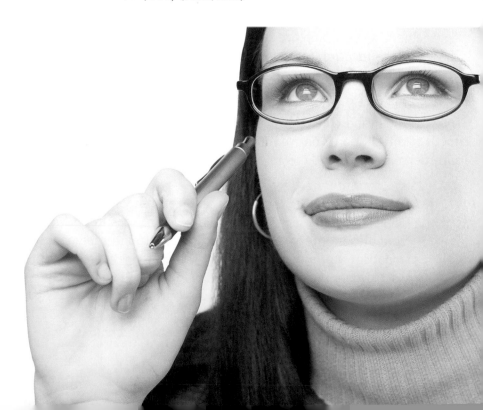

FOCUSED INTERVIEWING

Traditional interviewing is time intensive and standardized to meet employment regulations. There are ten traditional interviewing steps for most organizations. More effective, contemporary interviewing processes are needed to assist leaders in their quest for goodness-of-fit between applicants and the organization. To begin the transition to a more contemporary approach, consider the traditional processes and then compare with the proposed contemporary processes. The process must begin with a clear understanding of not only the basic credential of the individual, but also the skills and abilities that complement and enhance the current work of the unit. First, a white paper, as presented in Unit 5, Chapter 1 and later in this chapter, is needed to enhance the process. Interview questions, resume evaluation and reference checking can then be tailored to assess the applicant.

The list of steps for a contemporary approach to the hiring process seeks to decrease the time spent in reviewing documents and increase personal time with the applicant. Changes to each of the steps are not intended to create more work, but to decrease the time in some areas, sharpen the focus of the interviews to emphasize goodness-of-fit, and to increase the time spent with the applicant to experience the interpersonal and communication skills in a variety of situations. The most significant change is the addition of the audition—an experience to observe in person the abilities of the applicant.

Traditional Steps in the Hiring Process

1. Advertise for open positions.
2. Review resume/application for basic credentials and experience.
3. Conduct personal interview with applicant.
4. Interview with key stakeholders as a group.
5. Check references.
6. Validate credentials.
7. Conduct final interview.
8. Offer position/negotiate.
9. Complete process (physical exam/benefit selection etc.).
10. Establish goals/expectations during first evaluation.

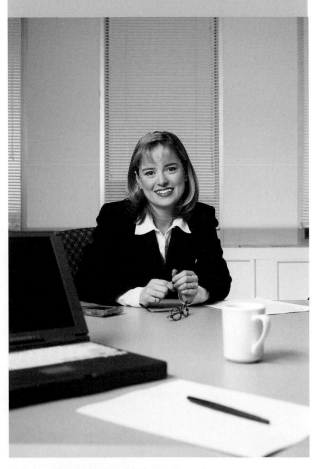

CONTEMPORARY APPROACH TO THE HIRING PROCESS

1. Advertise based on white paper.

2. Review resume/application for basic credentials, experience and congruence with white paper description and needs.

3. Conduct phone interview with applicant.

4. Interview with key stakeholders as a group, focusing on white paper.

5. Audition interview, focusing on applicant fit with needs of unit and organization based on white paper.

6. Check references.

7. Validate credentials.

8. Conduct personal interview to review interviews and feedback from team. Create a draft of goals and expectations.

9. Offer position/negotiate.

10. Complete process (physical exam/ benefit selection, etc.).

11. Finalize goals and expectations of position before first day of work.

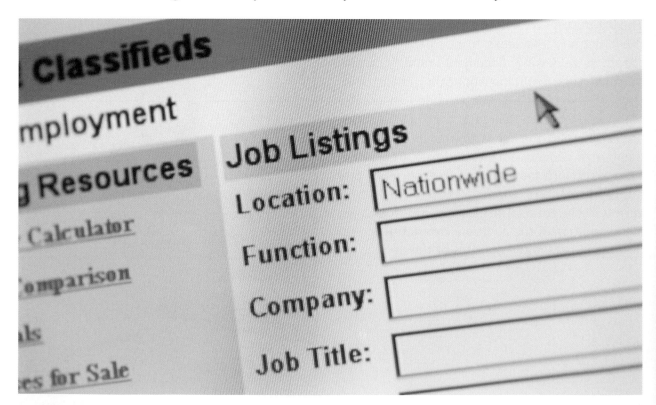

RESUMES, PORTFOLIOS, AND REFERENCES

Thoughts about Resumes

Historically, resumes are designed to describe one's experiences, education, and achievements. Professional goals, organizations, and awards are also included. The difficulty is that a resume tells a lot about the roles occupied by an individual and some outcomes, but much is missing. Seldom do resumes include process competencies, namely, the behaviors used to achieve those experiences and outcomes. Discovering core character traits of the applicant from the traditional resume is all but impossible.

It is unlikely that much will change in the traditional resume. What needs to change is how one identifies what is really needed about character and communication skills and works to get this essential information. Leaders can use the white paper as a template to evaluate a resume—which accomplishments and goals identified in the applicant resume will support and enhance the work identified of the unit and organization.

The Portfolio

The portfolio is a relatively new document to share contributions and special knowledge. Typically, it contains more information than the resume and is used by the professional as a document of one's professional experiences and achievements. Specific examples that support the resume such as copies of licensure, certifications, seminar attendance certificates, recognition awards, and publications are included. Letters from patients recognizing the quality of care, communication from peers regarding teamwork, and complimentary notes from supervisors serve to communicate one's effect on others.

In many ways, a well-prepared, focused portfolio can greatly assist both the applicant and the interviewers in the process. Documents in the portfolio can help to focus the discussion to better understand and recognize expert contributions of the applicant.

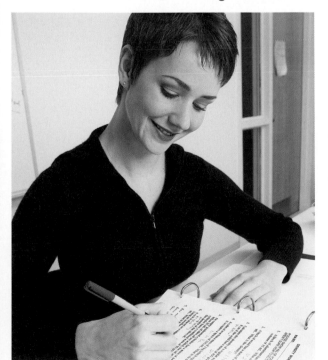

Definition: A portfolio is a purposeful, meaningful collection of one's work. The collection tells a story about the achievements and progress over time. Portfolios serve as windows on learning, enabling an audience to see a rich and complex view of accomplishments, supported by authentic samples of student work. If portfolios become nothing more than storage containers for work, their full potential is not realized.

REFERENCE CHECKING
A DILEMMA FOR ORGANIZATIONS AND LEADERS

The subjective nature of reference checking has rendered the practice annoying to most employers and nearly useless for leaders as a tool in learning about an applicant's character, personality, temperament, and ability to work with others. Yet the information specific to work ethic and interpersonal skills is invaluable is determining the goodness-of-fit between a prospective employee and the organization. Employers need accurate and reliable information about the technical and relational competencies of prospective employees in order to ensure a good fit with the organization. Current reference checking information for most employers has been limited to start and end dates of employment. Narrative information specific to competence and relationship skills is seldom if ever shared by previous employers in fear of future litigation.

Points to ponder:

- Should traditional reference checking be abandoned?

- Is it possible to shift the accountability to the applicant to provide reliable references specific to relationships and communication skills?

- What is the essential information about an applicant that is often lacking—information that one wishes he or she knew that would have affected the decision to hire?

- If one focuses reference questions on the desired characteristics identified in the white paper, can more valuable information be obtained?

- Be sure to check current licensure status and previous board discipline!

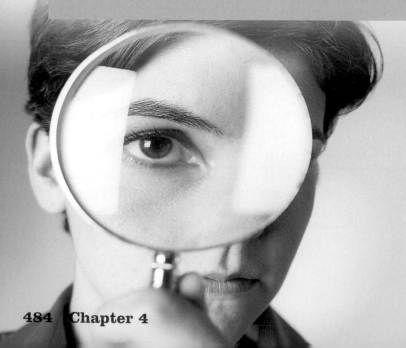

THE WHITE PAPER:
FOUNDATION FOR CREATING A FOCUSED INTERVIEW

The white paper created in Unit 5, Chapter 1, Assessing Your Organization, will be used to guide the development of a focused interview with the goal of determining what the applicant knows about the organization and how their skills would assist the team and the organization in furthering its goals.

My Health Care Organization, USA
The White Paper

We need you in our organization! Our organization is looking for individuals willing and able to commit to the best health care service possible. We are working to achieve Magnet accreditation and national recognition as a Top 100 Hospital in the country.

We are dedicated to evidence-based practice in a healing environment. Our facility is 5 years old; has all private rooms, which includes family space; and a moderate amount of technology and computerization.

Patient care: Our unit provides care to medical patients with primary diagnoses. More than 50% of our patients are Hispanic and most speak Spanish-only. Patient satisfaction is at the 87th percentile; our goal is to be above the 90th percentile by the end of the year.

Other satisfaction scores are:

Nurses' attitudes toward requests	78th percentile
Accommodations and comfort for visitors	92nd percentile
Noise level	88th percentile
Physician concern for patients	91st percentile
Adequacy of pain relief	94th percentile

Clinical outcomes:

Falls	3/1000 patient-days
Medication errors	<6/1000 patient-days

Safety: All departments have a unit-specific safety committee that has membership on a facility-wide safety committee. In addition to falls and medication errors, emphasis is placed on patient identification with the new bar-coding system, and hand washing to minimize nosocomial infections, which are currently fewer than three per 1000 patient-days.

The physical environment is very important in our organization. Adequate lighting, enclosed medication preparation rooms, and noise minimization are important. Employee safety is stressed through our no-lift environment, no-carpet environment, and motorized beds. Needlestick injuries were fewer than four last year; four minor back injuries occurred last year with no lost work time.

My Health Care Organization, USA
The White Paper (Cont'd)

Professionalism: 45% of caregivers are certified in their specialty and 28% belong to their professional organizations. Staff satisfaction is above average. Several areas of opportunity exist in the relationship between the staff and immediate supervisor. Overall satisfaction is 4.1 on a 5 scale.

Other scores include:

My immediate supervisor is a good coach	3.8/5
Change occurred as a result of the last survey	4.1/5
My opinions count in this organization	4.3/5

Patient care delivery model: The team model is used for patient care delivery and assignments. Each caregiver is expected to be autonomous in his or her own specialty and integrative with the team. No decisions are ever made in isolation. Daily assignments are made by a designated staff member familiar with the patients and the staff available to provide care. The levels of education include high school, college, and some graduate. Most nurses are associate degree prepared. The skill mix is 65% licensed and 35% non-licensed; 8% external travelers are used. There is no mandatory overtime. Employees participate in the creation of work schedules within defined guidelines. Current facility turnover is 9% and unit turnover is 12%.

Teamwork: The team consists of physicians/hospitalists, advanced-practice nurses, registered nurses, licensed practical nurses, nursing assistants, social workers, therapists, and nutritionists. Teamwork is assessed monthly using an electronic survey available to all employees.

Latest results are as follows:

My team functions at a high level	4/5
Everyone carries their share of the workload	3.5/5

Technology: Daily documentation is computerized for all caregivers except physicians. Medication administration is also computerized but not completely implemented. Clinical monitoring systems are electronic for vital signs and cardiac monitoring and are integrated into the documentation system. The goal of the organization is to be fully computerized and wireless in 3 years.

THE WHITE PAPER:
FOUNDATON FOR CREATING A FOCUSED INTERVIEW (CONT'D)

Examples of focused interview questions based on the white paper:

1. What is your understanding of a healing environment? How would I know if the environment is not supportive of healing?

2. Describe your experiences with evidence-based practice.

3. Share your experiences in leading, managing, or caring for patients with congestive failure, pneumonia, and diabetes. Share an accomplishment specific to these patient needs of which you are the most proud.

4. What do you believe are the greatest challenges in working with the Hispanic population?

5. How could you assist the team in improving "nurses' attitudes toward requests" and decreasing medication errors?

6. How would you ensure that pain relief adequacy was maintained?

7. Describe your involvement on committees focused on patient safety. How long were you a member? What were your responsibilities on the committee?

8. How would you ensure that your behaviors and work would contribute to a quiet environment?

9. Safety for patients, visitors, and staff is important in our organization—can you share a practice that you believe is absolutely essential to ensuring that the organization meets its safety goals?

10. Listening to others is important for everyone—staff and management. What approaches do you take that ensure you listen first and don't interrupt others before you respond?

11. If someone continually interrupted others, how would you address the situation? When would you do this?

12. What have you done when your workload was too high?

13. How would you assist the organization in reducing turnover?

14. Learning new technology for managers and caregivers requires time and patience—how have you been able to adjust to new technology?

15. Share your last three experiences with new computerized software, equipment, or hardware.

16. What advice can you give others to help them become competent with new technology?

17. Describe what you believe will be your greatest contribution to patient care outcomes if you are hired for this team.

18. How much time will be required before these results are realized?

MORE ON INTERVIEWING FOR EXCELLENCE

Facilitating an interview requires skill and artful sensitivity to the cues given by the applicant. Five general areas—collaboration, professionalism, compassion, initiative, and problem solving—are presented to assist leaders to delve into the interpersonal and communication skills of the applicant in a relatively short time. Finding the future stars for your team requires thoughtful planning and preparation. Asking the right questions is the first step in determining if there is a goodness-of-fit among the applicant, the team, and the organization.

Remember, the goal is to identify those who will assist your organization to be the star of health care. Consider these focused questions in your next interview. Also consider the relationship of these questions based on the white paper and the 14 Forces of Magnetism (FOM) to the needs and strengths of your organization or department. The FOM numbers following the focused interview questions refer to the Magnet behavior that could or should be elicited from the question.

14 Forces of Magnetism (FOM)

1. *Quality nursing leadership*

2. *Flat, decentralized structure*

3. *Participative management style*

4. *Supportive personnel policies and programs*

5. *Professional model of care*

6. *Quality care is personalized*

7. *Quality improvement is evident*

8. *Consultation and resources are available*

9. *Independent judgment is supported*

10. *Community involvement*

11. *Nurses are teachers*

12. *Professional image of nursing*

13. *Interdisciplinary collaboration*

14. *Professional development*

From American Nurses Credentialing Center, 2005

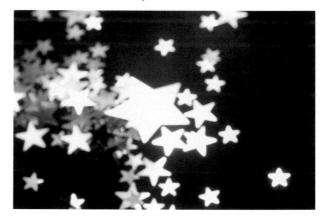

Three Interviews: Three Goals

1. **Individual interview**: The purpose of this approach is to validate what is already known from the resume and any other documents presented by the applicant.

2. **Group interview**: The purpose of this approach is to begin to learn how the applicant responds to multiple interview questions and values and respects all of the participants, and the level of comfort in the group setting.

3. **Audition**: The purpose of this approach is to learn about the applicant's skills in selecting an appropriate topic for the position, and presenting and interacting in the group setting.

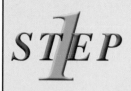

The individual interview

Goal: Determine if the individual presents the required credentials and experience for the position. Learn about the interpersonal skills, application of technical skills, and goodness-of-fit with the team and the organization.

Focus: Employer focused to learn about the applicant

Key Points: inform the applicant of the goal of the interview. Limit the time to I hour or less.

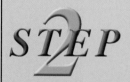

The group interview

Goal: Provide an opportunity for members of the team to learn more specific information about the applicant's overall skills, group management skills, and ability to respond to on-the-spot questions.

Focus: Shared focus among employer, team members, and applicant

Key Points: Prepare a series of questions for each member of the interview team to be sure that all areas of interest or concern are addressed. The questions should be reflective of the descriptions and accomplishments identified in the white paper.

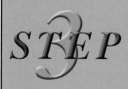

The audition

Goal: Provide an opportunity for the applicant to share a topic in which he or she excels to several members of the team. The applicant's organization, presentation of key information, and interactions with participants to verify understanding of presentation can be evaluated.

Focus: The focus is on the applicant to demonstrate knowledge, skills, and abilities for the position in an area of personal expertise.

Key Points: Share the goals of the audition with the applicant in writing. Provide specific instructions to the applicant for a 10-minute presentation using the preferred audiovisual aids. Be prepared to assist the applicant with PowerPoint setup etc.

Focused Interviewing:
Connecting Interview
Questions to Forces of
Magnetism

Professionalism

Compassion

Collaboration

Initiative

Problem Solving

Collaboration and Teamwork

The purpose of these questions is to learn about the applicant's typical day, how the applicant describes the work, the work processes, how others are considered in the assignment of duties, applicant's priority setting, and the ability to manage time. (Refer to p.486 for FOMs.)

1. Describe your most recent position. FOM: 11,12,14

2. What was your routine from the beginning of your day to the end? FOM: 5

3. What things do you need to consider when you are making a patient assignment? Assigning a project? How frequently do you check on someone after an assignment is made? FOM: 3,5,8,14

4. How did you organize your work? With whom did you work? FOM: 8,13

5. How often did you work beyond your planned end time? FOM: 9

6. How do you know if assignments are fair? FOM: 6,7

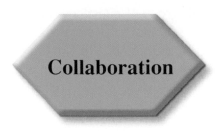

Collaboration

The purpose of these questions is to determine who is involved and how teamwork occurs from the perspective of the applicant, the challenges of complex assignments, the reality that work is often difficult to complete, and the ability to prevent problems rather than react to them.

1. Describe a situation in which you worked together or collaborated with several others to complete work. Who was involved? What did you contribute? What did you do when others did not complete their work? FOM: 3,8

2. Describe a situation in which you were unable to complete the work on your shift or to meet the agreed-on deadline. How did you communicate this to others? How often does this occur? FOM: 8,13

3. Describe a situation in which you were proactive in working with others to address poor communications. What prompted you to address the issue? Who was involved? How did others respond to you? Were you satisfied with the outcome? FOM: 7,13

4. Describe a situation in which you helped others learn new skills or new knowledge. Have you ever assisted others in overcoming barriers to sharing their information? FOM:11,14

5. Share a situation in which you help a new person get involved in teamwork. Why did you recruit this person? How did you identify the team members' strengths? FOM: 11,14

Collaboration—Coaching and Communication

1. Helping others learn new skills is often a challenge due to motivation, timing, and competing priorities. Describe a situation in which you experienced a challenge in educating either a colleague or a patient. What were the circumstances? How did you handle it? FOM: 8,11,4

2. Describe a situation in which you coached coworkers who disliked one another. FOM: 3,9,11,13

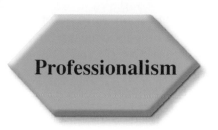

Professionalism

The purpose of this group of questions is to identify several behaviors specific to professionalism, the level of personal accountability for lifelong learning, the essence of professionalism from the very basic attribute of workplace attire, and the effect of cell phone use in public places.

Professionalism—Lifelong Learning

1. How do you remain competent in your work? Describe your learning during the past 12 months: seminars, coursework, journals, books, online information, etc. FOM: 14

2. Describe the benefits of a dress code. What is the ideal dress code for a health care facility? FOM: 4,5,6

3. When and where should cell phones be used? FOM: 4,5

Professionalism

1. Discuss a time when your integrity was challenged. How did you handle it? FOM: 1,8,12,13

2. What would you do if someone asked you to do something unethical or outside of facility policy? FOM: 1,8,9,12,13

3. Describe a time when you challenged someone in your workplace for an inappropriate practice. What was the outcome? FOM: 5, 8, 9, 12, 13

Professionalism—Accountability

1. Describe a time when you had difficulty taking responsibility for your actions. What were the circumstances? How did you handle it? How did it turn out? FOM: 8,9,14

2. Describe a time when someone looked to you for help in solving a problem. What were the circumstances? Why did people seek you out? FOM: 8,11,12,14

3. What motivates you to identify solutions rather than problems? FOM: 1,3,5,9,12

Compassion

Compassion—Motivation for Healing

1. Share your reasons for working in the health care field. What did you consider in making your choice? FOM: 1,3,7,9,11,12,13,14

2. Have you encouraged others into your field? FOM: 1,8,10,11,14

3. What gets you excited about your health care work? FOM: 1,6,9,11,13

4. Describe how you avoid becoming immune to suffering. FOM: 1,3,9,10,14

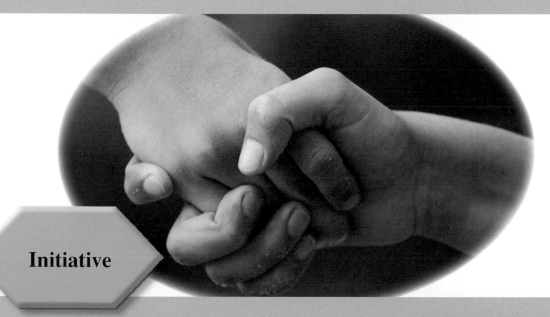

Initiative

1. Describe a time when you volunteered to help others without being asked. FOM: 1,5,6,8,9,12

2. How many times have you been late or absent in the past month? FOM: 5,12,13

3. How frequently do you change your assignment or modify your plans in a day? FOM: 1,3,6,7,9

4. Describe a time when you worked on a special project to further the work of the department or professional discipline. FOM: 8,12,13

5. Share an experience in which you reported a personal error and took accountability for your actions. FOM: 1,6,7,9,12

Problem Solving

1. What would you do if you were given an assignment that you could not complete in the expected time? Describe the circumstances of the last time this happened to you. What was involved? FOM: 1,3,5,6,8,9,12,13

2. Describe a time when you were able to be flexible with your work assignment. What were the circumstances? What were the results? FOM: 1,3,5,6,9,12,13

3. Describe a situation in which you solved a difficult problem. Who was involved? How did you go about discovering the facts? How long did it take to resolve the problem? What or who was affected as a result? FOM: 3,5,6,7,8,9,12,13

4. Once you have made a decision, what would make you change your decision if challenged? FOM: 1,3,5,6,7,8,9,12,13

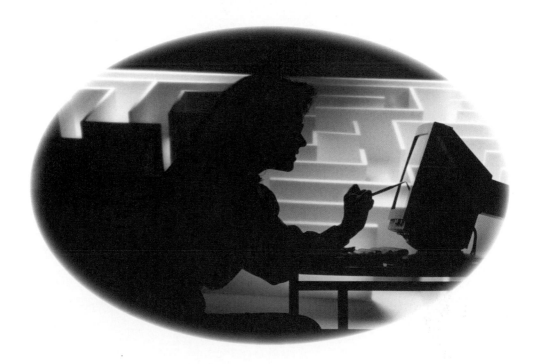

DISCOVERING TECHNOLOGY COMPETENCE

The use of technology is an expectation in health care organizations and presents different challenges to the multigenerational caregivers in the workforce. One's attitude toward technology is critical for success. If the current setting is not fully wired and computerized, most likely it will be in the next 5 years.

The interview process offers an ideal time to determine not only basic skills with keyboards, hardware, and software navigation, but also the level of technology competence and attitude toward computerization. The following questions are presented as a distinct group of items but can be easily integrated into the sections on initiative or problem solving. They focus on determining the level of skills, the applicant's sensitivity to the environment, and overall technology attitude.

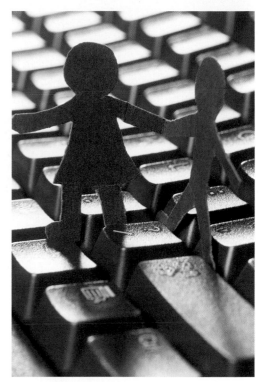

ATTITUDE MATTERS!

Technology Attitude

New generations of health care workers are adept with computers and expect to be competent in using clinical and management information systems. The important attitude that is needed is patience and adaptability to the ever-changing and not always functional systems in health care.

Positive attitude: Interested, always seeking better solutions, and potential effect on better patient care.

Negative: New systems and devices are seen as interferences in work processes. No system is ever quite good enough. Irritated with the shortcomings of any computerized system—quick to point out the problems of the system to anyone who will listen except to those who are able to address issues and improve the system.

COMPUTERIZATION AND TECHNOLOGY SKILL LEVELS

1. **Basic:** Able to use and navigate the keyboard and perform data entry

2. **Intermediate:** Able to document in selected systems, problem solve when system not fully operational, implement downtime processes, and enter data accurately

3. **Expert:** Advanced skills in using multiple clinical documentation systems as well as management information documentation; able to participate in evaluating software programs, devices for documentation and clinical assessments/monitoring, and implementing new and upgraded systems

Interview Questions

1. The use of computers is routine in most health care organizations. Describe your skills with the keyboard. What types of computer systems have you used in the past 2 years?

2. What considerations or precautions are necessary to be sure computer users do not experience fatigue or wrist injuries?

3. What other systems or devices can you use?

4. Would you describe level of technical skill as basic, intermediate, or expert?

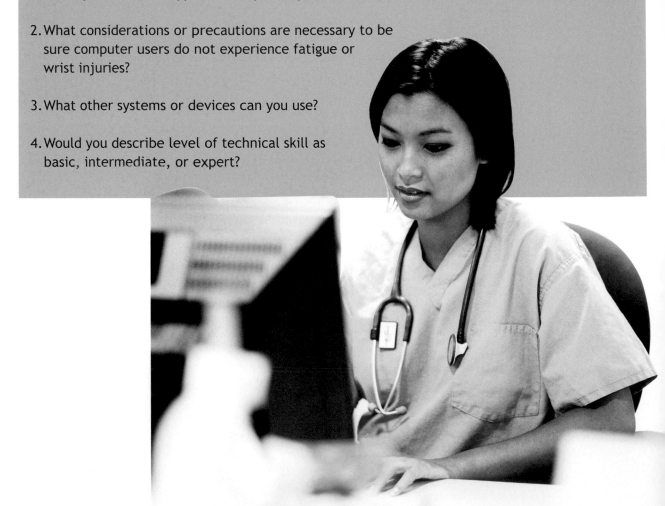

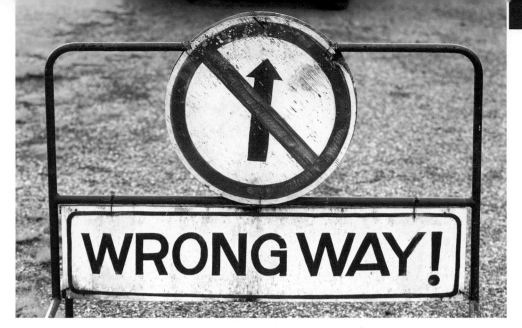

RED FLAGS IN THE INTERVIEW

Take note when the following situations are identified. Each instance by itself may not be problematic; however, when several behaviors and attitudes are identified, raise a red flag; this might not be a person who is a good fit for your team.

- Unable to share specific examples; responds to questions about specific situations with generalities.

- Unable to share times when a specific skill was evident; creativity, compassion, collaboration are all seen as vague ideas with little applicability to the real world.

- Confides that he or she often leaves work for others.

- Unable to share situations in which he or she disagrees with a decision but is still able to support the consensus. Discloses inappropriate responses to team decisions; criticizes decisions after supporting them.

- Has little experience working in teams; likes to work alone. Focuses on the negative aspects of teamwork; unable to describe positive outcomes of teamwork.

- Does not share information unless specifically requested. Does not link knowledge or skills shared with team performance, patient care, and increased productivity.

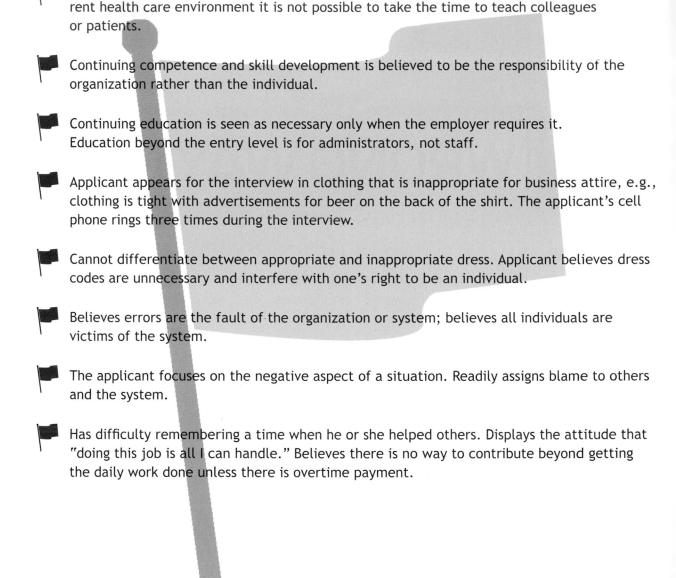

The potential employee believes strongly that education is important; however, in the current health care environment it is not possible to take the time to teach colleagues or patients.

Continuing competence and skill development is believed to be the responsibility of the organization rather than the individual.

Continuing education is seen as necessary only when the employer requires it. Education beyond the entry level is for administrators, not staff.

Applicant appears for the interview in clothing that is inappropriate for business attire, e.g., clothing is tight with advertisements for beer on the back of the shirt. The applicant's cell phone rings three times during the interview.

Cannot differentiate between appropriate and inappropriate dress. Applicant believes dress codes are unnecessary and interfere with one's right to be an individual.

Believes errors are the fault of the organization or system; believes all individuals are victims of the system.

The applicant focuses on the negative aspect of a situation. Readily assigns blame to others and the system.

Has difficulty remembering a time when he or she helped others. Displays the attitude that "doing this job is all I can handle." Believes there is no way to contribute beyond getting the daily work done unless there is overtime payment.

COMPASSIONATE CLOSURE

Not every applicant fits with every organization. Although there are significant shortages in many health care positions, there are also times when there is more than one applicant for the position or the one applicant does not pass the goodness-of-fit test. When the leader determines that the applicant will not be selected, organizations dedicated to excellence ensure that the end of the process is managed with dignity, respect, and honesty. Although not all applicants might be interested in interview feedback, the leader should at least offer to discuss the decision.

1. Be clear why the applicant is not selected. The often used message "other applicant more qualified" may be accurate, but is not very helpful to the applicant. Request participants in the interview process to identify areas specific to the desired goals: technical skills, experience, collaboration, professionalism, compassion, problem solving, and initiative. Share feedback with the applicant.

2. Discuss other opportunities with the organization if you believe there is a goodness-of-fit.

3. Offer recommendations to assist the applicant to enhance skills and modify behaviors if needed.

> *Note:*
>
> **The work of compassionate closure takes time and effort. It is a direct reflection of the leader's commitment to excellence, compassion for the individual, and belief in the potential for future opportunities for both the organization and the applicant to work together.**

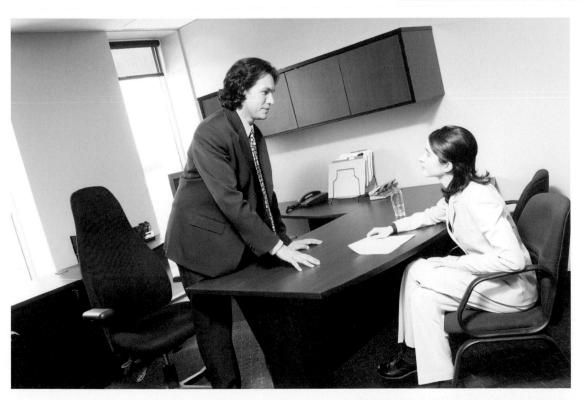

References

American Nurses Credentialing Center. (2005). *Magnet recognition program: Application manual.* Silver Spring, MD: American Nurses Publishing.

Jones, C. B. (2005). The costs of nursing turnover, Part 2: Application of the nursing turnover cost calculation methodology. *JONA*, 35(1), 41-49.

Vestal, K. (2005). Ensuring organizational sustainability. *Nurse Leader*, June 2005, 10-111.

Suggested Readings

Cherry, B., & Jacob, S. (2005). *Contemporary nursing: Issues, trends & management.* St. Louis: Elsevier.

Coleman, D. (1998). *Working with emotional intelligence.* New York: Bantam Books.

Nierenberg, R. J. (2003). The use of a strategic interviewing technique to select the nurse manager. *JONA*, 33(10), 500-505.

CHAPTER 5

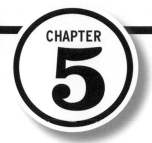

SOCIALIZING NEW EMPLOYEES

Employee retention is a complex process that begins with the first encounter with a potential employee and continues throughout the employee's association with the organization. Every encounter matters!

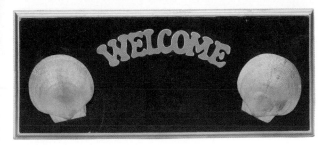

Key Points in Welcoming New Employees

1. *Time is of the essence.*

2. *Mentoring needs vary; socialize to generational differences.*

3. *Short- and long-term goals are essential.*

4. *Monitor the process to be sure the employee is a fit with the organization.*

The first days of a new job are filled with stress, anticipation, and uncertainty. Given the high cost of turnover, organizations cannot afford to lose well-qualified applicants because of a poor socialization and welcoming process. Socializing new employees transforms the new employee or new member of the team from an outsider to a fully functional, engaged member of the team in the shortest time possible.

Guiding the new employee in this process requires creating a partnership between the new employee and the selected preceptor or coach for the new employee.

In addition to the traditional processes of getting to know team members and learning the way around the facility, the socialization process is an opportunity to validate and confirm expected new employee skills. Even in the best of interviewing sessions, interpretations of expectations can vary widely from person to person. The socialization time is for reconciling differing perceptions that may have occurred during the interviewing process. Identifying and reconciling differences between what is needed and what the employee is able to do will improve and facilitate the new employee's success in the organization.

In this section, topics specific to supporting leader development of skills that enhance their ability to partner with new employees in the socialization process are presented. These include socialization, creating positive first impressions, planning for successful socialization, advice to new employees, proactive steps to avoid turnover, precautions to manage early information overload, and feedback to support retention of the right kind.

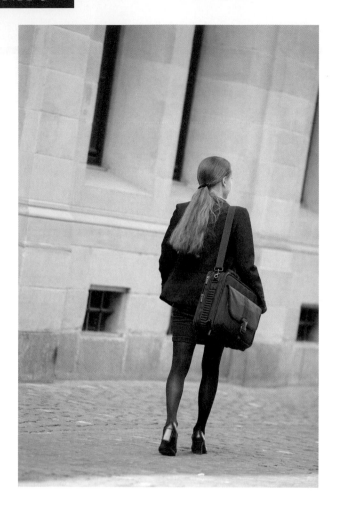

MY FIRST DAY AT WORK

First impressions do matter. The welcoming process or what later becomes the first impression, is a critical behavior in beginning employee socialization and long term retention. Consider the following two scenarios as relayed by recently hired employees.

A Good First Day

I arrived on the unit and was met by the unit clerk who welcomed me to the team. She toured me through the unit and introduced me to staff. Each person welcomed me to the team and offered to help in any way they could. She showed me to the office of the supervisor, and got me a cup of coffee. Shortly after, the supervisor came to greet me and begin my orientation. What I didn't know was that this supervisor also had forgotten that I was coming to the unit that day! The staff stepped up and made my welcome the most important task at hand. I am anxious to be a member of this team.

A Not-So-Good First Day

I arrived on the unit and no one knew who I was or what to do with me. An employee, somewhat frustrated with the situation, attempted to make me welcome by showing me the locker room. I was instructed to wait there and have a cup of coffee while she figured out what to do. I remained in the locker room while others came and went; no one spoke to me. Fifteen minutes later, a supervisor came in and explained that she had forgotten that I was coming. She had another commitment and would get back to me to begin my orientation within the hour. I felt like an intruder and a disruption to their work. I don't know if I want to come back tomorrow.

First impressions log:
Ask each new employee to share the positive experiences and suggestions for improvement. Encourage all team members to review the log and continue to create the optimal orientation experience.

Empowering New Employees

A basic tenet of transformative power is that people must obtain it for themselves; it cannot be given to them. No one can empower another person because the achievement of power that affects transformation can come only from self-action. The role of the leader and experienced employees is to create the conditions and support to empower each employee to become the best employee possible. Thus in socialization, leaders must become partners and coaches in the process rather than directors.

Goals of Socialization

Assist the new employee to:

• Become familiar with the mission of the organization and his or her role in the success of the organization.

• Understand the organizational priorities and become able to act with a sense of urgency.

• Create commitment to give personal best efforts and not hold back because of fear of failure.

• Develop comfort to freely contribute to organizational goals without worrying about who will get the credit.

• Be able to value others' thoughts and ideas and treat team members with respect and compassion.

• Share feedback openly with others without fear of reprisal.

• Uncover the joys of being a caregiver!

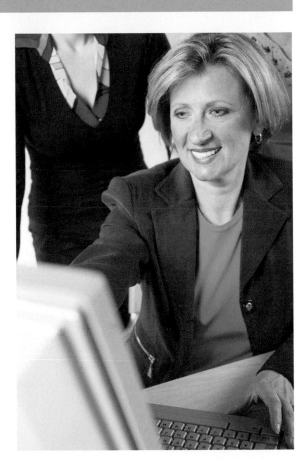

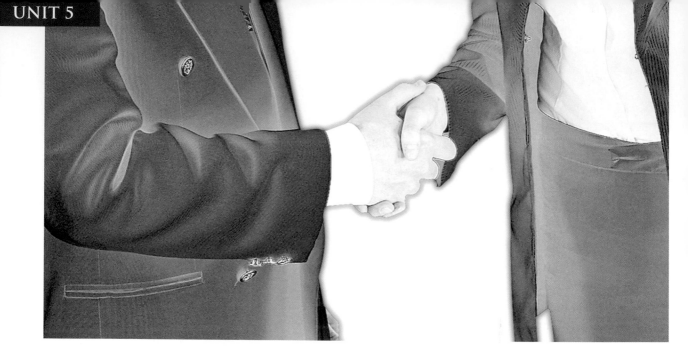

WELCOME TO OUR ORGANIZATION!
PLANNING FOR SUCCESS

Welcoming new employees requires preparation and focus. The following activities will assist leaders in working with the new employee to achieve great results.

1. Establish the relationship. Be sensitize to involving unit staff to support new employees, particularly those who were involved in the interview process. Not feeling welcome is a reason identified by many new employees for their early exit from organizations.

2. Be prepared. Assign a specific staff member to welcome the new staff member. Greet the new employee warmly. Be sure the unit clerk is aware who is coming and when. BE EARLY!

3. Customize orientation to ensure competence and allow staff to do their work as quickly as possible so they can feel valued.

4. Orient to the unit or department routine specific to socialization—report times, content of reports, breaks, lunch, and how to interact with the administrative assistant or unit clerk. Acceptance into the work group is important; new employees need to know they are welcome, know that staff are glad they are now a part of the team AND are willing to assist them in getting accustomed to the department as quickly as possible.

5. Introduce the new employee to support staff, coworkers, and supervisors as quickly and often as you can; redundancy is helpful because there are many individuals to meet.

6. Provide a list of names of team members and contact information.

7. Create a "check-in" plan—different individuals prefer differing levels of oversight and communication. Plan to check in at least every hour for the first few days—OVERCONNECT to be sure new staff are becoming less stressed, more comfortable, and receiving adequate support. Ask focused and purposeful questions:
   • What is going well for you?
   • What is not going well for you?
   • On a scale of 1 to 10 how do you feel you are contributing to the organization?
   • What would make it possible for you to achieve a level of 10?

8. Be sensitive to information overload. Assist the new employee to prioritize orientation information. Reviewing policies and documents and completing online competencies can be overwhelming to new employees. Select the most critical competencies and policies for review, then review progress each day. Encourage new employees to work on document review whenever there are gaps in the orientation activities. Be sure to discuss employee progress with document review and answer questions as they arise.

> **Note:**
> A simple "How are you doing?" is superficial and does not get the information you really want. Be specific and focused.

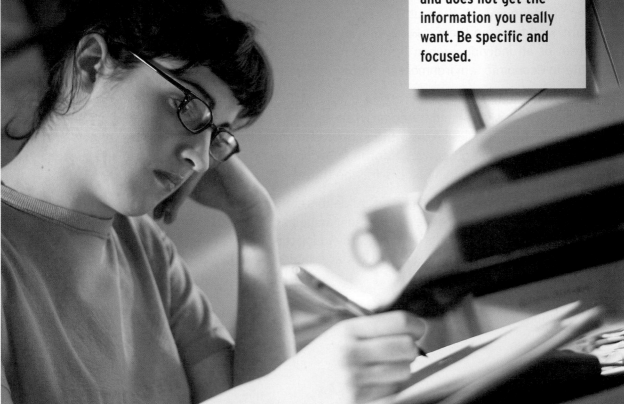

Weekly Check-in Guidelines

The importance of checking in with new team members on a regular basis to determine their progress in becoming integrated into the team cannot be underestimated. Consider the following guidelines as you work with new members of your team. It is always helpful to begin with what is going well—learning about the positive aspects of the work and why the new employee believes things are effective and going well. Using an appreciative inquiry (AI) approach begins positive role modeling for new employees and encourages them to use the same approach with others.

1. Share your experiences of what is going well for you.
2. Which new team members did you meet this week?
3. Who was most helpful to you?
4. What was the low point of the week?
5. What would you like to accomplish next week?
6. What do you think you have contributed to the organization at this point?
7. How can I (we) help you in reaching your goals?

APPRECIATIVE INQUIRY OVERVIEW

Appreciative Inquiry (AI) is about the search for the best in people, their organizations, and the relevant world around them (Cooperrider et al., 2003). It is about the discovery of what gives life to a system or an individual when they are most alive, most effective, and most constructively capable in economic, environmental, and relational terms.

Asking AI questions focuses on crafting questions that elicit how and why things are working well. The intent is to eliminate negativism and criticism and replace them with the spirit of discovery, dream, and design. Also the AI approach minimizes the potential for leaders to transfer personal goals and objectives to others; AI focuses on revealing the goals and successes of the new employee as building blocks for the future.

Taking all of these together as a gestalt, AI deliberately, in everything it does, seeks to work from accounts of this "positive change core," and it assumes that every living system has many untapped and rich and inspiring accounts of the positive. Link the energy of this core directly to any change agenda and changes never thought possible are suddenly and democratically mobilized.

ADVICE TO THE NEW EMPLOYEE

Whether one is a new leader or new staff person, several considerations will assist in making a smooth transition from applicant to a fully functioning member of the team:

- Be a follower first; your time to lead your own work will come quickly. Learning about the work and work processes will position you for success rather than working blindly with many missteps.

- Focus on priorities: Identify what needs to be accomplished early in the first weeks of employment.

- Resist the temptation to tell others how things were done at your previous employment—you are at a new place and their processes may be much better!

- Listen and learn during orientation.

- Be present and open-minded and at the same time avoid blindly accepting every thing you hear. Develop skills in listening first, then ask questions, discuss the issues to ensure clarity, and then—and only then—share alternatives to support the achievement of organizational goals. Regularly telling others how it was done in your previous organization can be annoying and create negative feelings in a new relationship.

- Listen some more and reflect on what you are hearing.

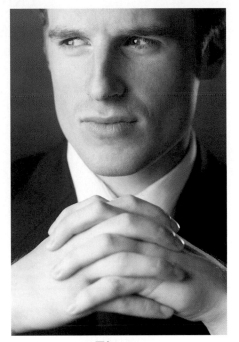

First:

Listen and

Learn!

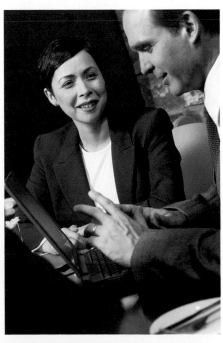

BE PROACTIVE: IDENTIFY AND ADDRESS TRIGGERS FOR TURNOVER

Preventing turnover can be accomplished by recognizing those common situations in which employees are known to become dissatisfied and consider leaving the organization. Integrate these feelings and potential experiences into the socialization process as a means to be proactive in not only addressing them, but also working proactively to avoid them. The following perceptions and feelings have been identified as triggers for turnover.

Loss of Control

Caregivers often feel they are powerless to stop processes they believe are less than satisfactory. Most common is the perceived lack of time one is able to engage with patients during procedures and treatments.

Reverse this experience by discussing opportunities to give feedback and get involved in groups to share ideas.

Devaluation and Disrespect

The holistic work of caregivers is often reduced to technical interventions, with the art and coordinative work being dismissed as nonessential. Only a portion of the caregiver's service is valued by the organization or society at large. Reverse this experience through emphasis on evidence-based practice. Encourage leaders and caregivers to be familiar with caring research and its economic value as well as linking positive patient care experiences with positive organizational outcomes, which are strongly influenced by caregiver interpersonal skills.

Overextension

Too often, caregivers are so stretched they are like rubber bands waiting to snap. They are pulled by leaders, patients, visitors, and peers. In attempting to meet myriad needs, there is little time for personal care.

Reverse this experience by encouraging employees to become comfortable with saying no when capacity is exceeded. The stream of incoming work will not stop. The skill of coaching upward is essential when overextension occurs.

Fragmentation and Frustration

As a result of overextension, caregivers often attempt the impossible—to meet all of the demands even though such attempts are unrealistic and impossible. One person, no matter how competent and hardy, cannot do the work of two individuals. Thus only partial, superficial work can be done; orders are missed, patient teaching is superficial, assessments are less frequent than standards require, and on and on. An important reality is that there will always be more work, more challenges and seldom enough time to do what is believed should be done.

Reverse the situation with an emphasis on priority setting and learning to say no. Most work can be ordered and life-threatening needs addressed with clear communication. Chaos and irritation of needs not being met usually result when there is no plan for resolution and others are left to guess when the needs will be met.

Diversity of Goals

Within one organization, many professions share common goals; physicians, nurses, pharmacists, and therapists all focus on health and healing. Within these common goals are diverse goals: differing roles, believed competing clinical areas, and expectations within one profession that often cause discord. Healers unwittingly compete with each other for resources, staff, equipment, and position for personal gain rather than the good of the whole organization.

In addition, horizontal violence (aka eating our young) continues to occur within professions, particularly nursing.

Reverse these behaviors, with an emphasis on respect and development of partnership skills to achieve effective teamwork.

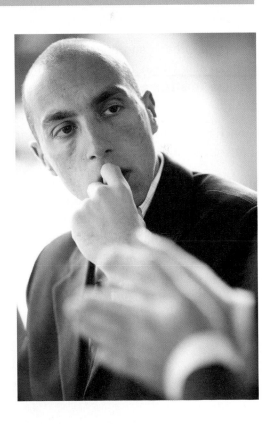

Focus on the Greater Good of Healing!

FEEDBACK FOR SUCCESS:
ORIENT, COACH, PERFORM, ORIENT, COACH, PERFORM

The partnership between the leader and the new employee requires ground rules specific to the rules of engagement; specific to when feedback will be given—what will be discussed, and the manner in which feedback is given.

The socialization process is optimal, creating the expectations from initial encounters that support the work of informing, coaching, and performance, a cycle that continually repeats as new work is introduced. During the process, feedback can be given for four reasons: performance, growth, upward communication, and on-the-spot performance.

Effective socialization includes both the instructional sharing of organizational processes and the initiation of healthy dialog in which the expectations for growth, excellence, and modification of behaviors are established.

Giving feedback and coaching processes aim to enhance the performance and learning ability of others. It involves providing information and includes motivation, effective questioning, and consciously matching one's management style to the coachee's readiness to undertake a particular task.

Coaching is an interactive partnership process and focuses on helping the coachee to help her- or himself; it does not rely on a one-way flow of telling and instructing.

To be a good coach you must believe that people want to do well, that they want to please the manager and grow professionally. Your role as a coach is to help others gain skills, abilities, and knowledge they need to increase their potential and improve their performance. In this section, four types of coaching are presented with multiple steps. These steps or processes often occur quickly in practice and may overlap. The distinction of each step is to instruct and assist the reader in gaining an appreciation of the complexities of the process.

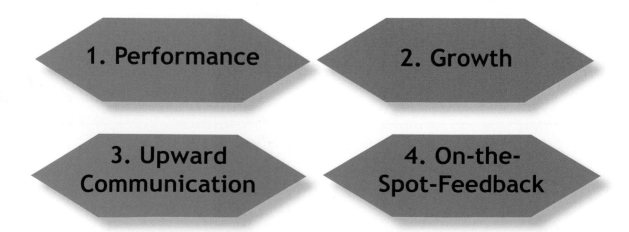

1. Performance

2. Growth

3. Upward Communication

4. On-the-Spot-Feedback

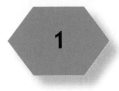

FEEDBACK FOR PERFORMANCE

The goal is to assist the employee in modifying behaviors to improve results. Examples include technical performance of skills, communication style, work planning and prioritizing, and timeliness.

Several steps are involved in providing feedback about performance. The following steps and scenario for performance feedback provide guidelines for the leader. Often, each step does not occur distinctly and sequentially, but may overlap or occur in a different sequence. Regardless of the sequencing, each step is important for effective outcomes.

Step 1. Describe the situation that you observed.

Include the interactions that were observed in the group meeting such as interrupting others many times. Describe your perceptions of the behavior. For example, "You seemed aggressive and irritated. Can you tell me what was going on?"

Note: Be cautious not to ask if the employee was indeed irritated or aggressive; the reality is that you, as a member of the team, experienced that feeling. The challenge is to get recognition from the employee that an adversarial exchange occurred and then to work with the employee to channel negative behaviors and nonverbal messages into more positive behaviors.

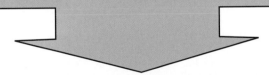

Step 2. Gather additional information and agree on objectives of the coaching session.

Would you share your thoughts on the experience? Were there other things going on? Is this a good time for us to talk about this and see if we can't figure out how to avoid this in the future?

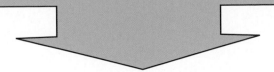

Step 3. Invite suggestions to achieve the goals.

How can you address this behavior? What new skills are needed? I understand that you are anxious to share your ideas with others and don't always agree with what is being said. Let's figure out how you can share your ideas, show respect for others by not interrupting them and encourage questions and discussions of other alternatives.

Focus this request on replacing negative behaviors with positive, respectful behaviors. Challenge the new employee to shifting from competing with others in the giving of information to a spirit of collaboration in which all members of the team learn from each other. Also, it is important to work to change one's own behaviors, not the behaviors of others.

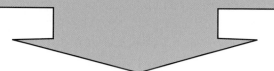

Step 4. Create a plan for action.

Be specific. Plan for new behaviors at the next group meeting. Assist the employee to review the goals and purpose of the meeting and then determine how the employee will be able to contribute to this meeting. Also, help the employee identify what to expect to learn from others at this meeting—a very important step in the process to changing behavior.

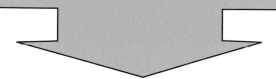

Step 5. Follow up.

After the next group meeting, discuss behaviors, share observations, and ask for feedback from the new employee. Thank the new employee for the willingness to modify behaviors to achieve excellence in the organization.

GROWTH

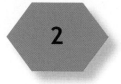

2

The goal is to assist the employee in developing new skills. Examples include new workflow skills, software applications, and participation on committees.

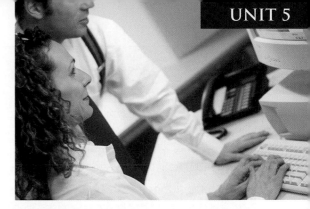

Continuing to develop skill is the goal of the majority of employees. Although it is difficult to develop new skills during the initial socialization, desired experiences and skills are often identified at this time. Leaders can work with new employees to create strategies to investigate opportunities and identify timelines and resources to support interests. Consider the following steps in helping new employees continue their journey of lifelong development.

Step 1. Describe the situation.

The new employee has identified an interest in becoming the leader of the patient safety committee. The new employee is experienced and highly qualified in this area. The current leader of the patient safety committee is competent and has served in this role for 5 years.

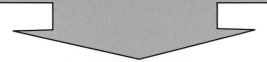

Step 2. Agree on outcomes of coaching session.

Coaching should encompass creating a plan to achieve the goal and identification of facilitators and barriers to achieve the goal. Another important outcome is the creation of a timeline for the achievement of this goal.

Step 3. Validate

The new employee would like to become a member of the safety committee, learn the structure and processes of the committee, and request support from the leader to learn about the committee. The employee would like to be involved in the leadership of the committee but does not intend to focus on being the leader until learning about the committee and its processes.

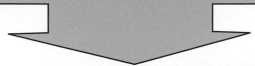

Step 4. Share leader assessment.

The leader should reflect on the goal and the potential for achievement within the current organization. Just because an individual desires to become leader of a group does not mean that the current leader wants to be relieved of responsibilities—nor does it mean that the current leader might be ready for a change! Regardless, the new employee is correct in wanting to become a member of the committee to learn about the processes and work currently in progress before announcing the desire for the leadership role. Thank the new employee for willingness to get involved, share expertise, and work within the culture of the organization.

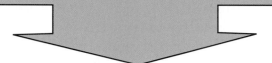

Step 5. Select a course of action.

Several activities can occur between the new employee and the coach. First, the leader can introduce the new employee to the committee chair and request permission for the new employee to attend a meeting as a guest. The next step is to secure membership on the committee.

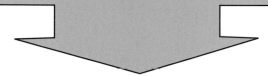

Step 6. Follow up.

Review experience as a member of the committee after each meeting. Identify contributions, relationships with members, and perceived credibility on the committee.

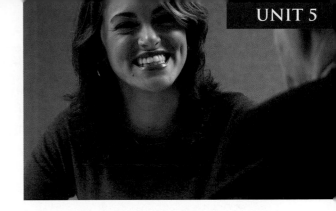

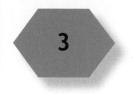

3 UPWARD COMMUNICATION

The goal is to assist the employee in sharing feedback, issues, and concerns with those in power. Examples include management of workload, disagreements with policy changes, and benefits.

Giving feedback to a person with more power, authority, and experience, for some is a comfortable expected behavior. For others, it is very stressful and may be one of the most challenging experiences. Sharing ideas and perceptions with members of the organization is important in creating high-performing teams. Sharing that information with those in position of power is especially important because these individuals are positioned to make changes and to affect significant numbers of individuals. Feedback provides opportunities to enhance the work of the team and the organization as a collective unit. In spite of the fact that not everyone wants feedback, the employee should always work to give open, honest feedback, both positive and negative. Failing to attempt to give feedback eliminates all possibility for change.

Risks of Upward Feedback

One's ideas may be rejected and have a negative effect on the relationship. Giving feedback requires careful positioning and timing to minimize the threat or perception of threat to the upward person. For the first few encounters, individuals should work with an experienced colleague in planning this feedback.

> **Step 1.** Describe the situation.
>
> At a recent meeting a leader recognized the accomplishments of one department and criticized others for failing to achieve the same standards. The leader believed that by encouraging competition, a core value of his generation, then employees would see it as a challenge and respond positively. Unfortunately, this approach demoralized the criticized team and embarrassed the successful team. The team members believe that criticizing the team in public has negatively affected the team's motivation.

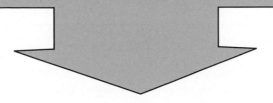

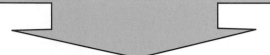

Step 2. Agree on objectives of the coaching session.

The goal is to share perceptions, identify that the discussion was unhealthy, and acknowledge that the department was already aware of the results and working on corrective action. A second goal is to request that this type of communication not occur in the future.

Step 3. Schedule a time for discussion.

Let the person know in advance that discussion about the recent meeting is requested. Spontaneous discussion of the concern with the leader rather than a formal meeting tends to lessen the significance of the message to be delivered. As one becomes more comfortable in giving feedback to leaders, less formality may be indicated.

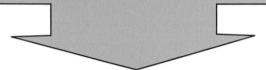

Step 4. Meet with the leader, present the issue, and request a change in behavior.

Prepare for the meeting by writing out issues concisely, asking for feedback from the leader. Be prepared to request changes. Presenting a complaint without ideas for change will be interpreted as complaining. Be sure to thank the leader for his or her time and willingness to listen.

Step 5. Request a follow-up meeting to discuss proposed changes.

This may not always be indicated, but one can identify other opportunities for discussion to continue building a relationship with the leader.

Step 6. Reflect on process for discussion with one's leader.

What went well? Would you do anything differently? Were there any surprises? Would you do anything differently the next time? Will there be a next time?

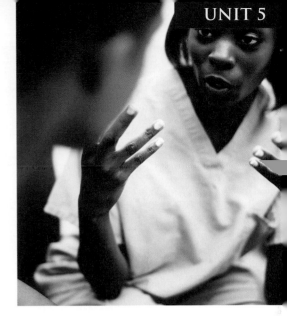

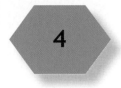

4

ON-THE-SPOT FEEDBACK

The goal is to assist the employee in immediately correcting behavior that is believed detrimental to safety or the organization's reputation. Examples include unsafe situations in which someone is loud, aggressive, and physically confrontational.

Giving feedback on the spot requires focus and compassion: focus for the safety of others and the reputation of the organization and compassion for those involved. This work is difficult for most individuals who are averse to conflict and making others feel uncomfortable. But this is the most humane approach to deal with challenging situations. Although the stress of the moment may be significant, the long-term effect of confronting the issue in a timely manner is much healthier than ruminating about an incident and discussing it with others at a later time. In such situations, time is of the essence, so each situation should be addressed quickly, safely, and diplomatically. Failure to address these situations could result in patient injury and negatively affect the organization's reputation.

Step 1. Describe the situation.

While walking down the hall, an employee was observed talking loudly and rudely to a patient while wheeling the patient in a wheelchair. The patient was also yelling and wanting to get out of the wheelchair.

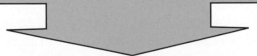

Step 2. Intervene to assess.

The priority in this situation is to stop the negative behavior and address the patient's needs. The next goals are to reverse the effect on the patient and inform the employee of the effect of such behavior. Tactfully request the employee to stop for a minute and then step aside out of hearing range of the patient and discuss the situation.

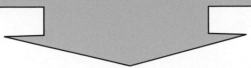

Step 3. Share assessment of the situation.

I observed you yelling at the patient and ignoring the patient's request.
This is inappropriate behavior.

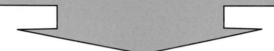

Step 4. Intervene to diffuse and correct the situation.

Reassure the patient. The patient is confused and disoriented. Request that the employee continue reassuring the patient while completing the transportation.

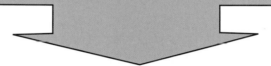

Step 5. Plan for follow-up.

Request that the employee notify you when the transport is completed. At this time, determine with the employee how to manage similar situations in the future without negative consequences.

Step 6. Follow up.

Check in with the employee in 1 or 2 days. Thank the employee for the willingness to discuss the situation and work to change behaviors to support patients in a positive manner. Recognize the challenges of patient care and the need for team members to support each other.

A Gentle Reminder...

In the first days of a new job or role, emphasis is on introducing the new employee to the social and political norms of the department and the organization. However, the emphasis must quickly shift to getting the work done once. Leaders will always be challenged to balance the processes of socialization with getting the real work done.

Too often the social relationships and the politics of the organization get more attention than the essential work. According to Zaleznik (1989), the subordination of real work to psychopolitics is the understandable but unintended outgrowth of two phenomena: evolution of large organizations and success of the human relations school of management.

Social systems are not the result of conscious planning, but rather exist as a result of human proclivities, of all the human unwritten contracts that grow up between a company and its employees. Hence, every organization has illogical underpinnings as well as logical ones.

Too often, leaders put interpersonal matters, power relations, and peacekeeping above the real work of the organization. When process takes precedence over substance, the work of the organization is at risk. The real work of providing services, assuring customer satisfaction, controlling costs, and developing new products cannot be set aside in favor of social rituals and the guise of empowerment. Leaders are accountable for creating the context for a system of cooperation which includes effective communication systems, effective decision-making processes, and the achievement of the purposes of the organization.

Don't Forget the Real Work

The real work of providing the optimal context for patient care, providing that care, and acting on ideas to improve services must be the principal preoccupation of health care workers.

Note:

Excessive psychopolitics drives out the real work—drives out the intellectual and emotional energy needed to do the real work. Focus on the work to be done and avoid the distractions of emotional, unfocused discussions whenever possible.

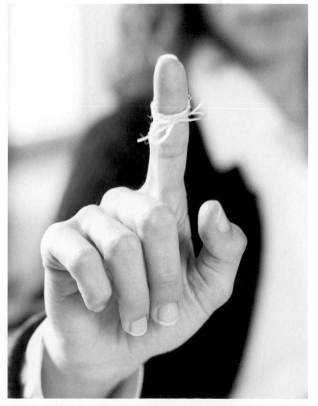

Socializing New Employees 519

References

Cooperrider, D. L., Whitely, D., & Stavros, J. M. (2003) *Appreciative inquiry handbook: The first in a series of AI workbooks for leaders of change*. Bedford Heights, OH/San Francisco: Lakeshore Publishers/Berrett-Koehler.

Zaleznik, A. (1989). Real work. *Harvard Business Review*, 67(1), 1-7.

Suggested Readings

Connelly, L. M. (2005). Welcoming new employees. *Journal of Nursing Scholarship*, 37(2), 163-164.

Jacobs, B. B., Fontana, J. S., Kehoe, M. H., Matarese, C., & Chinn, P. L. (2005). An emancipatory study of contemporary nursing practice. *Nursing Outlook*, 53(1), 6¬14.

Landsberg, M. (1997). *The tao of coaching*. Santa Monica, CA Knowledge Exchange, LLC.

UNIT 6: BUILDING THE FUTURE OF EXCELLENCE: MENTORING, LEARNING, AND LIVING LEADERSHIP

1. SYNTHESIS: THE NEW ROLE OF THE LEADER

2. MODELING AND MENTORING LEADERSHIP

3. MANAGING RISK AND VULNERABILITY

4. PRACTICE IN A WORLD OF UNCERTAIN EXPECTATIONS

5. BUILDING RELATIONSHIPS IN THE NEW AGE OF WORK

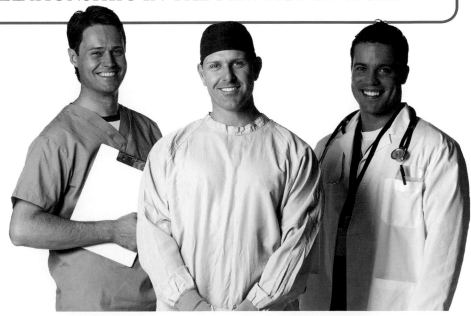

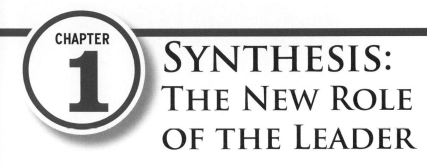

CHAPTER 1

SYNTHESIS: THE NEW ROLE OF THE LEADER

Synthesis of vital information is essential for leadership success in complex organizations.

Leaders with expertise in synthesis have learned to analyze situations, integrate multiple pieces of data, and assimilate elements of insight into the whole situation, which then guides the imagination and thinking of the leader in the process of expert decision making. In the broadest sense, synthesis involves scanning and sensing the environment, reflecting on past experiences, integrating the data from the scanning process with one's intuition and experience. Synthesis is an intermediate step in the expert decision making process and provides substance for interpretation and selection of a course of action.

The transforming leader has evolved from a leader focused on compartmentalizing and completing tasks in a linear fashion to a leadership style that is steeped in systems thinking and the interrelatedness of all variables. Leadership synthesis may indeed be the most significant distinguishing characteristic of expert leaders. Leaders recognized for their expertise have most likely developed an incredible ability to quickly synthesize the essential variables of a situation to quickly make effective decisions. Less skilled leaders struggle with analysis of facts and consideration of options.

> *Synthesis:*
> *The process or result of building up separate elements, especially ideas, into a connected whole, especially into a theory or system; the opposite of analysis.*
> *(Webster's Dictionary)*

This section provides leaders with an overview of the value and skills of synthesis, considerations in developing synthesis competence, the benefits and limitations of synthesis, and the application to complex situations as the means to achieve optimal outcomes and the most appropriate use of resources. Developing skills of synthesis is an ongoing and meaningful process of the learning journey of all leaders. Leaders must continually challenge themselves and their colleagues to develop high level skills of synthesis.

SYNTHESIS 101

> *Note:*
>
> *Synthesis is about linking collateral efforts into the whole; everything matters!*

Three processes are identified in leadership synthesis; scanning the environment, reflecting on one's experiences and intuition, and integrating information. They are presented as distinct events within the process of decision making for presentation purposes only. In reality, the activities of scanning, reflecting, and integrating may occur simultaneously and seldom in a predictable linear fashion. In this model, synthesis ends when interpretation begins.

Developing expertise in leadership synthesis requires experience and practice. Consider the music of a symphony orchestra that reflects the technical skills of tonal creation on instruments, years of individual practice, more practice as a group of musicians, and intuitive sensitivity to travel with the music as it emerges from those musicians led by a most skillful orchestra leader. Musicians reflect on experience as they intuitively know how to go with the flow of the music. The synthesis of technical skills, fine equipment, experience, sensitivity, presence, intuition, and leadership results in the sought-after incredibly pleasing melody.

Health care leaders, similar to orchestra leaders or accomplished chefs, are able to achieve incredible outcomes from the effective synthesis of multiple ingredients, equipment, and most important, human talents. The expert chef achieves culinary excellence through baking, in which multiple ingredients are combined in a certain order and manipulated to produce a culinary delight. Similarly, the leader evolves from the very specific and mechanical skills of developing meeting agendas to the skillful facilitation of group processes. Health care leaders are continually challenged to bring disparate processes and work products together to create and support optimal decision making to synthesize multiple realities into one comprehensive reality.

The expert leader through finely honed skills of synthesis produces results that serve only to enhance the quality and timeliness of services.

> *The creation of mosaic pottery is a synthesis of raw materials, a process that integrates amalgamation, skill, and artistic ability, and a firing process that results in a unique product. Similarly, leaders, when confronted with the challenging situations, gather data from multiple sources, place it into the current context of the organization, and call on their past experiences and intuition to make decisions that are timely, well regarded, and cost effective.*

> *The survival of the human species hinges on our ability to develop a holistic framework that recognizes the interrelatedness of all knowledge.*
>
> *Richard Barrett*

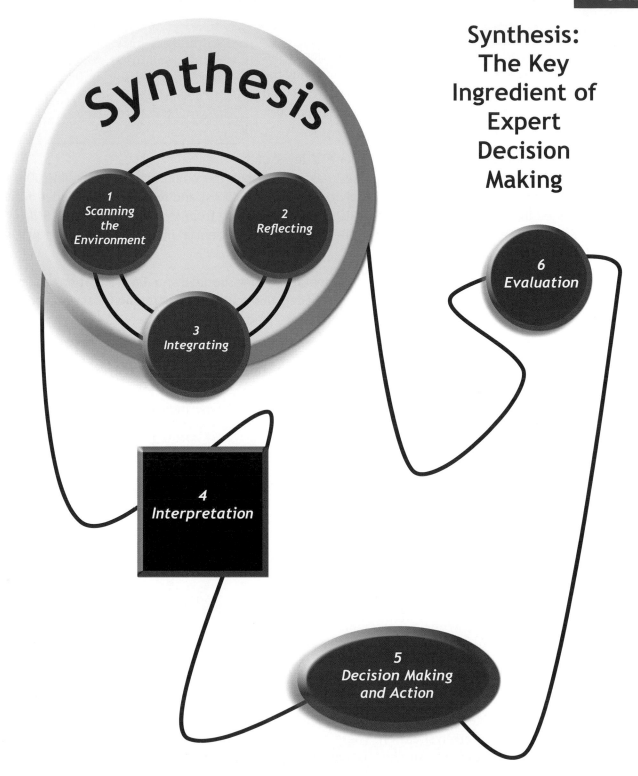

Synthesis:
The Key
Ingredient of
Expert
Decision
Making

1. Scanning the Enviroment

Synthesis is much more than rearranging information to put a new twist or spin on a situation; it is about identifying the appropriate information from multiple sources that will support the creation of solutions and approaches appropriate to the given circumstances.

> Synthesis is about external sensing, scanning the environment, integrating multiple sources of data, and reflecting on the information.

Sensing and scanning the environment require a level of consciousness that allows the leader to take in as much about the environment as possible. Data from multiple sources are involved in the activities of synthesis. First and foremost, the leader must become skilled in sensing the environment, listening and learning from the current activity. *Stilling one's mind* to be open to what is going on in the environment is essential in this process and requires discipline, practice, and commitment.

There is no template or format in which environmental scanning should occur. Each situation requires different considerations identified by the expert leader, who scans the environment based on previous experiences, knowledge of the current environment, and desired outcomes.

2. Reflecting

Once the environment is scanned, the leader and the team reflect on past experiences, consider how current events resonate with the past events, recall successes that reinforce good processes, and avoid negative experiences. Consideration is also given to how individuals will react in new circumstances—positively or negatively.

3. Integrating

The process of integration is the assimilation of the data collected during the scanning phase and the addition of reflective hypothesis and intuition; all of the relevant research, values, perceptions, experiences, intuition, and the political, technological, economic, and social data. The ever-present challenge of this phase is developing skill of which data to include and which to exclude to effect the best decision. The effective integration is not a lone activity—full integration of work and efforts of all members of the group is required.

Data integration also considers those phenomena that are outside of knowledge boundaries and necessarily requires trust in the process and the nature of life events—complex and not always explainable! Barrett (1995) explains that certain phenomena lie outside these belief systems and the boundaries of our knowledge; miracles cannot be explained by science or religion, synchronicity cannot be explained by psychology or science, and spirituality is outside the realm of religion and psychology. Yet all are possible in the course of events. The leader realizes that not all events are knowable and explainable and that no amount of analysis could uncover the rationale for the events or specific outcomes of a given situation. These phenomena or potential phenomena are continually integrated by the expert leader who has become an expert synthesizer.

DEVELOPING SYNTHESIS COMPETENCE: SCANNING THE ENVIRONMENT, INTEGRATING, AND REFLECTING

The depth and range of considerations examined in the synthesis process are significant. Each of the following portrays one or several of the phases experienced within the synthesis process.

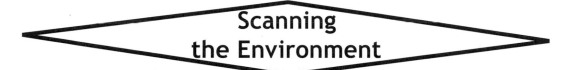

Scanning the Environment

Scanning: Critical listening to what others are saying and not saying.

Scanning: What qualitative and quantitative research evidence is available?

Scanning: Economic considerations—What resources are available now or will be?

Scanning: Events occurring in the organization and in others' lives; competing initiatives, holiday scheduling challenges, etc.

Reflecting

Reflecting about this situation and other similar situations of the past; how does this compare with past experiences?

Reflecting and intuiting about future events

Reflecting and integrating: Considering personal values/ethics/viewpoints. How do these guide decision making? Are they congruent or oppositional or is it uncertain how they are aligned? Is personal presence expected or is electronic communication preferred?

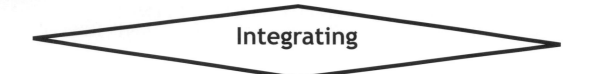

Integrating

Integrating and reflecting: What are the anticipated positive and negative outcomes?

Integrating: What is the right time for action or no action?

Integrating: Consider unrelated events that occur in the environment as well as the level of activity in other areas that could or could not support another initiative.

Integrating and reflecting: Considering organizational values/ethics/viewpoints. How do these guide decision making? Are they congruent or oppositional or is it uncertain how they are aligned?

Integrating empirical knowledge about the nature of the patient care experience; what is it like and how will actions affect the desired patient care experience?

Integrating: Considering the goals of the organization across the system from the organization as a whole, to the team, to the department, to the unit, to the individual.

Synthesis
Scanning, Reflecting,
and Integrating

INDIVIDUAL TRANSFORMATION: FROM ANALYSIS TO SYNTHESIS

Leadership synthesis is an advanced skill that evolves with experience, knowledge, and a heightened level of consciousness. Effective leadership synthesis skills evolve more quickly in some individuals than in others, and for some, the ability to synthesize rather than simply process in a linear manner is never achieved. Given the incredible benefits realized from leadership synthesis, aspiring leadership experts are encouraged to examine the essence of synthesis and work with colleagues to develop high levels of effective synthesis. Failing to take the time to contemplate situations and synthesize ideas in favor of quick, poorly researched decisions can result in short-lived solutions, loss of engagement by disregarded employees, and increased cost to the organization.

Developing leadership expertise in synthesis mirrors the skill acquisition process identified by Dreyfus and Dreyfus (1986) and Benner (1984) for acquiring clinical expertise; individuals move from novice across the continuum to the expert level. The five stages of the skill acquisition model—novice, beginner, competent, proficient, and expert—provide an excellent perspective from which to appreciate the developmental process and the expert's overall depth of the skill. The significance of this work is the correlation of the expert level and the work of leadership synthesis. Effective synthesis skills developed by the leader represent achievement of expert status. Aspiring leaders are challenged to reflect on their progression of skill development and current level of achievement from this perspective.

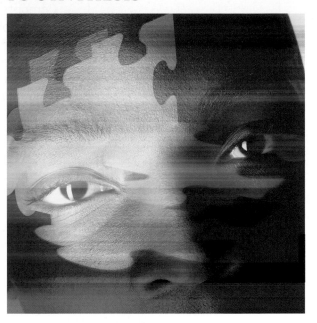

1. NOVICE

1. Novice: Learning the work begins with identifying the tasks to be done free from a specific context. The learner's work is primarily mechanical and focuses on describing and defining synthesis and the associated processes.

2. ADVANCED BEGINNER

2. Advanced beginner: As the novice gains experience in real situations, he or she begins to recognize the phenomena and the situational aspects. The learner begins to practice synthesis with the oversight of a coach or mentor in this stage. The activity is now both mechanical and experiential.

3. COMPETENT

3. Competence: Performance is characterized with detached planning, conscious assessment of elements or variables that are salient to the situation, and analytical, rule-guided choice of action, followed by an emotionally involved experience of the outcome. The activity is less mechanical, experiential, and linked to the context or setting in which the work occurs.

4. PROFICIENT

4. Proficient: Variables that present themselves as salient are assessed and combined by rule and maxim to produce decisions. Proficiency requires a transition from reflecting on situations and variables as a detached observer and ceases to look for principles to guide actions. Involvement at this level moves beyond the need for detached, conscious planning. The focus is experiential and intuitive.

5. EXPERT

5. Expertise: Situations are recognized from the broad range of experiences, and action is taken without calculating and comparing alternatives. The expert sees intuitively what to do without applying rules and making judgments, and does not deliberate. The process and work are intuitive. Synthesis skills are fully integrated into a unit of work.

BENEFITS OF SYNTHESIS

In this section, the benefits of synthesis are identified. These benefits are significant for individuals, teams, or organizations and can be directly related to the overall productivity and quality of organizational performance. Examples of some of the specific benefits follow:

Synthesis prevents partial solutions.

Synthesis prevents quick fixes and short-term solutions that are quickly undone.

Synthesis decreases resource misuse.

Synthesis prevents disenfranchisement of stakeholders by ensuring that those involved in a decision are considered and involved.

Synthesis increases the likelihood of sustainable solutions for complex situations.

Note:

Every act of synthesis creates a unique result and cannot be generalized to other situations. Each synthesis event is unique due to the specific information considered, the specific time it occurred, and context in which it happened.

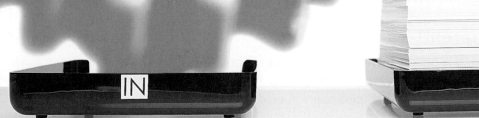
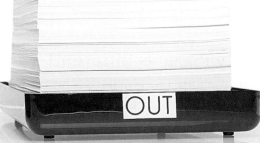

LIMITATIONS OF SYNTHESIS

Leadership synthesis is not the universal solution for all situations and challenges in organizational life. Like any commodity or entity, too much or too little can result in less than desirable outcomes. For example, attempting to extract models or templates for decision making from the process of synthesizing is counter to the notion of synthesis. No two situations are alike. The synthesis process is guided by the common processes of scanning, reflecting, and integrating but is always unique given the wide range and combination of variables.

> There is no template for effective synthesis, only guidelines as to how to ensure one is engaged in the process. Each situation is unique and cannot be re-duced to a template or model.

> Significant time is required to develop effective synthesis skills, to develop the skills of scanning, integrating and reflecting on the information at hand. Less time is required to develop skills to make decisions based on templates and policies.

There Is No Secret Magic Synthesis Formula

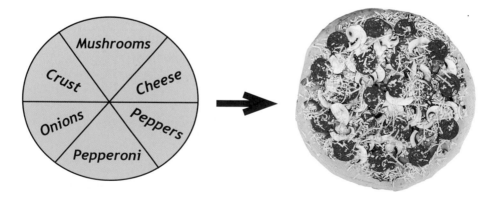

Every Pizza Is Different!

In its simplest form, making a pizza involves synthesis. First, one scans the environment for available ingredients; second, the ingredients are integrated into the desired pizza; and finally, one anticipates and reflects on the expected culinary product!

THE ABSENCE OF SYNTHESIS

When expertise in synthesizing information is not present, the result may be tolerable in the short term, but eventually the factors not considered must be reckoned with. Synthesis always includes critical assessment, critical thinking, critical analysis, and synthesis of the events surrounding a situation. Lack of synthesis is exemplified in compartmentalization, closed processes in which certain individuals are included, or fragmented and incremental processes.

Synthesis is absent when only one metric is used for decision making; other related variables are not factored in. For example, when the hours per patient day (HPPD) metric is believed to be the primary metric for performance, the assumption is flawed given there are multiple other variables that affect staff performance and patient outcomes. This assumption and conclusion are specific only to a single staffing metric that results in a level of financial performance, nothing more.

Note:
The absence of synthesis reduces decision making to a mechanical and rigid process.

VVhen the process of evaluating variables from a fixed template becomes the norm, the routine combination of specific and unique variables occurs without reflection and integration. The higher level intellectual processes of reflection and integration do not occur; decision making is limited to scanning the environment for specific data elements to insert into an algorithm.

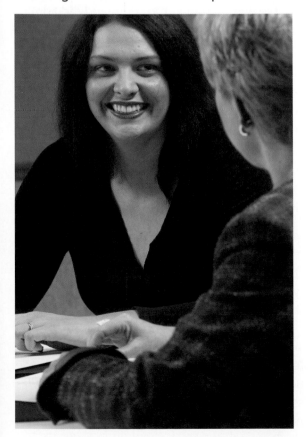

The Hiring Process: A Synthesis Exemplar

The hiring each individual is a unique and distinct process that is guided by specific principles for interviewing, evaluating candidates, and making offers for employment. Each interview experience is distinct from all other interviews. The synthesis process includes:

- Scanning of the application, feedback from the interview process, interactions with other colleagues.

- Integrating the available information, needs of the applicant, and congruence of the applicant skills with the culture.

- Reflecting on the effect of the potential employee on the team and the organization.

LIVING SYNTHESIS

Three situations, reacting to patient complaints, developing new programs, and creating evidence for current practice are examined to illustrate the value of synthesis.

CASE STUDY 1: REACTING TO A COMPLAINT

Background

The patient complained to the administrator that the nurse did not provide any care for him all day including administration of medications. The nurse has documented that she did give the medications and remembers giving them to the patient while the patient's daughter was present. In this situation, synthesis occurs quickly and includes the following considerations.

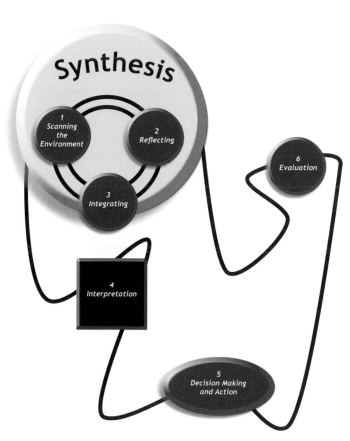

Scanning the Environment...

In this situation, the administrator identified who was involved: the nurse, other team members, the physician, and family members. The story was relayed by the patient without the daughter.

The daughter informed the administrator that the nurse was indeed in the room and did administer the medications. The patient was unable to recollect the events. The patient was insistent, but also known by his family to be forgetful.

Reflecting...

The administrator considered other experiences with this unit and nurse that were positive. Concern was expressed for the patient's failing memory and dignity. The goal was to regain the patient's trust in the nurse and be sure that no additional stress occurred.

Integrating the Information...

in this somewhat simplistic example, the integration involved the information from the key players: the patient, daughter, and nurse. Information about the unit, the nurse, and the need for patient trust were reflected on. All of the information was explainable and understandable. The administrator determined that the situation was not major; no information was missing and no harm had occurred—moving almost seamlessly into the interpretation phase of decision making.

CASE STUDY 2: PLANNING FOR A NEW TECHNOLOGY

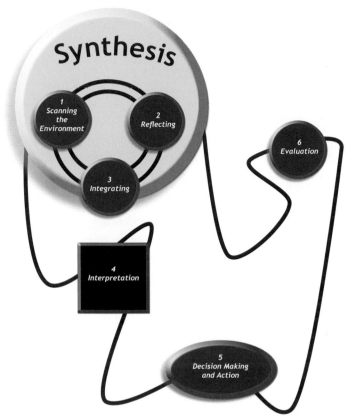

Facilitating Collective Synthesis

Synthesis is not only about individual synthesis, but also synthesis of the wisdom of the team. The collective integration of the wisdom of many members of the team serves to create better outcomes than any one individual could hope to achieve. The collective efforts of many individuals are integrated into systems thinking, self-management, servant leadership, problem solving that is not in isolation, and the collective search for opportunities within that collaboration. The synthesis model reflects high-level brainstorming and can be used as a guide in the integration of collective thinking, resulting in optimal results.

Background Information

The organization is planning to develop a fully electronic, wireless environment to document patient care. A plan that integrates improvements in patient outcomes and patient safety is needed to begin the transition. The organization believes selection of the metrics and from which to declare computerization a success is critical. The selected metrics must be specific to the stewardship priorities of the organization: the work, survival, and sustainability.

In this work, the leaders of the organization recognize that in order to integrate technology into mainstream health care, the synthesis of leadership skills, knowledge of the patient care experience, and goals and capabilities of the proposed technology are needed. Leaders are concerned that during the planning and selection processes there is a risk of technology driving the processes of patient care, rather than patient care processes driving technology.

Leaders are cautious of technology that increases the time spent away from the patient or requires more and redundant activities from the patient. Also, leaders are aware that sustaining and supporting the individuals who use the technology will require resources. It is hoped that the technology will provide faster, more efficient communication, easier management of data, and improved organization of information for decision making. These benefits assist the organization in developing resources and marketing their services more succinctly and effectively.

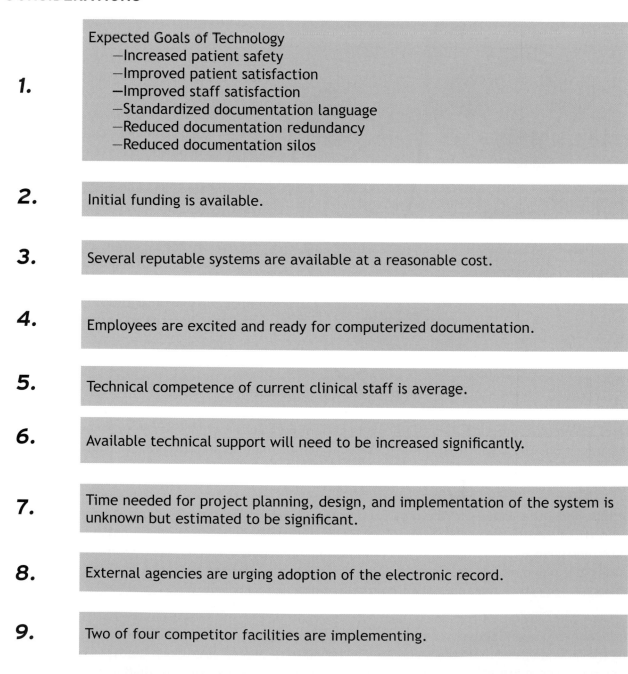

SCANNING THE ENVIRONMENT..._The need to identify the metrics to be used in evaluating the value of the technology selected is the issue at hand._

CONSIDERATIONS

1. Expected Goals of Technology
   —Increased patient safety
   —Improved patient satisfaction
   —Improved staff satisfaction
   —Standardized documentation language
   —Reduced documentation redundancy
   —Reduced documentation silos

2. Initial funding is available.

3. Several reputable systems are available at a reasonable cost.

4. Employees are excited and ready for computerized documentation.

5. Technical competence of current clinical staff is average.

6. Available technical support will need to be increased significantly.

7. Time needed for project planning, design, and implementation of the system is unknown but estimated to be significant.

8. External agencies are urging adoption of the electronic record.

9. Two of four competitor facilities are implementing.

10. The tentative timeline is 18 months.

REFLECTING

The orchestra leader facilitates the creation of an essence that is not recognizable in the individual components of the musician, instrument, or a partial group of musicians. Health care leaders are called to do similar work. The leaders posit:

"Can the integration of the new electronic technology become seamlessly integrated into the health care experience?"

If so, what resources are required?

Is this necessary to know, before metrics are selected?

Given that planning time is typically minimized in traditional projects, will the team be able to support the extensive planning that is needed for this project?

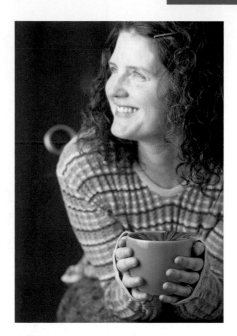

More Reflections

The health care experience requires human connection and caring behaviors. Whereas technology might have the capacity to improve processes and timeliness, the essence of health care embodies the touch of a human, a therapeutic, compassionate encounter that supports the healing process. One might be able to engage, educate, and intervene roboticallywith 21st century technology and cure the patient's disease, but one cannot hold the hand of the dying patient, comfort the family, or provide timely support without human presence.

One might be able to complete online coursework and collaborate with colleagues in online discussion groups, but one cannot appreciate the nonverbal response and critique of physical encounters to determine when behaviors are very effective or grossly inappropriate unless there is another individual physically present and sensing the nonverbal as well as the verbal communications. Human presence and involvement are the fundamental characteristics of the nurse-patient encounter.

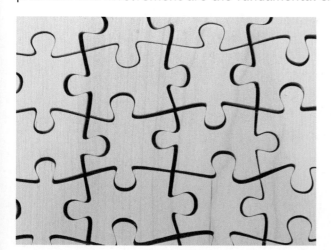

Integrating the Information...

Computerization should provide individuals with data and information that can be synthesized into learning and knowledge. The organization and resources are present with some limitations that are not insurmountable. Intuition and reflection indicate that data are available and the team could probably select metrics based on the identified goals of the project. Also, additional metrics could be developed as the project progresses. The synthesized information can be interpreted and actions taken to move forward with the work.

CASE STUDY 3: CREATING EVIDENCE FOR PRACTICE

Patient Care Delivery Models and Metrics

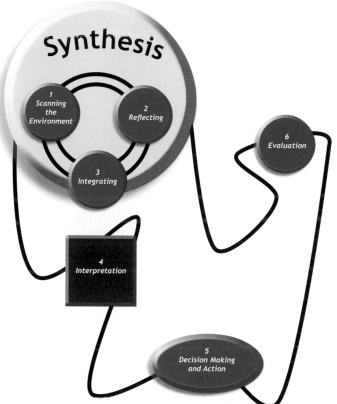

Synthesis

1 Scanning the Environment

2 Reflecting

3 Integrating

6 Evaluation

4 Interpretation

5 Decision Making and Action

Background

Chief metrics officers (CMOs) have been intro-duced into health care organizations to assist leaders with collecting and interpreting data. Further, in many organizations, CMOs have moved from staff-support positions into deci-sion-making positions.

Consider the situation in which the leadership team was requested to consolidate several middle manager job titles or positions into one standardized job description by the CMO to simplify the productivity analysis process. Fewer job titles would enhance the data analysis. The CMO also proposed that standardizing eight roles into one would result in significant savings.

Unfortunately, examination of the patient out-comes and staff satisfaction data specific to the varying roles was not included in the analysis. The leadership team was challenged to respond to the request for standardization of roles.

Scanning the Environment...

Wide variations among the eight units exist in the following:
- Roles and accountabilities of the eight identified roles
- Span of control varied from 8 to 30
- Skill mix varied from 45% to 80% licensed
- Clinical support was available only on the day shift
- Advanced-practice nurses were available in two areas
- Overtime percentage averaged 5% for all units
- External labor percentage varied from 0% to 10%
- Core staff percentage
- Years of service with organization
- Shift lengths
- Patient care needs intensity
- Financial or productivity

Leaders have identified the following clinical outcomes but have not linked the outcomes to the specific patient care delivery model roles and accountabilities.

- Patient satisfaction at the 95th percentile

- Patient safety: falls and medication errors less than regional norm

- Pain control at level 3 or better

- Nursing satisfaction at 95th percentile

- Zero sentinel events

- Fewer than five codes per month

- Employee injuries fewer than five per year

- Salary expense per patient-day

- Turnover percentage less than 8%

- Cost of risk management claims less than 5%

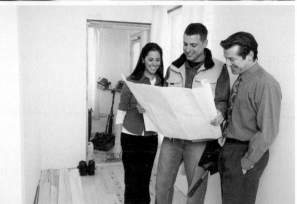

Reflecting...

Are we asking the right question?

Is the question really about the multiple roles?

Or is it about the patient care delivery model that has been created in each of the eight areas?

Is there another issue?

Is there lack of understanding of patient care delivery models by the CMO?

There is no empirical research-based evidence for the current eight roles.

There is an opportunity to use evidence-based practice in the examination of this issue.

The CMO has a need to make a difference and accomplish the standardization.

Clinical leaders have not addressed this kind of challenge in the past.

There is a need for a win-win solution to this dilemma.

Integrating the Information...

Data from the scanning process and the intuitive reflecting on the issues provide a complex situation that needs to be addressed to achieve a win-win for the organization. The lack of evidence for decision making by either the CMO or the leaders creates an initiative to examine each of the eight roles and the outcomes produced before decisions are made to consolidate or retain the eight positions.

References

Barrett, R. (1995). *Spiritual unfoldment: A guide to liberating your soul*. Alexandria, VA: Unfoldment Publications.

Benner, P. (1984). *From novice to expert: Excellence and power in clinical nursing practice*. Reading, MA: Addison-Wesley.

Dreyfus, H.L. & Dreyfus, S.E. (1986). *Mind over machine: The power of human intuition and expertise in the era of the computer*. New York: Free Press.

Suggested Readings

Bazerman, M.H. & Chugh, D. (2006). Decisions without blinders. *Harvard Business Review*, 84(1), 88-97.

Drexler, D., & Malloch, K. (2005). Cultural transformation through computerized documentation. *Nurse Leader: From Management to Leadership*, 3(4), 32-36.

McInnes, L. (2005). To synthesise or not synthesise? That is the question! *Worldviews on Evidence-Based Nursing*, 2(2), 49-51.

Stetler, C.B., Brunell, M., Guiliano, K.K., Morisi, D., Prince, L., & Newell-Stokes, V. (1998). Evidence-based practice and the role of nursing leadership. *JONA*, 28(7/8), 45-53.

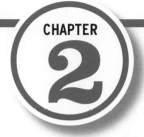

CHAPTER

2

MODELING AND MENTORING LEADERSHIP

Leadership is a learned behavior that reqquires knowledge, experience, and the assistance of successful leaders.

No leader can expect to be fully self-sufficient. Feedback and counsel from trusted, competent colleagues specific to improving the quality of one's work life, learning to prioritize effectively, and advancing one's career is essential in the journey to leadership excellence. The role of the mentor is designed to assist leaders in this work. The mentoring process provides the opportunity to continually seek open, honest, and timely feedback as well as share one's experiences and wisdom. Expert leaders serve regularly in the role of both mentor and mentee; they are always giving of themselves to others and learning from their interactions with others.

Mentoring Is Forever

The need for mentoring is ever present. Initially, aspiring leaders are best served with a more formalized relationship with a single mentor and commitment to structured processes. As the leader evolves, less formal and structured support is needed. New and different levels of mentorship with different emphases are identified. The frequency and intensity of mentoring change throughout one's career based on the role and context of the work. Experienced leaders often have informal mentoring relationships that are not formal—the leader seeks guidance from any mentor. When experienced leaders assume new roles or responsibilities, the need for more formal mentoring reemerges, focusing on enriching and accelerating the integration of the new work into the leader's role.

In this section, specific areas of focus for successful mentoring are presented to assist aspiring and accomplished leaders. The areas of professionalism, building relationships, creating the context for evidence-based practice, visioning and strategic planning, inspiring others, lifelong stewardship, and addressing the tough stuff of leadership are presented. These areas are selected to assist mentors and mentees in specific areas of leadership that one can expect to encounter in the lifelong mentoring journey designed for sustainable leadership excellence. To be sure, this is not an inclusive list of mentoring topics.

MENTORING

The focus of mentoring is on the mentee and the quality of the relationship between the mentor and the mentee. A mentor begins with guiding the mentee to develop skills in listening carefully, selecting reading materials, applying ideas, and observing. This work is always focused on supporting mentees as they progress in their personal development journey to discover and live in the role that is the best fit for them, the role in which they are most successful.

Mentors do not encourage mentees to adopt their own behaviors or to emulate their behaviors. Instead, effective mentors realize that the world is changing too fast to repeat their successful behaviors of the past, and work with mentees to develop their own style of leadership. Mentors realize that the future requires new and creative behaviors for success—behaviors that the mentee is empowered to create.

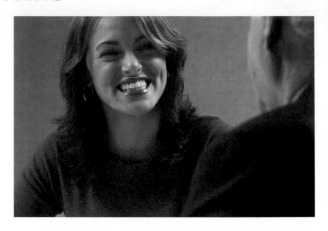

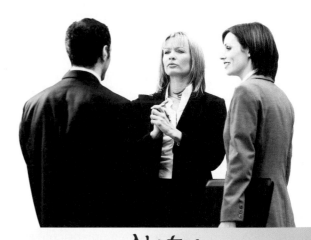

The Goals of Mentoring

- Assist others to become more accomplished.
- Assist others to be the best they can be with their own knowledge, skills, and talents.
- Instill accountability and confidence in others so that individuals are ultimately able to teach themselves and to assist others to use their own skills and knowledge to make decisions.

Note:

The mentor enables mentees to find their own essence or presence of professionalism as a leader and to become a living vessel representing the character of strong leadership with vision, willingness, capacity, and commitment to the work of the organization.

MENTORING CONCEPTS

Mentor

A mentor is a wise and trusted adviser who guides others on a particular journey. A mentor provides support, challenge, and vision.

Mentoring

Mentoring is the process of a more accomplished person assisting others to develop expertise and learn new skills based on the mentor's personal, tapped wisdom, reinforcing self-confidence, supporting real-life situations, and sharing personal experiences when appropriate.

Concepts Related to Mentoring

1. **Trainer**
One who gives private instruction and promotes particular behaviors as the ideal. In the trainer-trainee relationship, the trainer is the leader of the process and the trainee is a follower.

2. **Preceptor**
One who gives commands, makes rules; a teacher or instructor. In this relationship, the preceptor directs the pupil or new person in activities. The student is dependent on the preceptor.

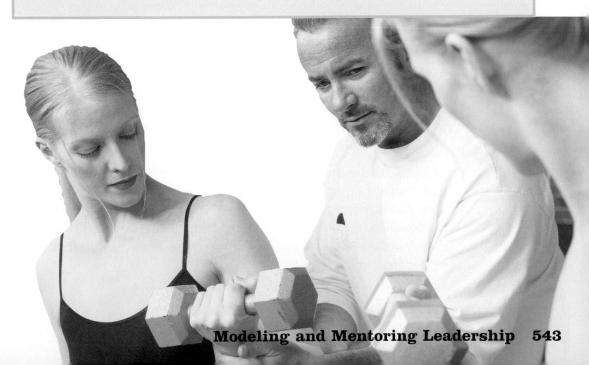

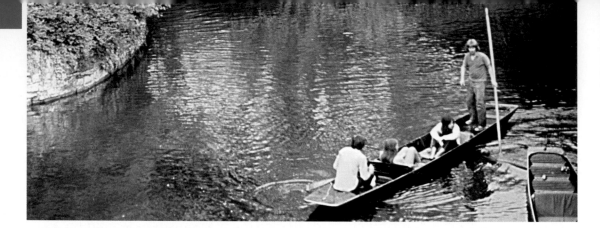

3. **Guide**

One who directs, steers, or points another person; a tour director. In this relationship, the guide is the leader of the process and others are dependent on the guide.

4. **Coach**

One who assists others to develop viable solutions, prioritize them, and then act on them; a coach works to assist healthy people to achieve their goals and when behaviors are unhealthy, refers the person to counseling. In this relationship, a partnership is formed between the coach and the one coached.

5. **Supervisor**

One who oversees or is considered the boss. In this relationship, competent individuals work nearly independently with the oversight of the supervisor.

6. **Consultant**

An expert who is called on for professional or technical advice or opinions; one who has much training and knowledge in a special field. A consultant is usually outside the client organization; someone who helps others profit or learn from their own experience. In this relationship, both the consultant and those using the consultant are independent and partnering to create better solutions that neither could do independently.

BE THE BEST!

There are seven areas of focus for the leadership mentoring process; professionalism, relationship building, evidence-based leadership, visioning and planning, inspiring, lifelong stewardship, and the tough stuff. Each mentee will learn and develop skills based on the areas of interest and the opportunities to experience situations specific to the topics in one's organization. Four overall thoughts are presented here.

- Mentors must avoid creating a clone of themselves in the mentoring relationship.

- The mentor must avoid moving from a mentor to a therapist; the mentor focuses on guiding healthy behaviors, a therapist focuses on correcting unhealthy behaviors.

- Communication between the mentor and mentee must be direct and honest, avoiding insincere and inaccurate messages.

- The mentee must be open to listening to but not replicating ideas without careful consideration.

Mentoring for Excellence: 7 Key Areas of Focus

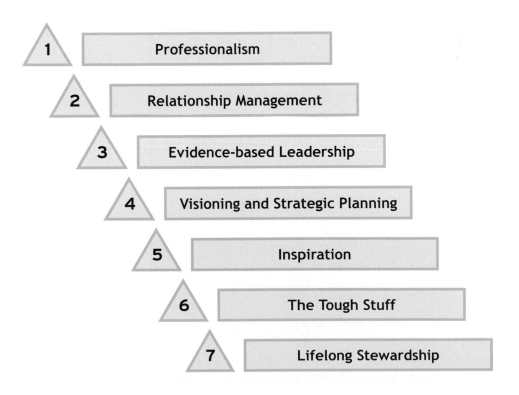

1. Professionalism
2. Relationship Management
3. Evidence-based Leadership
4. Visioning and Strategic Planning
5. Inspiration
6. The Tough Stuff
7. Lifelong Stewardship

1 MENTORING FOR PROFESSIONALISM

The first area for mentor-mentee focus is professionalism. Although there is always discussion as to who and what is professional, there are fundamentals as to attire, communication, and attitude. Professionalism of leaders is traditionally exemplified by the degree of behaviors present related to these three areas. Mentors can assist emerging as well as experienced leaders in ensuring the highest degree of professionalism through lifelong examination of and reflection of these areas.

ATTIRE

Much has been written about dressing for success and professional attire in the workplace. Each person has developed an understanding of what attire is professional and appropriate for the workplace, but the primary consideration must always be the customer, client, patient, or family to be served.

In health care organizations, the goal must be to ensure cleanliness and support of the control of spread of infections, and minimize distractions to the patient to support a patient-family centered focus rather than attention to the dress of the caregiver. Clean, conservative attire best facilitates and supports an emphasis on the patient and family. Wild prints, exposed skin, excessive jewelry, and colognes shift the emphasis and attention to the caregiver rather than the patient.

The workplace should not be considered appropriate to make fashion statements—display new fashion styles, extensive jewelry, or strong colognes. The first impression made with patients and their families should be positive and one in which the organization is portrayed as competent, safe, and focused on the work of patient care.

In the mentoring dialog, mentors and mentees should proactively examine their attire and be assured that personal appearance is not a hindrance to effective communication. Wise leaders ensure their personal presentation to team members continually exemplifies the highest level of professionalism as a mark of respect not only to one's individual reputation, but also for the leader's organization and community.

Professional Attire

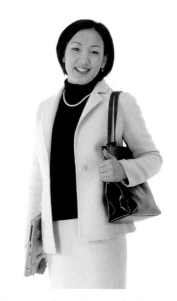

Unprofessional Attire

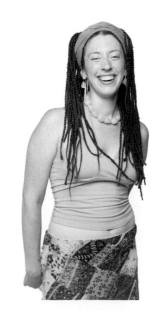

COMMUNICATION

The style of communication varies widely among individuals. The role of the professional requires communication behaviors that facilitate teamwork and respect individuals for who they are. Examples of principles that mentors and mentees should focus on include the following:

- Is responsive; timeliness is the norm
- Is not verbally hostile, abusive, or dismissive
- Is assertive rather than aggressive, unless safety is threatened
- Proactive rather than reactive: Avoids being passive to minimize personal rejection or conflict
- Requests rather than demands action
- Uses humor appropriately
- Reality based: Shows compassion for imperfection and the limitations of others; avoids placing blame
- Avoids spin or coloring the facts to avoid the real issues
- Avoids verbosity; focuses on streamlined and simplified communication
- Works to close the gap between differing factions within the organization: staff and management; physicians and nurses; etc
- Emphasizes principles and values; avoids insincere and misunderstood scripting

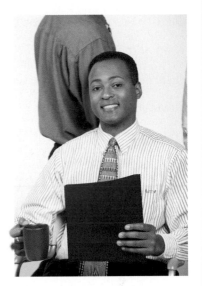

Attitude Is Everything!

In addition to physical presence, a leader's attitude is important. Attitude, or the manner, disposition, or inclination as to how one approaches and reacts to situations, further defines one's level of professionalism. One of the simplest descriptions of positive or negative attitudes is often expressed from the perspective of the glass: the half-full glass indicates a positive, optimistic, and hopeful attitude; the half-empty glass indicates a negative, pessimistic, and defeated attitude. A mentor can be helpful in assessing and reflecting the mentee's attitude.

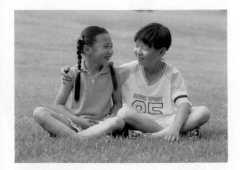

In the mentoring relationship focused on professionalism, the following supportive and nonsupportive behaviors are a means to reinforce a positive attitude toward leadership and to reverse the identified negative indicators. Each of these indicators describes expressions of attitudes seen in most workplaces, including health care organizations.

SUPPORTIVE ATTITUDE INDICATORS

- Competent and confident in abilities

- Fair, open, and honest; willing to stand up for beliefs

- Respectful: reacts with dignity and civility in all situations

- Reality based: recognizes personal limitations as well as those of others

- Kind and compassionate

- Internally motivated for learning and self-development

- Advocate for employees

- Not arrogant or insolent

- Resilient for the future

- Assumes toughness when needed that enables others to emerge from devastating situations without losing hope

- Persistent in achieving difficult goals

- Hardy: maintains healthy behaviors and worklife balance

- Curious and passionate about life

- Inquisitive: capacity for wonderment

- Values followers who are independent thinkers, actively engaged, and able to complement and support the work of the organization

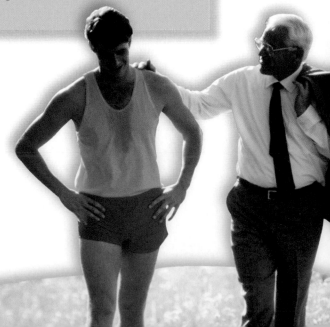

Nonsupportive Attitude Indicators

- Overly critical of others in private and in public

- Angry and aggressive

- Selfish: ensures personal comfort and safety first

- Negative: believes others are also disillusioned and only willing to do what is needed to get by

- Disinterested in reading professional journals and exploring new and radical ideas

- Inconsistent: changes convictions and support routinely depending on individuals involved

- Aloof

- Unsure of competence: lack of confidence in abilities

- Disillusioned with the health care system

- Conflict averse: gives in routinely to others to avoid making difficult decisions

- Transfers negativity: believes others are also disillusioned and only willing to do what is needed to get by

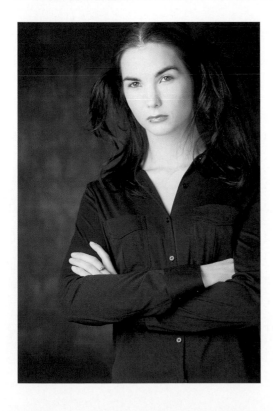

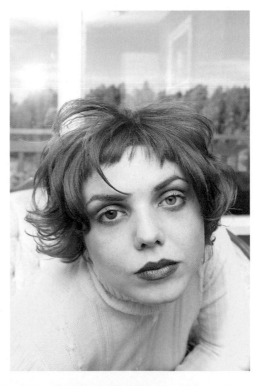

2 MENTORING FOR RELATIONSHIP MANAGEMENT

The second area of mentor focus is relationship management. Mentors have learned that all leadership work is based on relationships and that individuals become successful based on their relationships with others. Successful leaders have learned that relationships can either enhance one's ability to get the work done or hinder it.

For example, relationships may advance the work of the leader and the organization, invigorate and renew one's personal spirit and passion, stifle the work of the leader and the organization, or do nothing to affect one's well-being. Everyday, the quality of those relationships enhances or hinders one's effectiveness and can be considered the lifeblood of sustainable excellence.

Mentors are well positioned to share experiences of positive and negative relationships and most important to brainstorm with the mentee to identify relationships that will support and enhance the work of leadership. Four types of activities around relationships and their effect are presented for discussion (Ambrose & Moscinski, 2002).

Enhance Existing Relationships

Leaders should consider continuing and enhancing existing relationships when an individual:

- Supports the overall work of the organization and professional role
- Offers new ideas and information
- Is comfortable in engaging in discussions representing differing values
- Is able to challenge assumptions and beliefs
- Is able to see situations from another's point of view
- Portrays high personal integrity
- Accepts and incorporates feedback in a nonresistant and nondefensive manner
- Accepts responsibility for failure or errors
- Does not need reminders about academic responsibilities to patients or to other health care professionals in order to complete them
- Is available for professional responsibilities (i.e., required activities, available on clinical service, responds to pager)
- Takes on appropriate responsibilities willingly (not resistant or defensive)
- Takes on appropriate patient care activities (does not "turf" patients or responsibilities).

Ending Existing Relationships

Goals and purposes of relationships change; few relationships remain the same year after year. In one's worklife, relationships that were once mutually beneficial and facilitative of the work change when an individual moves to another location or organization. Also, the values and interests of individuals change over time thus decreasing common bonds and goals once shared. The mentor can assist the mentee in assessing changing relationships and modifying priorities with certain individuals when changes occur. Shifting the focus of the relationship and the time allocated to it becomes an effective time management strategy. Consider ending relationships with individuals when:

- Values and goals are no longer congruent.
- The individual is no longer in your area of work interest.

Avoiding Relationships

Leaders are encouraged to avoid relationships in which individuals are known to:

- Bully and harass others.
- Engage in routine gossip.
- Differ considerably in values/work processes specific to the respect of individuals and integrity.
- Be unreliable and need constant reminders to complete work.

Forming New Relationships

Leaders should consider forming new relationships to:

- Reach out to disciplines outside of health care but within the community such as school boards, legislators, and banking professionals to expand knowledge of the community.
- Gain greater insight into one's own discipline through university affiliation or membership in a national organization.

3 MENTORING FOR EVIDENCE-BASED LEADERSHIP

The third area for mentor focus is evidence-based leadership. Guiding leaders in the creation of an organizational context that supports and expects decision making on the basis of evidence and value is a complex, multifocal ever-changing process that is never done (Malloch & Porter-O'Grady, 2006).

Leading on the basis of evidence requires an understanding of existing organizational structures, workload management principles, and models of outcome measurement. For both experienced and new leaders, creating the context for evidence can be a radical shift from traditional leadership behaviors, values, and outcomes of measurement practices. Making decisions based on evidence is theoretically supported in discussions among leaders and their team members and in the classroom. It is the translation and integration of evidence-based practice into leadership work that requires attention and persistence.

Mentors can assist mentees in discovering what can be considered evidence and in making leadership decisions based on this evidence through role modeling and providing support with the following activities:

- *Develop organizational commitment within the governance infrastructure of the organization's mission, vision, and values.*

- *Ensure time for all team members to engage in the dialog and transformation work to achieve evidence-based practices.*

- *Identify points of access to resources for evidence references.*

- *Ensure financial support for evidence-based practice initiatives.*

- *Develop adequate evaluation tools to examine and measure the quantitative and qualitative effect of evidence-based practice with one's organization.*

- *Acquire skill to know when to rely on intuition and experience when the evidence is not available or readily accessible.*

- *Recognize the resistance to evidence-based practice and developing strategies to remove barriers and address the resistance as the means to achieve practice excellence.*

Note:

Evidence: The basis for belief or disbelief; things helpful in forming a conclusion or judgment

4 MENTORING FOR VISIONING AND STRATEGIC PLANNING

The fourth area of mentor focus is strategic planning. Mentors can be especially helpful in assisting leaders in the visioning and strategic planning processes for the organization.

Planning and visioning occur all the time—the leader must encourage regular discussions about the future and then integrate these ideas into the formal plans of the organization. In this way the work of strategic planning is always alive and contemporary. Everyday, leaders and staff are envisioning a better future that includes improved processes, new technology, and new behaviors based on the degree of effectiveness of existing processes.

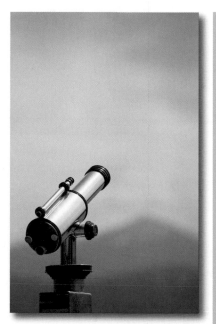

Note:

The goal of strategic planning is to transform the institution to support current practices in a safer, more effective, and therapeutic manner. The transformed culture must comprehend and value the human condition of imperfection, the passion of healers, and the never-ending need for health care services.

Planning for Future Considerations

- Avoid the temptation to limit planning to an annual, formalized process. Mentors can be particularly helpful in assisting mentees in managing competing priorities of getting the daily work accomplished and keeping an eye on the future—a very fine balance!

- Focus the work: Segment the work of visioning and planning into discrete initiatives, then integrate into the whole for the formalized processes of planning:
  - Succession planning and workforce development
  - Equipment planning
  - Physical space planning
  - Culture transformation needs
  - Patient care delivery models
  - Intellectual capital development

- Engage in participative processes: Create the infrastructure of participative strategic planning that involves members of the team in the visioning and planning processes. Skilled mentors encourage mentees to nourish the skills and relationships of team members to share and connect their ideas and efforts in the work of creating a better future.

- Question proactively: Routinely asking what is working, what is not working, and what would make it better is essential to lifelong growth and organizational sustainability.

- Integrate both short- and long-term planning processes throughout the organization. The leader carefully nourishes the skills and relationships necessary to assist others in connecting their own efforts with the grand work of creating a better future.

- Be prepared and ready with ideas and proposals all the time!

5 MENTORING FOR INSPIRATION

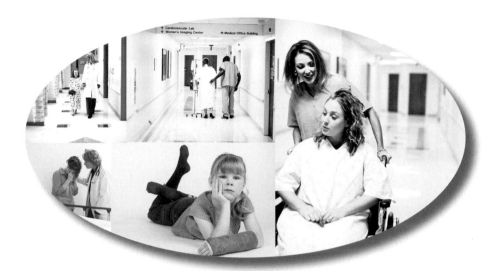

The fifth area of mentor-mentee focus is developing inspirational behaviors that guide or stimulate others to action. Mentoring the leader to become an inspirational force for caregivers is perhaps one of the most challenging aspects of the mentoring role. Mentoring for good relationships, communication, and using evidence is concrete and objective. Guiding the mentee to become an inspirational leader authentically engaged in creating an optimal context of health care begins with mentor role modeling. Teaching others to be inspirational requires commitment to lifelong caring for others.

The work of leading a healing organization is filled with a range of emotions from the joy of the birth of a healthy baby, to the trauma of accidental injuries, the uncertainty of financial performance, and the joy of high staff satisfaction. Leading in this emotionally charged environment requires first, awareness of this complexity of emotions, and second, a strong desire to continually assist and guide the team to function effectively.

INSPIRE FOR...

Recruitment:
- Inspire compassion and commitment in others to become interested in the work of healing—to join the professions of health care.
- Inspire interest in both the work of healing and caregiving.

Some leaders, like caregivers, never tire of the work of health care and the ability to affect others, who at times are morose over the inconsistent commitment of members of the health care team, the lack of resources for full access to health care, and poor health care practices of many of the citizens. Some vacillate between feeling very good and actualized from the work of health care and the challenges of the work. All leaders are called to role model behaviors that inspire or stimulate others to be the best they can as health care workers. This work quickly extends to become an effective recruitment and retention tool. Other employees and team members are encouraged and stimulated to provide quality care. Each mentor and mentee should identify examples of inspirational activities and their effect on the organization's work.

INSPIRE FOR...

Retention: for employees to remain and thrive in the organization:
- Inspire compassion and commitment to continue the work of healing.
- Inspire confidence, loyalty, and hard work based on the vision.
- Inspire others to continue to excel in good times and to revitalize in times of challenge; assist others to find meaning in negative events.
- Inspire healers to integrate personal and team time for reflection as the means to better understand, enrich relationships, and revitalize.
- Inspire others to find hope in the expression of core values—especially in life-changing events.

INSPIRE FOR...

Teamwork: to be a great, fully engaged member of the team:
- Inspire others to move from an organization of individuals to a team of individuals focused on the work of the system.
- Inspire and encourage others to move from completing tasks to becoming professionals fully engaged in the work of healing.
- Inspire accountability for professionalism standards across the generations for workers.
- Inspire an aura of therapeutic serenity!

INSPIRE FOR...

Growth: to learn more, give more and be more to enhance the organization:
- Inspire others to assist the emotionally incompetent to achieve levels of emotional competence; to become fully engaged in the work of healing.
- Inspire a love of technology; assist colleagues to see the incredible potential of a fully wired electronic system to manage the inherent challenges; moving forward in an uncertain world.

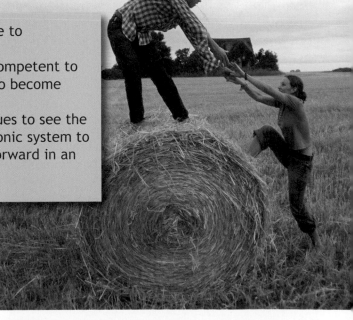

Modeling and Mentoring Leadership   555

6 MENTORING FOR THE TOUGH STUFF

The sixth area of focus for the mentor-mentee is the work of addressing those difficult situations filled with conflict. These are often referred to as the tough situations encountered in the leadership role that are typically relational, recurring, and deeply rooted in personal value issues.

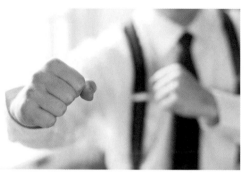

Learning to understand and address the trials and tribulations of organizational life requires persistence, commitment, integrity, and a trusted colleague! For some leaders the ability to respond effectively to difficult situations is straightforward, for others, confronting difficult situations seldom comes easy and is usually filled with angst and trepidation.

Working with a mentor to address these situations helps the mentee avoid unnecessary missteps and additional stress. No strategy can fully remove the stress associated with such issues; however, strategies to increase the understanding of the issue, clarifying who really owns the problem, and reframing the situation can assist in more effective resolution of the issues.

Seldom is a difficult situation limited to a single event. Addressing difficult situations would be much easier to manage if there were no history with an individual, if one did not ruminate about the situation, and all recent experiences with the involved individuals had been positive.

The goal of the mentor-mentee relationship in managing tough situations is to transform difficult relationship problems into situations that are managed fairly and in a timely manner. Mentors know what has worked for them in the past, the importance of timing, and how to reframe difficult conversations from personal experience in addressing similar situations. These experiences should always be considered informational rather than directional for the mentee. The mentee needs to integrate the information into his or her own personal style and comfort level in a way that is humane, focused, and goal oriented.

Addressing the Issues

Five areas in which tough issues typically arise include lack of prioritization, poor communication, lack of collaboration, lack of diversity, and lack of integrity. Examples of behaviors in each issue and steps to identify and address are presented.

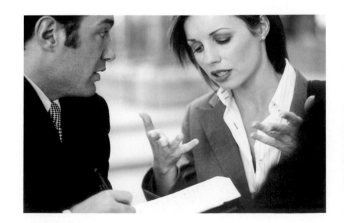

FACE THE TOUGH ISSUES STEP BY STEP

Lack of Prioritizing
- Failing to meet deadlines
- Repeatedly breaking appointments
- Continually extending beyond the allocated time
- Overloading schedules

Poor Communication
- Inapprpriate interpersonal encounters
- Antagonistic and apologetic without results
- Rude, interrupting, and reacting before all the information is provided

Lack of Collaboration
- Manipulative, hard bargaining
- Avoiding issues; tunnel vision

Lack of Diversity
- Avoids conflict at all costs; does not want to consider other viewpoints
- Limits team membership to selected similar colleagues

Lack of Integrity
- Fails to address the poor performance of a colleague who has become a friend
- Routinely offers insincere empathy
- Fails to identify the underlying issue before reacting

When Addressing the Tough Issues, Follow these Steps:

1 Confirm the issue or situation with those involved.

2 Reframe when possible.

3 Suggest correction.

4 Negotiate to advance the organization.

5 Retreat if there is a stalemate.

6 Revisit to achieve resolution.

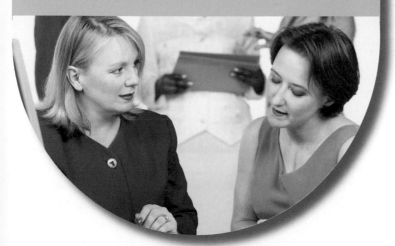

Modeling and Mentoring Leadership   557

7 MENTORING FOR LIFELONG STEWARDSHIP

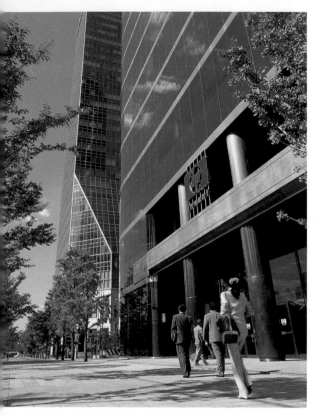

Effective leaders achieve excellence through innovative programs, sound strategies, and effective systems. In addition, the ultimate achievement of the leadership excellence is the creation of an organizational infrastructure and culture of excellence that lives on long beyond the presence of the individual leader. Too often the successful organizational culture is linked strongly to an individual and when the individual leaves the organization, the culture unravels quickly. The importance of leadership that is able to create a sustainable culture based on values and community needs cannot be underestimated.

Mentoring for lifelong stewardship that values an organization's success and survival is about assisting others to focus on the team and the organization. This may seem contradictory in the early development of leaders who are working to define themselves and their contributions. But the goal of mentoring is to assist the leader through the phases of identifying personal leadership style and contributions and transcendence to the ultimate steward of the organization and its resources.

Mentors and mentees are encourgaged to study situations in which the culture is tied too closely to an individual to begin to understand why things seem to fall apart when the leader leaves the organization. What leaders leave behind should not depend on their continuing presence. When the organization falls apart, the leader has failed to endow the organization with the qualities needed to transcend previous achievements and continue the mission-based culture of the organization, not the values of the most recent individual in the top leadership position. The success of the organization should not be based on a powerful personality but what is left behind—commitment and drive to continue the work of the organization.

Leadership Success: A Legacy without a Personal Crown!

Many innovations and new ventures are documented and published in local papers and national journals. When these innovations are attributed to the leader, the individual leader achieves significant recognition for the accomplishments of the team. The challenge for the leader is to avoid the temptation to accept the recognition as an individual and to ensure that the recognition is for the team and the organization as a whole. For health care leaders, the result of good leadership is excellent patient care and recognition by the community and national organizations for the achievement.

STRATEGIES TO AVOID PERSONAL CROWNS

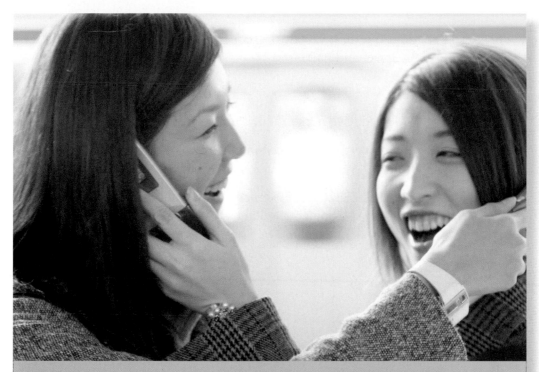

Avoid rhetoric and emphasis on personal satisfaction for specific performance. Avoid requesting that work is performed to make you or the leader happy—this infers that good work product is related to another's personal happiness—the work product satisfaction is related to the value it adds to the organization.

Monitor dominating strong personalities who provide little time for dialog with others in the organization. Work with those who are overly directive and controlling to meet personal schedules and goals. Encourage routine assertiveness and dialog with members of the team.

Avoid too much hierarchy in which the division between levels of employees is emphasized. Language or approaches that identify my team and your team and their accomplishments tend to separate the work into disparate groups who are in fact working toward the same goals.

Continually ensure that leadership is shared and encouraged among all employees so that the culture is self-sustaining. Consider rotation of project assignments to diffuse power and develop less experienced team members.

References

Ambrose, L., & Moscinski, P. (2002) The power of feedback. *Healthcare Executive*, Sept/Oct, 56-57.

Malloch, K., & Porter-O'Grady, T. (Eds.). (2006). *Introduction to evidence based practice in nursing and healthcare*. Sudbury, MA Jones and Bartlett.

Suggested Readings

Bellack, J. P. (2005). The RWJ executive nurse fellows program, Part 2. *JONA*, 35(12), 533-540.

Chinn, P. L. (2004). *Peace and power: Building communities for the future* (6th ed.). Sudbury, MA: Jones and Bartlett.

Melnyk, B. M., & Fineout-Overholt, E. (2005). *Evidence based practice in nursing and healthcare: A guide to best practice*. Philadelphia: Lippincott Williams & Wilkins.

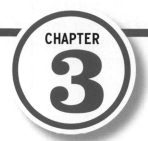

CHAPTER

3

MANAGING RISK AND VULNERABILITY

The health care environment continues to evolve and adapt to the knowledge and technology of the information age. Taking risks is inherent in the role of the leader and requires skills that guide the leader to embrace rational and avoid irrational risk taking.

Learning to not only thrive in the health care environment but also develop these skills in others, is a lifelong journey—the essence of contemporary leadership. Just as one uncertain situation is embraced and managed, another one is present. The feelings of vulnerability that accompany each risk-taking experience need to be recognized and embraced willingly, rather than avoided. Taking risks requires a view of the world that is steeped in openness to new ideas and comfort with the reality that not everything works as intended, no matter how well thought out the plan might be. Taking risks and being vulnerable is not about irresponsibility or incompetence, it is about living in reality.

> **Risk**
> The possibility of suffering harm or loss; danger;
> the quantifiable likelihood of loss or less than expected returns

Note:

Action does not always bring happiness, but there is no happiness without action.

> **Vulnerability**
> Exists when taking an action creates the potential for loss that could exceed the potential gain

Risk can never be eliminated. Leaders can only work to understand, strategize, and manage risks to the best of their ability. There are rational and irrational risks. The work of the leader is to study the environment, reflect on experience, weigh and balance the options, and select the most appropriate course of action. In this section, the experiences and feelings associated with risk taking, the relationship of organizational trust to risk taking, an overview of rational and irrational risk taking, and five strategies to minimize risk are presented.

THOUGHTS ON RISK TAKING

Risk Taking and Patient Safety

The safety movement has created a paradoxical situation for leaders; standardization has been identified as a characteristic of high-reliability processes and the need to challenge long-standing processes that may not be as safe as once believed. The safety movement is as an excellent guide for the leader to differentiate rational and irrational risks. Balance of organizational stability and growth can be facilitated with greater confidence through achieving the highest level of patient and organizational safety possible.

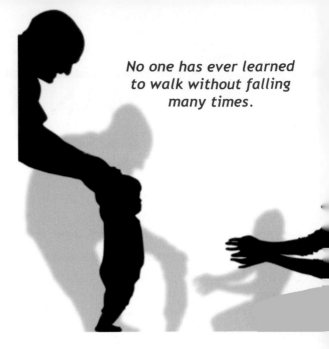

No one has ever learned to walk without falling many times.

Increasing System Reliability for Rational Risk Taking

The goal of the safety movement is to increase the safety of the the organization and simultaneously integrate safety into strategic planning, operations, resource allocation, and evaluation criteria. The overall goal to minimize risk and ensure organizational stability is closely linked to the level of trust in the organization. Creating an organization based on trust is important in ensuring organizational stability and simultaneous support for rational risk taking.

Trust implies that one individual is vulnerable to the actions of another. The greater the trust, the more positive are the expectations that individuals have about others' intentions and actions based on established roles, relationships, experiences, and their interdependencies. Trust is one individual's willingness to be vulnerable to another based on the belief that the latter party is competent, open, concerned, and reliable, thus rendering risk taking more rational and realistic.

Organizations that have high levels of trust recognize the benefits of adaptive organizational structures, strategic alliances, responsive virtual teams, effective crisis management, and reduced costs associated with litigation.

When trust is lost, feelings of betrayal, stress, and vulnerability emerge.

High Reliability Culture Values

- Trust, openness, and high reliability
- Support for new evidence
- Safety
- Creativity to survive in the future

Key Concepts: Increasing System Reliability

Major theories specific to improving safety and organizational reliability have been identified by researchers (Marias et al., 2004) as important to effecting a change in organizational culture: normal accidents theory (NAT), high reliability organizations (HROs), and systems accident theory. Key concepts of these theories are identified.

Normal Accidents Theory (NAT)

Accidents are inevitable.

Redundancy is necessary to improve safety.

(Perrow, 1999)

Tightly coupled system: A highly interdependent system in which each part of the system is tightly linked to many other parts. Tightly coupled systems respond quickly, which can be disastrous.

Loosely coupled system: A decoupled system that has fewer or looser links between parts and therefore is able to absorb failures or unplanned behaviors without destabilization.

High Reliability Organization (HRO) Characteristics

- Performance and safety are organizational priorities.

- Simultaneously decentralized and centralized

- Organizational learning from multiple sources including error evaluation

- Extensive use of redundancy (Weick & Sutcliffe, 2001)

Interactive complexity: The presence of unfamiliar or unplanned and unexpected sequences of events in a system that are either not visible or not immediately comprehensible

Reliability: The probability that a component satisfies its specified behavioral requirements over time and under given conditions

Redundancy: The ability to provide for the execution of a task if the primary unit fails or falters

Systems Accident Theory or Nonredundancy Approaches

Reduce complexity.

Reduce or eliminate the likelihood of hazards.

Address technical, organizational, social, political, and financial uncertainties.

(Leveson, 2004)

Safety is an emergent or system property, not a component property.

(Marias et al., 2004)

Minimizing Risk: Millionaire Style

1. *Call a friend.*

2. *50/50: Eliminate two options.*

3. *Ask the audience.*

RISK TAKING AND IRRATIONAL NEGATIVE FANTASIES

Often leaders have become paralyzed or deterred to take action in uncertain situations due to negative fantasies about what might happen. In reality, there is little if any chance for such fantasies to be realized. Perhaps themost common negative fantasy in health care is that one will be fired for taking risks and speaking up. Individuals worry that speaking up will have a negative outcome on their reputation, their ability to communicate openly and honestly with others, and the security of their position.

The reality is that individuals are seldom involuntarily removed from their jobs for speaking up and taking risks. Involuntary termination is more about incompetence, substance abuse, poor attendance, and dishonesty.

Negative Fantasies

My dad will kill me if I...

I'll get fired if I say something...

No one will like me if...

The nurses will quit if...

Leading Reasons for Termination of Employment

- *Is not competent to do the job*
- *Does not meet scheduling requirements*
- *Substance abuse*
- *Resigned in lieu of discharge*
- *Unprofessional conduct*
- *Falsified records*
- *Unacceptable attendance*
- *Failed to keep licensure current*

(S. Hughes [Human Resources Director, Banner Health], personal communication, October 2005.)

The Myth of Job Security

Job security is a myth. No job is guaranteed forever—or even until next month! Jobs are eliminated due to downsizing, the need for new skills and locations, and different delivery model structures, none of which are related to the activities of risk taking.

The workplace environment changes frequently—new leaders, new colleagues, new work, and so on. The workforce is continually modified, thus the focus should always be on being employable rather than being employed!

RATIONAL RISK TAKING: TAKE RISKS FOR THE RIGHT REASON!

Risk taking is not viewed as a classical leadership behavior, nor is it traditionally welcomed and encouraged. Instead, it is viewed negatively. It increases the organization's exposure to unforeseen hazards and to the loss of net income. Playing it safe and being a hardworking employee is the more preferred behavior.

Taking the initiative rather than clinging to the same old routine is now the work of the contemporary leader. This requires that one exposes oneself to failure rather than staying with mediocrity and embracing opportunities rather than retreating from them. The role of the leader is to inspire creativity and hard work and to challenge the past as the means to a better future. The work of inspiration requires not just inspirational phrases but inspirational behavior. Risk-disposed leaders motivate others by showing what can be done, not merely by sermonizing about opportunities. They need to exhibit candor and vulnerability, be able to identify value in marginally successful efforts, and be willing to allow others to take risks and experience success and failure.

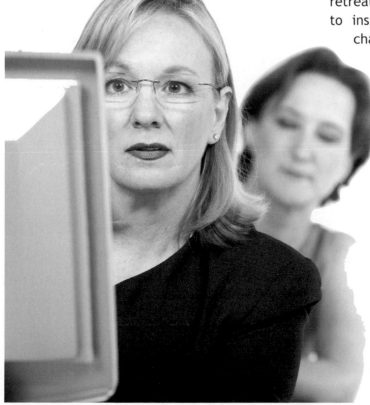

ZERO RISK DOES NOT EXIST: RISK IS ALWAYS PRESENT!

Vulnerability exists when taking an action creates the potential for loss that could exceed the potential for gain. One cannot escape the reality of risk and the associated feelings of vulnerability. The work of the leaders is to recognize this reality over and over and ensure that all members of the team recognize the realities and benefits of living in a risk-filled environment. The goal for all leaders is to examine each situation and embrace those risks that are irrational.

Risk exists when you...
- *Take action*
- *Don't take action*
- *Tell part of the story*
- *Tell the whole story*
- *Withhold information*
- *Blow the whistle*
- *Don't blow the whistle*

The course of events usually begins with recognizing that one is vulnerable; then the risk is embraced, new behaviors are tested as one stretches current capacity, the new reality is experienced, evaluation occurs, and the process begins again.

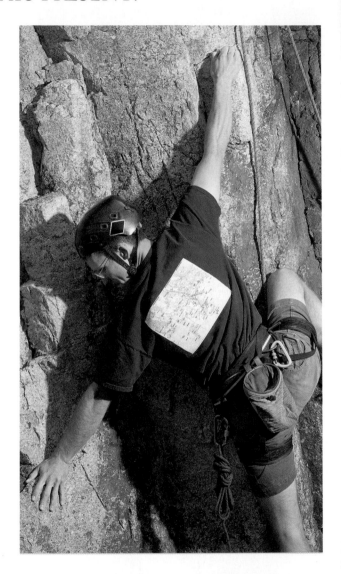

Failure to Take Risks Can Lead to:
- *Injury*
- *Regret*
- *Unnecessary rumination*
- *Extinction*
- *Living in the past*

Note:
It is much easier to be critical than correct.

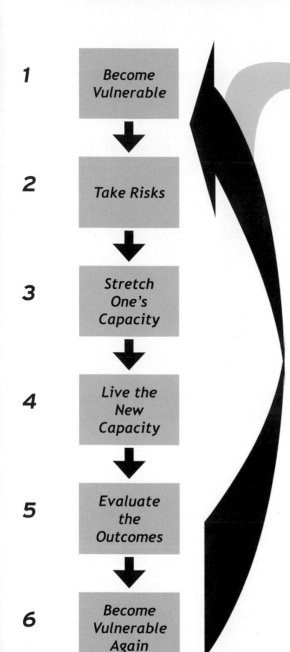

1. Become Vulnerable

2. Take Risks

3. Stretch One's Capacity

4. Live the New Capacity

5. Evaluate the Outcomes

6. Become Vulnerable Again

both positive and negative outcomes result from risk taking.

When the risk taken results in a less than optimal outcome, the work becomes that of course correction and remediation. The new knowledge gained from the unsuccessful effort is critical to continuing success; this information serves to inform others of a course of action that should not be repeated.

Addressing Negative Outcomes

1. Acknowledge the outcome.
2. Correct negative outcomes quickly; ensure personal safety.
3. Apologize to those affected by the outcome.
4. Review the goal and the selected process and identify areas of vulnerability .
5. Be sure the work is still the right thing to do. Determine if the goal is still appropriate.
6. Modify the process to avoid further negative outcomes.
7. Never be reluctant to abandon the goal and the process if safe and effective processes cannot be determined.

Although decisions made under conditions of incomplete information sometimes fail to have a positive outcome, leaders must be willing to risk changing course if there are good reasons to do so. No one knows the future for certain, as shown by the many mispredictions perpetrated by supposed experts.

Punitive approaches should be considered only when an individual has repeatedly disregarded advice and directions to modify actions. Punishing individuals for outcomes that involved many factors and many individuals is futile and demoralizing. Punishing discourages individuals from future risk taking that could benefit the organization.

Note:

No person was ever honored for what he received. Honor has been the reward for what he gave.

Managing Risk and Vulnerability   567

TRUE AND FALSE?

Determining when to take a risk is seldom straightforward. Learning to fly an airplane is steeped with risk but also supported by extensive safety processes. In addition to one's personal comfort and competence with risk taking, the context in which the risk is taking place can be supportive or not supportive. The same risk may be viewed and managed quite differently in different organizations; some view it as positive, others as negative and disruptive. Leaders are encouraged to assess their perceptions of risk taking and risk takers and work to create a culture that is open, trusting, and supportive of new ideas.

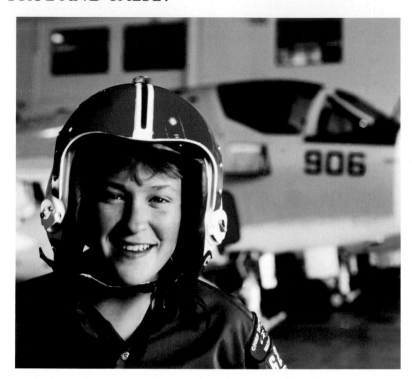

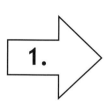

1.

The more risks you take, the more secure your job is.

True, with every risk, you grow professionally and learn information that is helpful to both yourself and the organization.

In an organization supportive of creativity and growth, this is certainly true. In a risk-averse organization, this is probably false.

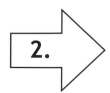

2.

The more risks you take, the greater the probability of being fired.

True, if taking risks compromises the organization's financial status and reputation when new approaches don't work.

This is true in risk-averse organizations and false when rational risks are taken and the organization is supportive.

The more risks you take, the better the organization will be.

True, when each new attempt supports a culture dedicated to finding new and better ways to accomplish the work and more efficient ways of doing business that will increase the profitability and sustainability of the organization.

This is false when risk taking overshadows the ability of the organization to accomplish the work at hand. There is a need for balance between operations and stretching the limits of current processes.

3.

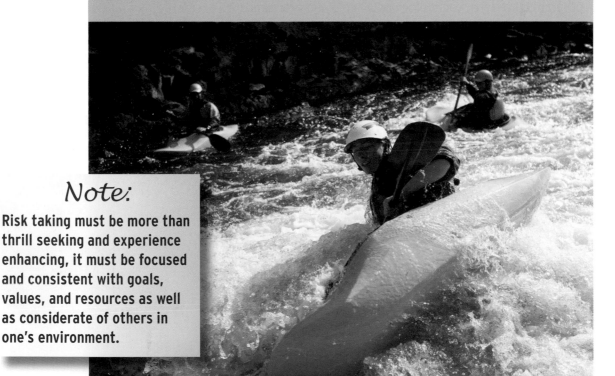

Note:

Risk taking must be more than thrill seeking and experience enhancing, it must be focused and consistent with goals, values, and resources as well as considerate of others in one's environment.

The more risks you take, the less others will like you.

True, when one is perceived as always rocking the boat, threatening the security of the status quo, and never allowing others to enjoy the present.

This is false when others in the organization view your willingness to try new approaches as an important contribution to the sustainability of the organization.

4.

Managing Risk and Vulnerability 569

FOUR RATIONAL RISKS

The contemporary leader is able to discern rational from irrational risks and advance the work of the organization. There are four areas in which risk is considered rational: advancing the organization, developing skills, mandatory reporting, and whistle-blowing. Each area serves a different purpose.

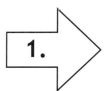

1. Advancing the Organization

Every organization strives to not only survive but thrive. In ensuring contemporary services, numerous programs, systems, technology advances, and products are considered by the leadership team. The leader is routinely faced with choices about clinical programs, initiation and expansion of new services, hiring, firing, selecting equipment, and prioritizing which issues will be addressed and which issues can wait. Choices that are rational and minimize risk are made on the basis of core values, respect for others, the safety of individuals, strategic goals of the organization, and available resources.

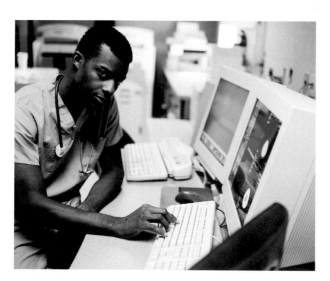
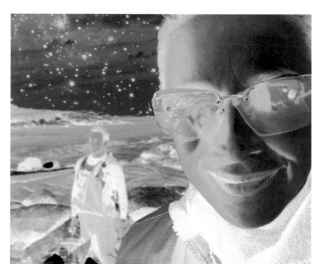

2. Developing Skills

Regardless of current competence, everyone needs new skills to continue to exist in a changing environment. Learning opportunities and acquiring new knowledge and skills that are rational include those skills specific to job performance and one's personal preferences. Considerations should be given to personal physical capability, resources, and family obligations to support rational risk taking. Many leaders continue to develop computer program skills in public speaking, sports, art, and personal protection such as judo.

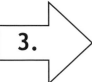

3. Mandatory Reporting

Many state licensing agencies require licensees to report the unprofessional conduct of other licensees to the licensing board. Protecting the public from licensees who commit repeated errors, abuse alcohol or drugs, and/or are incompetent to do the work often requires professionals to identify issues and take risks to speak up and address the situation. This action is not an option in many states and requires collegial support. Examples include unprofessional conduct, repeated medication errors, boundary violations, and theft from patients. Mandatory reporting is a rational risk required by statute.

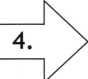

4. Whistle-Blowing

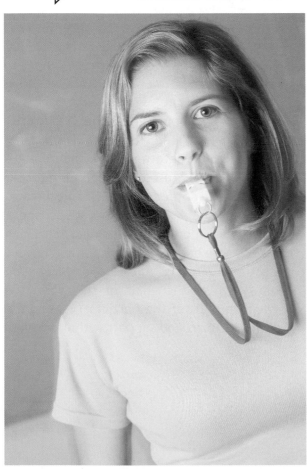

Whistle-blowing is about righting a wrong that is believed to be deceitful or results in the mistreatment of others. The need for whistle-blower protection arises when the culture of the organization does not support open communication, differing opinions, and rational risk taking. Individuals believe they have not been heard on an issue or that public interest is compromised and there is danger to the public or the environment. The intent of the federal whistle-blower act, also known as the False Claims Act, is to combat fraud and corruption and to protect those who exposed information from wrongful dismissal, allowing for reinstatement with seniority, double back pay, interest on back pay, compensation for discriminatory treatment, and reasonable legal fees. Despite whistleblower legislation, this approach is considered a rational risk and involves personal and professional risk regardless of the outcome.

IRRATIONAL RISKS

Irrational risk taking may not always be readily apparent; however, the following categories can be used as guidelines to identify and avoid irrational risks.

History of Failure and Oppression

The last attempt did not work and no one cares anyway. Just because it did not work last time does not mean that one is forever doomed to fail. New energy, new ideas, new products and new technology can create success from past failure.

Poor Judgment

Walking in traffic is an example in which the risk of injury to oneself and to others is present and probable. This action is irrational and similar to the leader who continues to hire employees in the midst of a financial crisis. The organization incurs additional financial obligations, and the positions of new employees will most likely be eliminated.

Unrealistic Expectations

There is very little potential for success. Attempting to implement one more program when the staff is already overwhelmed and frustrated is not rational.

There Is No Known Benefit for the Action

Planning education programs for which there is no audience and establishing committees when the work can be done by email are irrational actions because resources are put at risk for no value.

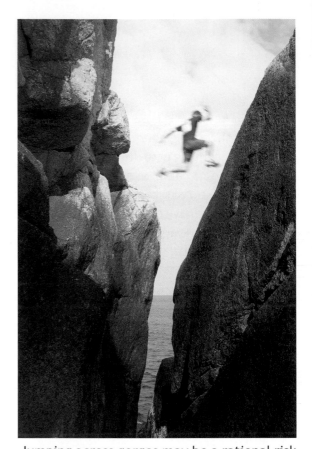

Jumping across gorges may be a rational risk for the skilled mountain climber and irrational for the unskilled individual. The work of the leader is to determine if the appropriate conditions are present to support the risk: performance objectives, skills, and climate. In organizations, similar situations apply. Experience in addressing conflict, changing patient care delivery models, or adding new electronic systems must be embarked on knowledge of the goals of the work, the available skills of the participants, and the other activities and support within the environment.

THE LEADERSHIP GOAL IS TO DEVELOP STRATEGIES TO MINIMIZE RISK

In this section, five strategies to minimize risk are presented: speaking up with evidence, selecting the perfect time for action, upward communication, accelerating competence, and apologizing with a flair.

1. Speak Up Boldly with Evidence

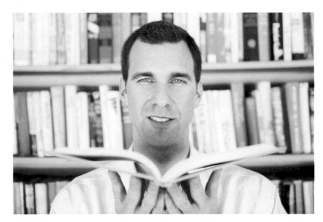

The first strategy to minimize risk is to speak up with evidence or rationale for action. The best safeguard to avoiding poor outcomes is that of using data, evidence, and rationale though processes. When there are significant variations in practice patterns, multiple opinions about the best solution, and little use of technology to validate the assumptions, there is a need for evidence that is based on rigor, experience, and values. It is these conditions of uncertainty that precipitate evidence-based practice initiatives and reduce the risks involved in attempting new strategies.

- **Data, data, data!**

- **Rationale for actions helps to make the case.**

- **Recommend a plan to develop the evidence if necessary.**

If the following scenario, validated for the health care industry, were used to support the need for staffing model and pay practice changes, the response would be much different than limiting the rationale for changes to that of turnover and dissatisfaction without specific metrics. Although these data may seem overstated to some, there is now opportunity for leaders to validate such data in their own organizations. A model with specific and significant metrics is available from which to examine salaries, productivity, turnover, and cost of care.

Evidence: Reframing the Cost of Turnover

The annual cost of turnover (hiring, training, and reduced productivity) represents about 5% of the annual operating budget. Stated differently, according to Waldman and colleagues (2004) it would be revenue neutral to offer each departing nurse (who chose to stay) a staying bonus equal to 86% of his or her annual salary or give every nurse on staff a 33% retention supplement every year!

(Waldman, et al., 2004)

---

2. Timing and Tinkering: Selecting the optimal time

The second strategy is timing—always an important consideration. Not every risk must be addressed immediately; sometimes waiting is prudent. Levels of workload, the availability of key participants, and the overall climate of the organization need to be considered before taking risks. Classical leadership behavior encompasses strategic planning and the purposeful review of ideas. With recent advances in information technology, these processes are becoming increasingly outdated. The emphasis now includes short-term incremental strategies similar to the concept of tinkering, introduced by Abrahamson (2000).

- Plan ahead; be prepared.
- Consider what is going on.
- Consider who is present.
- Consider how important the message is; is this the hill to die on today?

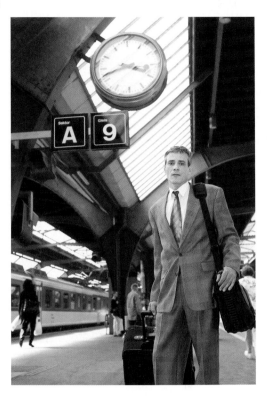

Risk-disposed leaders develop a high level of self-discipline that allows risk to evolve. A strong sense of commitment can be more valuable than intelligence, education, luck, or talent. Leaders adept at taking risks neither surrender nor overreact to crises; they regroup and return. They take stock of the situation, often pulling back temporarily while they plan the next steps. They realize that sometimes it is best to put aside personal feelings and let bygones be bygones. They focus on the present and the future, both of which offer perils and possibilities, rather than on the past, about which nothing can be done.

Notes on Tinkering

- Tinkering offers an opportunity to learn how to take risks.
- A little tinkering and a lot of expertise allows a small group to make changes with big goals in mind and to evaluate the changes efficiently.
- Team members' skills are stretched with little risk to the organization.
- Support for constant tinkering minimizes the chance that the organization will drift into inertia. Risk becomes the norm, change is internalized as essential for survival, and employees gain experiences and develop new skills.
- Tinkering becomes the expectation, the status quo—team members seriously challenge assumptions and ask questions not out of idle curiosity but by looking carefully at current dogma and raising issues that open the door to substantial improvements.

3. Encourage Upward Communication

The third strategy is about focused communication that gains the attention and support of decision makers. Top-down communication remains the most common type of communication in an organization. Cultures with shared leadership structures reinforce and support lateral communication more effectively than traditional organizations; however, the need for upward communication remains. Greater emphasis is needed to ensure upward communication and that leaders know what is going on in the organization so they can support the best decisions. The first step is to realize that leaders cannot and do not know everything and, second, to learn to share the appropriate information that affects the operations and reputation of the organization. Learning what information to share and when to share it evolves with experience and commitment to core values.

Decreasing Fear, Increasing Trust, and Upward Communication Checklist

1. Have the right people been involved in making decisions? If not, identify who should be involved and why. Avoid the temptation to complain and mumble, "If they only had asked me. ..."

2. Are the goals and values of the organization respected? If a decision does not seem consistent with the goals and values, take two actions. First, identify what specifically is not consistent with which value. Second, identify what you would like done to improve congruence with values.

3. Don't get lost in the process—if something is not working, give it up, even if it means retreating and regrouping. Identify that the work is off course and needs correction. It is easy to lose sight of the original goal.

4. Identify when work-arounds are created that avoid the real issue. New policies that add workload to all employees are often created for isolated, aberrant behaviors. Challenge leaders to address the issue rather than create another policy.

5. When decisions are made on biased or impartial Information, offer the additional information. Offer the information not to one-up another, but to achieve the best decision with all of the information.

Words of Wisdom!

- Leaders don't always know what is going on—not because they don't care, but because of limited time to be involved in everything.
- Leaders are not mind readers!
- New ideas are continually emerging—ear thermometers, electronic documentation improvements—and leaders need to be aware of them.
- Leaders are not always ready to hear your information—that should not stop the effort to communicate.
- Learning to frame, reframe, and avoid giving up easily is essential if you believe the issue is of value.

LEARN TO SHARE THE RIGHT INFORMATION

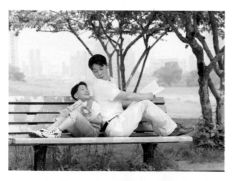

If I said everything I was thinking...such as...

— I don't like Chinese food.
— I don't like to hike mountains.
— Your outfit is weird.
— That's too expensive.
— He complains all the time.

...I wouldn't have very many friends. I wouldn't have anyone to go on vacation with!

Sometimes discretion is the best approach!

When team members withhold information, leaders must discover why the information was withheld and how to create the conditions that will support openness. One should never need permission to speak up about issues of safety and security. Further, it is often a moral imperative that one does speak up and address these issues. Failing to speak up may result in harm or inappropriate use of resources that could have been prevented.

Consider the following situations:

- The housekeeper did not inform the nurse of the patient's nausea and vomiting.
- The nursing assistant did not report a high blood pressure.
- The registered nurse did not call the family about a change in the patient's condition.
- A pharmacist did not call a physician about an unauthorized drug substitution.
- The respiratory therapist did not inform the next shift about incomplete treatments.
- The director did not inform the administrator about an employee theft of patient property.

For each of these situations there is a reason. While not always easy to discern, the leader begins with knowledge gaps first. Does the individual know that an action was expected? Providing information and setting new expectations becomes a straightforward solution. If the individual was withholding information deliberately, then the leader must determine the reason before change in behavior can be expected. If the employee was fearful about discipline, the leader can work to encourage more open communication. Not all situations are quickly resolved; however, they need to be addressed.

4. Accelerating Competence

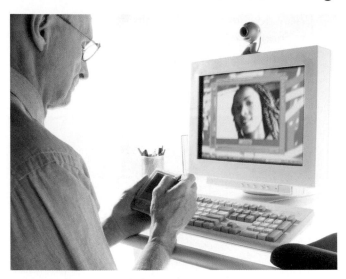

The fourth strategy is to increase one's competence quickly as new equipment, technology, and processes become available. The more one can learn about new approaches, the more competent one is to not only evaluate the innovations but also to determine if the new approach is right for the organization. Further, this approach reinforces evidence-based principles as the supportive rationale for change. Assuming a posture of risk avoidance and waiting for others to test and critique new approaches decreases the leader's ability to sustain an organization that is contemporary and able to integrate processes and equipment into the work of patient care.

Leaders need to be able to discern innovations that add value and those that serve as obstacles to the work. Creating more work to streamline processes that ultimately decreases productivity and the timely achievement of quality outcomes, is not a rational approach.

Create Competence Quickly in...

- *Electronic communication with wireless voice pagers.*
- *Computerized documentation.*
- *Scanning documents.*
- *Eliminating or minimizing paper use.*
- *Principles of genome therapy.*
- *Creative employment contracts for staff and providers.*
- *Schedule bidding.*

New Systems Bring New Challenges

Ten years ago no one could have identified the effect of 200+ emails a day or the strategies to manage them! In spite of large volumes of messages, few users are giving up the email system; rather they work to plan days for email time and filter out unwanted messages.

Timing Matters

Implementing the second-best idea now is a better strategy than doing the best thing a week from now. It is a bigger risk to delay making decisions than to make marginal ones.

(Executive Leadership, National institute of Business Management)

THE RISK OF CPOE

The value of computerized physician order entry (CPOE) has been identified; however, the resulting benefits create new and unanticipated issues. Although some studies indicate reductions in errors of 80%, new errors can also be introduced, rendering the organization more vulnerable for other errors. New errors of dosing, discontinuing, and renewing on the basis of established rules have been identified following implementation of CPOE. System downtime further fragments the hoped-for seamless record. The leader is challenged to pursue the journey of computerization of the health record to a level that is unknown and untested, to pursue a journey filled with risks of provider alienation and uncontrolled costs, and ultimately improve the entire process of providing patient care.

Leaders of health care organizations must be thoroughly enmeshed in the CPOE processes and highly knowledgeable about when to forge ahead with the efforts and when to retreat and regroup in the transformation to a fully integrated electronic health record.

Form New Partnerships

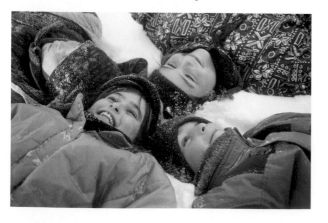

Dare to Move to a Virtual World

How does one enmesh oneself in the world of technology and still retain the human touch? Moving aggressively to greater levels of technology is about advancing into uncharted territories.

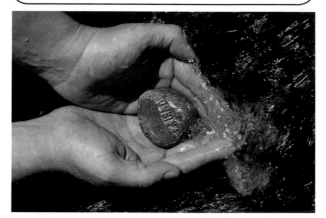

Accelerating Competence through Teamwork and New Partnerships

In times of high risk and uncertainty, the leader must first focus on effective communication through highly skilled teamwork. The greater the teamwork and support for creativity, the more ideas that will emerge. Encouraging all members of the organization to share and develop their leadership skills requires passion and engagement in the richness of the collective decision-making process.

Further, competence can be developed by reaching out beyond the normal network of colleagues to others with related skills. Developing relationships beyond traditional health care disciplines can provide new insights and greater depth of understanding. Embracing environmental psychologists and human factors experts to assist in team collaboration and communication can greatly enrich work processes. Florists and musicians and potters also give new meaning and understanding to the work of healing—and serve to sustain the focus on healing and avoid the tendency to focus on technology or publications.

5. Apologize with Flair

The fourth strategy is to apologize quickly and appropriately when an error or misstep is recognized. Resiliency is the key. Leaders must be resilient and able to regroup and move on when things don't go as anticipated. Recognizing negative situations and acknowledging them with others can be therapeutic. It is far better to acknowledge the misstep than to ruminate endlessly. This approach avoids leaving others to wonder about your competence and assists you to get back on the right path.

About Errors, Missteps, and Mistakes

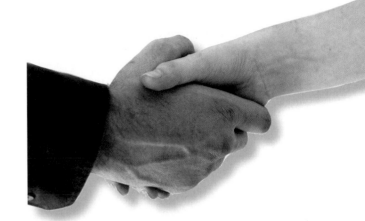

- Recognize that mistakes happen! Right the wrong as quickly as possible.

- Be sincere and apologize when appropriate.

- Use humor only when appropriate.

- Admit you were wrong—avoid the silent treatment.

- Don't try to rationalize and blame it on someone else.

- Say you are sorry when you are.

- Shake hands and make up!

Address the Missteps: It Happens!

- You hired an individual without checking references and when the references are finally available, they are not positive.

   -Action: Confront the issue, face the employee with the information, and seek assistance from human resources to reverse the hiring decision.

- You gave the wrong medication.

   -Action: Admit the mistake, inform the patient and the physician. Give the correct medication.

- You called the wrong physician.

   -Action: Acknowledge the mistake and call the right physician. It happens—usually at the worst possible time!

- You wrongly accused someone before you had all the information.

   -Action: Apologize to the individual as quickly as you learn the correct information.

References

Abrahamson, E. (2000). Change without pain. *Harvard Business Review*, 78(7), 75-79.

Geneen, H., & Powers, B. (1997). *The synergy myth and other ailments of business today*. New York St. Martin's Press.

Leveson, N. G (2004). A new accident model for engineering safer systems. *Safety Science*, 42(4), 237-270.

Marais, K., Dulac, N , & Leveson, N. (2004). *Beyond normal accidents and high reliability organizations: The need for an alternative approach to safety in complex systems*. Cambridge, MA: Massachusetts Institute of Technology. Retrieved February 7, 2006. from littp://esd.rnit.eduisymposium/patspapers/rnarais-b.pdi.

National Institute of Business Management. (2005). Executive leadership: Why the best leaders take action first and ask questions later. McLean, VA. Retrieved July 16, 2006 at http://www.nibm.net/newsletters.asp

Perrow, C. (1999). *Normal accidents: Living with high-risk technologies*. Princeton, NJ: Princeton University Press.

Waldman, J. 0., Kelly, F., Aurora, S., & Smith, H. L. (2004). The shocking cost of turnover in health care. *Health Care Management Review*, 29(1), 2-7.

Weick, K., & Sutcliffe, K. (2001). *Managing the unexpected: Assuring high performance in an age of complexity*. San Francisco: Jossey Bass.

Suggested Readings

Manollovich, M. (2005). Promoting nurses' self-efficacy: A leadership strategy to improve practice. *JONA*, 35(5), 271-278.

Sheridan, S. E., & Hatlie, M. J. (2005). Measured impatience. *Patient Safety & Quality Healthcare*, 2(2), 8-11.

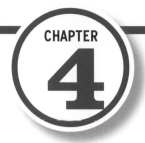

CHAPTER 4

PRACTICE IN A WORLD OF UNCERTAIN EXPECTATIONS

The work of leaders is about working in uncharted territory and creating an infrastructure for the best decision-making processes.

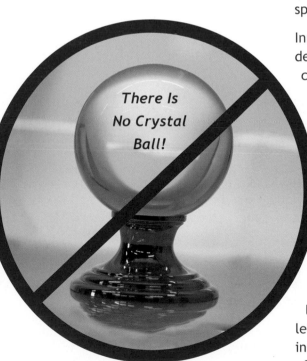

There Is No Crystal Ball!

Change is an inevitable reality, a topic familiar to leaders and managers. Discussions about the challenges of change certainly are not new for the experienced leader. What is new and more challenging than ever is the speed of change and its associated complexities and chaos. With new technology and rapid dissemination of information via the Internet, the speed of change can be overwhelming at times.

Innovations by their very nature do not have clearly defined outcomes, only anticipated outcomes. Health care system complexity along with innovation is a source of the increasing uncertainty. Contemporary leaders must manage the anticipated outcomes of new knowledge, technology, and process interactions with as little negative effect on the organization as possible.

In this section, the complexities of uncertain expectations are explored. Several strategies are offered to assist leaders not in creating an algorithm to manage uncertainties, but rather behaviors, principles, and guidelines for consideration as one traverses the world of complex leadership. Six topics are discussed to assist the leader in managing uncertainty: the process of selecting and supporting advocates for innovation, the role of core values, the importance of an anomaly, challenging assumptions, creating new metrics, and modifying or course correcting when outcomes are not those originally anticipated.

Practice in a World of Uncertain Expectations 581

UNCERTAIN EXPECTATIONS

The source of uncertainty can be external, internal, or both. The external source of uncertainty is about the work to be done and is usually associated with stakeholder expectations, the attributes of the organization's structure, the processes of leadership and patient care, or the outcomes of the system. The internal source is about personal capacity and willingness to address the unknown.

The issues can be described in two questions, "What is the work that needs to be done in this uncharted territory?" and "Will I be able to do the work if I am not certain of what it is?"

External Sources of Uncertainty

Health care stakeholders' (patients, payers, caregivers, and policymakers) expectations change as new information and innovation emerge. Each group has expectations about what service is provided, who will provide it, where it will be provided, and how much it will cost. Given the numerous individuals involved and affected by any health care process, the uncertainties are innumerable.

The structure is also a source of uncertainty. Organizational structures are continually evaluated and reshaped to better match the work to be done. Roles are added, modified, or eliminated to improve performance and outcomes. Each change is accompanied by anticipated but unknown outcomes. Published research and the experiences of other leaders can suggest what the outcomes might be; however, the result of each modification of the organizational structure is unique. No formula or algorithm exists to predict the effect of these complex dynamics, thus uncertainty abounds.

When innovations occur, organizational processes are affected. Process improvements include changes in the numbers and types of staff members, the work to be done, and the level of acuity of patient needs. All of these present uncertainty.

It is important to note that leaders have the dual accountability of ensuring processes that support a stable workforce and consistent processes to achieve quality outcomes and continually modifying processes to be consistent with innovations—a daunting challenge!

WHAT AM I SUPPOSED TO DO?

SOURCE OF UNCERTAINTY

─ORGANIZATIONAL STRUCTURE, ROLE DESIGNATION, EDUCATIONAL REQUIREMENTS, SPAN OF CONTROL

─WORK PROCESSES, TEAMWORK, RESOURCE AVAILABILITY

─EXPECTED PATIENT, CAREGIVER, ORGANIZATIONAL, AND COMMUNITY OUTCOMES

The approach to outcome analysis can also contribute to uncertainty. Often single metrics are selected to consider effectiveness. When different metrics or different groups of metrics are selected for analysis, additional uncertainty is introduced, and the number of conclusions increases. Leaders must identify the metrics that reflect the true value of the work.

Internal Sources of Uncertainty

The second source of uncertainty is internal, one's personal capacity for tolerating the unknown.

Leaders may be competent and capable of managing the realities of the current environment but quite uncertain about their personal ability to adapt to new expectations. The challenges of family responsibilities, relationships with colleagues and friends, and financial resources all influence personal capacity for thriving in uncertain times.

It is often difficult to consider new roles, new relationships, or new skills that may be required as the result of innovation when one is comfortable and satisfied with the current work and level of income. What is certain, of course, is that there will be change in all of these areas.

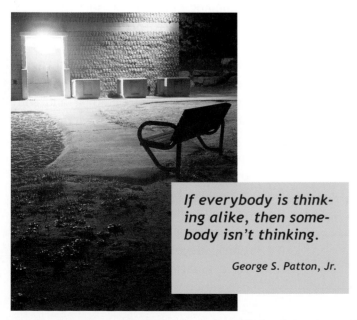

If everybody is thinking alike, then somebody isn't thinking.

George S. Patton, Jr.

Uncertain Expectations

WILL I BE ABLE TO DO THE NEEDED WORK?

- BALANCING WORK AND FAMILY LIFE, KNOWLEDGE, RELATIONSHIPS, AND FINANCIAL NEEDS

- PERSONAL INTELLECTUAL CAPACITY TO MEET THE CHALLENGES

- COMFORT WITH CONFLICT

- SKILLS TO MEDIATE AND NEGOTIATE

- WILLINGNESS TO CHANGE

Practice in a World of Uncertain Expectations 583

STRATEGIES

The leader's spirit of lifelong inquiry and the value of exploration of uncharted territory is fully realized in the work of the information age. Indeed, lifelong inquiry is fraught with uncertainty.

The spirit of inquiry is more than working to discover new processes, mindsets, and new technology; it is about discovering and integrating the best new ideas into current work processes. The assumptions of inquiring leaders are immersed in the belief that uncertainty is necessary for the evolution of processes and for convergence of the best resources. Indeed, current processes will be effective only as long as the environment and resources remain stable.

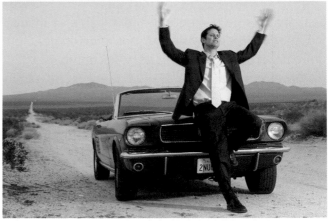

Strategy 1	*Identify and support advocates for innovation.*
Strategy 2	*Manage by values.*
Strategy 3	*Respect and value the anomaly.*
Strategy 4	*Challenge assumptions and clarify expectations.*
Strategy 5	*Reframe and revise metrics for evaluation; develop aggregate metrics.*
Strategy 6	*Develop course correction expertise.*

Leaders who are venturesome, daring, and innovative require support in managing uncertain expectations. Six strategies are presented to assist leaders in managing the uncertain expectations of the ever-changing health care environment. These strategies are useful in guiding and supporting leaders in managing uncertain expectations: seeking out those with innovator and early adopter characteristics for support and development, managing by values, respecting and valuing the anomaly, challenging assumptions and clarifying expectations, developing aggregate metrics for evaluation, and developing course correction expertise.

Strategy 1	*Identify and support advocates for innovation.*

Creating Partnerships for Innovation

Before innovations can be adopted throughout an organization, individuals must first be involved and committed to the new work. The diffusion of innovations process described by Rogers (2003) has described the accountability of leaders to internally and personally adopt innovations before the critical mass diffusion processes across the organization can occur.

Leaders are encouraged to identify those individuals who are innovators and early adopters (Rogers, 2003) of change as well as the characteristics of leaders able to support the development of new expectations and metrics for changing work. Greater numbers of colleagues dedicated to innovation are able to create a critical mass of energy and effort dedicated to thriving in uncertainty that is channeled into the productive work of confronting, monitoring, and modeling innovative behaviors whenever possible.

Innovators

- *Venturesome*

- *Control of financial resources to absorb possible loss from unprofitable innovation*

- *Ability to cope with a high degree of uncertainty about the innovation*

Early Adopters

- *Integrated part of the system*

- *Serve as role models or other members*

- *Respected by peers*

- *Successful*

Note:

Leadership stagnation or leadership focused solely on maintaining the present is a significant threat to managing uncertain expectations.

Ten characteristic competencies of leaders in managing uncertain expectations can be reviewed and compared with existing job performance expectations to reinforce supportive leadership behaviors. These characteristics can guide leaders in the development of other leaders to gain expertise in this area.

Leadership Characteristics Supportive of Managing Uncertain Expectations

#1 *Is experienced and competent in current role and aware of limitations*

#2 *Is approachable; able to see situations from another's point of view*

#3 *Has personal accountability; maintains personal high standards and high expectations; recognized for high personal integrity*

#4 *Is responsive and maintains open lines of communication*

#5 *Is willing to take risks*

#6 *Has good business savvy; able to create and evaluate outcome metrics*

#7 *Values education and professional development*

#8 *Prefers to work in team environment; empowers and encourages other to act*

#9 *Values diversity; brings people of different backgrounds together*

#10 *Expects organizational accountability; sets high standards and holds people to them*

Strategy 2	*Manage by values.*

Most organizational values reflect the essence of their basic beliefs about people and health care and the principles by which they operate. These values clarify for all members of the organization how to behave and treat others. They are the basis for evaluating management practices and bringing them into alignment with core values when needed. Each innovation may challenge the team, thus core values refocus discussions and make difficult decisions with sound rationale.

The second strategy for the leader in managing uncertain expectations is to focus on managing by values. As every organization faces increasing complexity, the focus of the leader and team members must be on work deeply rooted in core values, the guiding and determining force in managing uncertain expectations resulting from innovation.

Innovations should be considered first from the core values related to the essential stewardship responsibility for quality work, survival, and profitability. Beyond the essential stewardship responsibilities, attention to ethical decisions, responsiveness, and lifelong learning from experiences also guides the leader.

RESPONSIVE

- Identifies needs and delivers appropriate service
- Ensures effective evaluation and feedback processes
- Follows through on commitments

ESSENTIAL STEWARDSHIP

- The work of health care
- Survival to continue the work
- Profitability to sustain growth

ETHICAL

- Fair and equitable treatment of employees
- Business integrity
- Communicate complete and accurate information

LIFELONG LEARNING

- Competent caregivers
- Support for education or professional development
- Support for research

Strategy 3	*Respect and value the anomaly.*

Anomaly: Deviation from the normal or common order or form or rule

I can't understand why people are frightened of new ideas. I'm frightened of old ones.

John Cage

Note:

Putting the brakes on to avoid change is irrational; no on can stop the future from occurring!

The third strategy is to respect and value the anomaly. Innovations associated with unknown or uncertain outcomes are considered out of the ordinary or anomalous to the existing paradigm. Leaders are expected to be open-minded, flexible, and willing to embrace and incorporate new behaviors. The anomaly is recognized as a potential vehicle to a better future. Anomalies present challenges that are inherent in the nature of the change process and opportunities to design and mold future systems.

The work of the leader is to continually challenge the status quo to encourage new ideas and better ways to provide health care.

Resistance to anomalies is not uncommon. The digital world could be considered an anomaly as a move from paper to electronic documentation emerged. Virtual health care services in which there is no physical contact between the patient and the provider is another. Once the anomaly gains acceptance and is believed to be the preferred way to do work, the leader begins the adoption process to integrate the anomaly into the emerging paradigm.

A note of caution is given by Kuhn regarding significant changes to an existing mental model or paradigm. According to Kuhn (1996), the mere presence of an anomaly is not by itself sufficient for a paradigm change. New expectations then follow the adoption pathways of awareness, interest, evaluation, trial, and implementation as described by Rogers (2003).

Overview

From Modification ➡ *to innovation* ➡ *to anomaly* ➡ *to transformation*

Another approach to gaining understanding of the realities of uncertainty is to consider the world from what is happening in the current work, from modifications resulting from process improvements, to innovation, to anomaly, and then to transformation and creation of a new paradigm reflecting the innovations. Using the work of Kuhn (1996), existing practices reflect the known paradigm, performance improvements or modifications reflect the second class of phenomena, and innovations reflect the third type in which an anomaly emerges.

According to Thomas Kuhn (1996), there are three types of phenomena about which a new theory might be developed.

1. The first consists of phenomena already well explained by existing paradigms.

2. The second type consists of those whose nature is indicated by existing paradigms but whose details can be understood only through further theory articulation. These are the phenomena to which scientists direct their research much of the time, but that research aims at the articulation of existing paradigms rather than at the invention of new ones.

3. The third type are the recognized anomalies whose characteristic feature is their stubborn refusal to be assimilated to existing paradigms. This type alone gives rise to new theories. Paradigms provide all phenomena except anomalies with a theory-determined place in the scientist's field of vision.

Strategy 4	*Challenge assumptions and clarify expectations.*

The fourth strategy for the leader is to challenge assumptions and clarify expectations. It is about challenging the assumptions of existing processes, mindsets, and technology applications as a key strategy to achieve excellence. Challenging assumptions serves to ensure that resources are allocated appropriately and are aligned with organizational goals.

This leadership work is also about coaching others to recognize the importance of continual examination of the work coupled with the need for experimentation and exploration of uncharted territory. Leaders who are able to balance these often competing priorities can achieve higher levels of performance without misuse of resources.

Ask These Questions

- Are the processes still effective? Challenge basic patient care work of admission content, daily whole body assessments, frequency of vital signs. Challenge basic leadership processes such as annual performance reviews and in person meetings.

- Is this still the work that needs to be done? Should it be eliminated, modified, or expanded?

- Is there evidence of value from the work? How does the consumer know there is value from this work?

CHALLENGING ASSUMPTIONS: EXAMPLES FOR CONSIDERATION

Ask Yourself—Are These Assumptions Still Valid?

1. *A meeting cannot occur without physical presence of participants.*

2. *Minimum staffing ratios will guarantee patient safety and caregiver satisfaction.*

3. *Shift change cannot occur without face-to-face physical presence of oncoming and off-going caregivers .*

4. *Annual budgeting is the most effective, reliable method for estimating resource use.*

5. *Strategic planning is worth the time and effort managing resources.*

6. *The optimal route for medications is intravenous.*

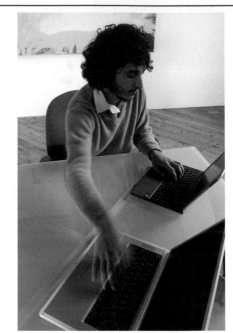

Challenging assumptions: Is multitasking really improving productivity?

Ethnopharmacology: Challenging Assumptions about Current Prescribing Protocols

An innovation that requires leaders to challenge current assumptions specific to medication prescribing and dosing is ethnopharmacology, the study of ethnicity and drug response. Genetic and cultural factors are believed to influence a given drug's pharmacokinetics (its absorption, metabolism, distribution, and elimination), pharmacodynamics (its mechanism of action and effects at the target site), and patient adherence and education. Adopting principles of ethnopharmacology requires identifying supporters of these beliefs, and developing expectations and metrics to determine if this information does improve costs and outcomes. What assumptions about patient information must be challenged?

1. Is there a need for new information such as cultural history?
2. Is there a need for body/basal metabolic rate data?
3. Is there a need for DNA testing?
4. Is patient weight still necessary?
5. What data that are currently collected could be eliminated?

More on Challenging Assumptions:

RAILROADS AND ELECTRONIC HEALTH RECORDS: IS HISTORY REPEATING ITSELF?

Consider the following story of the initial resistance to the railroad. Are there similarities to the current adoption of the electronic health record?

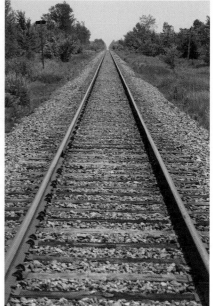

Railroad Resistance*

In the early 1800s, the lack of reliable low-cost transportation was a major barrier to American industrial development. The stagecoach was the primary form of transportation. At best, 12 passengers and their luggage could travel at 4 miles an hour!

The opposition to railroads was widespread. Various groups such as highway and bridge companies, and owners of stagecoaches and ferries, worked to create laws that would prohibit trains from carrying freight. A group of physicians in Boston warned that the jarring produced by trains traveling at 15 or 20 mph would lead to head concussions.

The 1842 petition brought before the Boston legislature to support railroads was opposed by town members for these reasons:

1. The railroad will result in incalculable injury to the town. There will be sacrifice of private property if any portion of the pathway for the railroad track is located in highly populated parts of the town. Also, railroads near public highways will forever obstruct communication among townspeople and continually endanger the lives of those near the railroad tracks.

2. If the railroad must proceed, construction should be located over the marshes and creeks bordering the harbor and river, and as remote as possible from all other roads.

Supporters for the railroad noted: Another transportation initiative, the "big ditch" (aka the Erie Canal) sparked an economic revolution. Before the canal was built, it cost $100 and took 20 days to transport 1 ton of freight from Buffalo to New York City. Following the advent of water transportation, the cost fell to $5 a ton and transit time was reduced to 6 days.

This section excerpted from Mintz (2004).

While resistance stems from financial, social, and technical realms, the work of the leader in examining the electronic health record as a significant innovation is to challenge the assumptions of current processes, clarify expectations as the knowledge evolves, and work to align these expectations with available resources.

RAILROADS AND ELECTRONIC HEALTH RECORDS: IDENTIFYING AND ADDRESSING RESISTANCE

If consumers expect a comprehensive EHR, how does an organization address the uncertainties and inadequacies of the current system? When is the level of risk acceptable given the unknown value of the innovation? Small and large innovations require clarification of the assumptions peculiar to the innovation and the expectations for improvement. In addition to understanding assumptions and expectations, much can be learned from the rationale for resistance to innovations and comparison with other innovations. Resistance specific to competing priorities, newly created obstacles from the innovation, and negative fantasies about what might happen are common to the introduction of the railroad and the EHR.

Innovation	Purpose/ Expectation	Rationale for Resistance	Comments
Railroad	• Create more reliable, low-cost transportation	• Concerns about loss of land for housing • Competing priorities of shipping industry, roads, bridges, waterways • Negative fantasies about head injuries • Decrease available housing • Physical safety hazards	Challenging assumptions about the perceived effectiveness of the current system and analysis of benefits and costs can assist resistors to understand the effect. Small incremental programs to test or pilot innovations can also be helpful. In addition, more innovations may need to occur to manage one innovation, e.g., new security models for the electronic record.
Electric health record (EHR)	• Legible, retrievable integrated standardized health record that is accessible by several providers at several locations	• Significant cost • Steep learning curve • Loss of provider autonomy • Information security • Competing priorities for health care building • Technology limitations / functionality/inadequate application interfaces	

| Strategy 5 | *Reframe and revise metrics for evaluation; develop aggregate metrics.* |

The greatest difficulty is to identify and measure what really matters: which metrics are the critical variables that indicate value, service, and cost outcomes accurately and comprehensively. Multiple related metrics are required to explain the causality of relationships; seldom does one variable explain one outcome. By its very essence, the complex and dynamic nature of health care renders it resistant to simple linear cause-and¬effect metrics. For example, no one intervention is accountable for the resolution of a patient's pneumonia; diet, fluids, medications, and activity all contribute to the resolution of the chest congestion. Similarly, the hours per patient-day (HPPD) metric cannot be linked simply and traced to the activities of a single unit leader; the competence of staff, level of illness of patients, number of interventions required, and availability of equipment and supplies all affect the level of HPPD.

It is seldom readily apparent which combinations of metrics provide the desired information. Further, as health care continues to evolve, the evidence and metrics change.

Another important issue is that focusing on the combinations of metrics or aggregate metrics has advantages and disadvantages, supporters and nonsupporters. The work of the leader is to identify the critical variables, build the case for the selected combination of variables and their associated metrics and document their results.

Metrics for Excellence: Magnet Criteria

The 14 Forces of Magnetism provide guidance for metric modeling and the most comprehensive template of nursing characteristics for excellence. This serves as a template for a collective or aggregate profile for better performing organizations; however, more data are needed to determine the strength and contribution of each of the forces. Although many of the metrics supporting Magnet excellence can be compared and benchmarked externally, many metrics are internal to the organization.

There are four important questions the leader should ask:

1. What are the metrics?

2. What is the relationship of the selected metric to the mission of the organization?

3. What other metrics/ variables directly affect this metric?

4. What are the appropriate internal and external benchmarks? For the metric(s)?

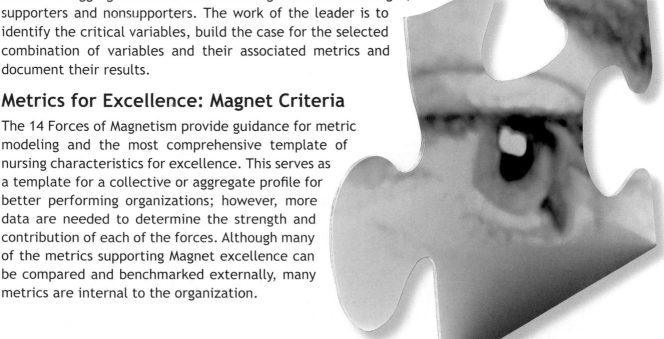

CREATING NEW METRICS FOR NEW WORK

Evolving Expectations

With each modification of work, the outcome expectations change. New mindsets, new approaches, and new resources evolve as expectations change. Consider the evolution of two processes: creating and managing one's personal calendar and documenting. It is important to note that as the innovation evolves and becomes more defined, expectations evolve reflecting the intent of the innovation. This evolution of expectations is an integral part of the process of adopting innovations.

Personal Calendar: Evolving Expectations and Metrics

Innovation	Expectation (intent)	Metric
Manual handwritten calendar	Summary of information	Appropriate space allocation for entries
Dayplanner	Organized summary of information associated with notes/addresses	Compact, portable notebook, appropriate space allocation
Electronic calendar	Computerized, editable, accessable by multiple individuals, able to archive and retrieve information	Real-time availability, accessable to selected individuals to facilitate scheduling; decrease time in calendar management
Interconnected, Internet-accessed calendar	Wireless, Internet access	Accessibility from multiple devices and multiple locations

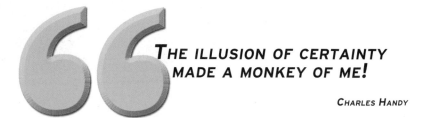

THE ILLUSION OF CERTAINTY MADE A MONKEY OF ME!

CHARLES HANDY

DOCUMENTATION: EVOLVING EXPECTATIONS AND METRICS

Innovations to improve the process, quality, and storage of information have evolved over time. Each innovation is associated with new expectations and new metrics. The challenge is to review and revise the expectations, then modify the metric to reflect the outcomes.

In this table, the evolution of documentation from the paper and pen to the mass storage device or memory stick, associated expectations of the innovation, and the metrics to evaluate the innovation are identified. Each change or innovation requires reconsideration of the expected metrics to identify the real value of the innovation. It is important to note that continuing to use the same expectations and metrics for paper and pen handwriting for voice recognition would be an incomplete realization of the benefits of voice recognition technology. Metrics must reflect the expectations.

Innovation	Expectation (intent)	Metric
Paper and pen to record information/handwriting	Documentation of the information that can be retrieved	Amount of paper or ink used Amount of time to document
Electronic writing/typing	Documentation of the information Retrieveable from paper file Legible Correct spelling	Amount of paper Cost of device and keyboard technology Decreased time for documentation
Computer programs for data or word processing to include storage devices: 3-inch floppy disk Zip drive/ CD/ DVD Mass storage device/memory stick	Large file data storage Portable High-speed access Retrievable from multiple access points File back-up device Device compatibility	Data storage capacity Cost of hardware and devices and software Size of devices Productivity; number of pages produced
Voice recognition documentation	Elimination of typing Device compatibility Increased speed for documentation	Productivity Number of pages produced Cost of recording/interface devices

More on Expectations and Metrics...

Not all innovations require new metrics. Some changes in health care work result in new expectations for greater involvement of individuals or higher performance targets while the specific metric remains the same. For example, changing from nurse-administered pain medication to patient controlled analgesia (PCA) pumps does not change the expectation for pain control; rather the intent of the change is to improve the level of achievement or performance of the specific metric. Patient satisfaction with pain control and comfort should be better with the PCA than with nurse-administered pain interventions.

New metrics are needed when innovations are introduced. In most cases, multiple interrelated metrics are required to adequately reflect the value of the innovation. Two examples of innovations with changing expectations but no new metrics and one example, accommodating family presence, which does require a new metric, are presented in the following table.

> *If you have built castles in the air, your work need not be lost; that is where they should be. Now put the foundations under them.*
>
> Henry David Thoreau

Improvement or **Innovation**	Expectations	Metrics
PCA pump for pain relief	• Improved patient involvement in pain management • Increased pain control	No new metrics • Adequacy of pain management • Patient satisfaction with pain control • Cost of equipment/pharmaceuticals • Cost of caregivers
Room service for hospitalized patients and thier family	• Patient control of diet, time of meals, selection of food, and family participation	No new metrics • Patient satisfaction with meals, timeliness, and quality of food. • Cost of room service • Family satisfaction with meals
Accommodating family presence at the bedside and participation in care	• Families are not only welcome but also expected to participate in patient care. • Accomodations are comfortable and include furniture for resting, Internet access, Internet education.	Current metrics for family satisfaction are used. New metrics are needed for: • Quality and adequacy of Internet access. • Cost of the devices/service. • Cost of furniture accomodations.

COMPARING METRICS

Multiple structure and process variables interact to produce safe medication administration. Working to decrease preventable adverse drug events (PADEs) without additional changes to structure and/or process variables could be futile. For example, increasing nursing hours of care without adding electronic processes to support patient identification and ensure legibility of orders could result in no change in the number of PADEs. To effect change, combinations of variables known to affect the structure and processes are needed. In this table, scenario 1 is optimal for patient excellence based on the structure and processes available.

Preventable Adverse Medication Events (PADEs): Multiple inputs, Processes, and Metrics

Structure	Processes	Metric	Expected level of performance
SCENARIO #1 • Electronic health record • Enclosed medication preparation rooms • Bright task lighting of at least 1400 lux • Single-bed rooms • Decentralized pharmacists • Positive patient identification	• Computerized physician order entry with standard order sets • Computerized medication administration documentation • Bedside documentation • Patient/medication bar-coding	• Number of PADEs • Nursing hours of care per patient-day • Pharmacist hours per patient-day • Total cost of care per patient-day • Number of verbal orders • Turnaround time from order to dispensing for first dose, non-stat medications	• Fewer than 4 PADEs per month or 0.001 error per 100,000 doses • Nursing hours less than 6 per patient-day • Pharmacist hours less than 0.2 per patient-day • Cost of patient-day <$240 <2% verbal orders • Turn around time (TAT) <60 min for first dose, non-stat medications
SCENARIO #2 • Manual documentation system • 75% single-bed rooms • Centralized pharmacy services • Overhead lighting less than 1400 lux	Manual documentation at central station • Handwritten physician orders • Manual order transcription • Visual patient name identification	• Number of PADEs • Nursing hours of care per patient-day • Pharmacist hours per patient-day • Total cost of care per patient-day • Number of verbal orders	• Fewer than 20 PADEs per month or 0.005 error per 100,000 doses • Nursing hours less than 6.2 per patient-day • Pharmacist hours less than 0.25 per patient-day • Cost of patient-day <$300 • <10% verbal orders. • TAT <3 hours for first dose, non-stat medications
SCENARIO #3 • Electronic medication administration record • 75% single-bed rooms • Centralized pharmacy services • Overhead lighting less than 1400 lux	• Manual documentation at central station • Handwritten physician orders • Manual order transcription • Electronic documentation/reconciliation of medications • Visual patient name identification	• Number of PADEs • Nursing hours of care per patient-day • Pharmacist hour per patient-day • Total cost of care per patient-day • Number of verbal orders	• Fewer than 15 PADEs per month or 0.004 error per 100,000 doses • Nursing hours less than 6.1 per patient-day • Pharmacist hours less than 0.22 per patient-day • Cost of patient-day <$275 • <10% verbal orders. • TAT <2 hours for first dose, non-stat medications

| Strategy 6 | *Develop course correction expertise.* |

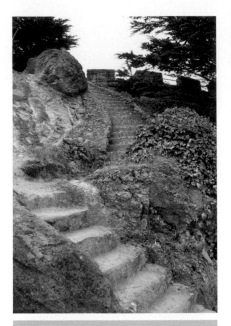

Expectations for success are not always realized for a variety of reasons. The wise leader works to minimize the time spent ruminating about the unsuccessful events and focuses on developing new solutions and course corrections to achieve the desired outcomes. According to Rogers (2003), rejection of an innovation may occur anytime along the adoption process, which includes awareness of the innovation, interest, evaluation, trial, and then adoption. Discontinuance is a rejection that occurs after adoption of the innovation. There are two types of discontinuance:

- Disenchantment discontinuance, which is a decision to reject an idea as a result of dissatisfaction with its performance.

- Replacement discontinuance, which is a decision to reject an idea in order to adopt a better idea.

Given the inevitability of rejection or discontinuance of a new work process, emphasis needs to be on making course corrections with evidence and rationale, then realizing the information and lessons that can be learned from the experience. Before implementing course corrections or new strategies, the team must be sure that the values of the work continue to be congruent with the organization, then challenge the assumptions of the work processes that went awry and clarify expectations that new processes have a high degree of potential for success.

> *The essence of optimism is that it takes no account of the present, it is a source of inspiration, of vitality and hope where others have resigned; it enables a man to hold his head high, to claim the future for himself and not to abandon it to his enemy.*
>
> *Dietrich Bonhoeffer*

Leadership Crucibles:
Learning from Significant Events

Bennis and Thomas (2002) have described the experiences that come to shape behaviors as a leadership crucible. The leadership crucible is the essence of a specific experience that includes trial and error and a point of deep reflection that forces one to question who they are and what matters to them. The leader examines values, questions assumptions, and hones one's judgment skills, resulting in stronger and more self-assuredness about values and purpose. Reflecting on these significant life events assists the leader in managing disappointments and accelerating course correction.

> *The essence of being human is that one does not seek perfection.* George Orwell

ANALYZING THE UNCERTAINTY

1. Begin with describing the area of uncertainty. Is it an internal uncertainty, an external uncertainty, or both?

2. Is it new technology? Or new work? Or something else?

3. Am I concerned about my knowledge of the issue and my technical skills?

4. Am I concerned about my willingness to be involved with the new work?

5. Am I concerned about the effect on my income?

6. Are core values being challenged?

7. Who else is uncertain about the new work?

8. How can I decrease the uncertainty?

Be Wary of Unfocused Activity

When you are not sure where you are going, it has been said that any path will take you there; further, if you don't know what to do, action rather than inaction makes it look like progress is being made when in fact it is only activity that is present and no useful, value-based outcomes result.

References

Bennis, W., & Thomas, R.J. (2002). Crucibles of leadership. *Harvard Business Review*, 80(8), 3-11.

Kuhn, T. S. (1996). *The structure of scientific revolutions* (3rd ed.). Chicago: University of Chicago Press.

Knox, S., & Charrity, J. (2002). Transitions in American hospitals: The necessary reshaping is taking place. *JONA's Healthcare Law, Ethics, and Regulation*, 4(1), 13-17.

Mintz, S. (2004). *The roots of American economic growth*. Digital History. Retrieved February 13, 2006, from www.digitalhistory.uh.edu/database/subtitles.cfm?TitlelD=79.

Rogers, E. M. (2003). *Diffusion of innovations* (5th ed.). New York: The Free Press.

Wheatley, M. (1994). *Leadership and the new science: Learning about organizations from an orderly universe*. San Francisco: Berrett-Koehler.

Suggested Readngs

Handy, C. (1996). *Beyond certainty: The changing world of organizations*. Boston: Harvard Business School Press.

Morgan, G. (1993). *lmaginization: New mindsets for seeing, organizing and managing*. San Francisco: Berrett-Koehler.

Vance, C., & Larson, E. (2001). Leadership research in business and health care. *Journal of Nursing Scholarship*, 34(2), 165-171.

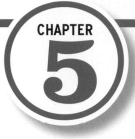

CHAPTER 5

BUILDING RELATIONSHIPS IN THE NEW AGE OF WORK

*In a quantum world, relationships are not just interesting;
they are all there is to reality.*

Margaret Wheatley (1999)

The work of health care is fundamentally based on relationships with employees, patients, and members of the community. These relationships range from mere acquaintances to friend to colleague to partner and may be collaborative, participative, or autocratic.

No leadership work can occur in the absence of connections with others. Relationships are essential in coaching, mentoring, conflict resolution, and problem solving.

In this chapter, an overview of the advantages of healthy relationships, discussion of four characteristics of healthy relationships—self-awareness, shared values, trust, and involvement—are presented. Issues and strategies specific to the work of healing, multigenerational workforces, the integration of information age relationships with the work of health care, and strategies to support relationships that ensure technology supports the work of health care are presented to stimulate dialog among developing as well as experienced leaders.

From Local to Global Communication

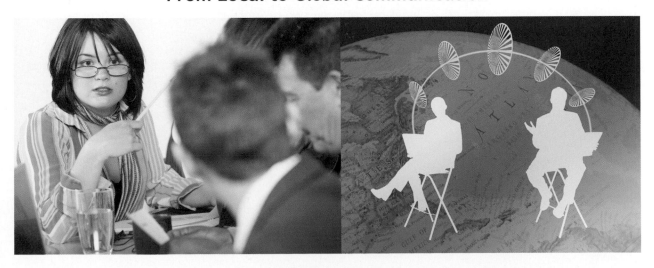

WHY SHOULD WE WORK ON OUR RELATIONSHIPS?

The work environment is dynamic and constantly changing!

1. Healthy, effective relationships require care management, much like our most sophisticated equipment. Just like tuning in TV channels, rotating antennas, filtering noise and artifact from the most sophisticated cardiac monitoring equipment, leaders are challenged to calibrate the relationships within teams to work together in much the same way you would calibrate your most sophisticated technological equipment or monitoring system.

2. The unprecedented speed of introduction of new technology and computerization of work processes have accelerated the dissemination of new information rendering once reliable relationships now inadequate. The breadth and depth in relationships has expanded dramatically to integrate the greater complexity of computerized work processes. The speed of processing has opened the vista from local operations to global realities and from face-to-face interactions to virtual reality. Leaders must continually examine and remodel the structure of the organization, policies, available resources, and skill level of members of the organization to ensure contemporary effectiveness.

3. New models of communication and expectations that fully integrate the advances in human and technological processes are needed for two reasons. The first is to ensure that effective communication is occurring to support organizational performance and second, that the human experience is driving the work rather than the technology driving work processes.

4. Given these challenges and the very nature of health care, which is based on relationships, creating and sustaining healthy relationships remain a priority.

Relationship Definitions

- A particular type of connection existing between people related to or having dealings with others. A logical or natural association between two or more things; connection, correlation, interdependence, or link.

- The commitment of two or more people to supporting each other in the pursuit of a common goal.

- An abstraction belonging to or characteristic of two entities or parts together.

(American Heritage Dictionary, 2003)

The ability to develop and manage relationships between individuals and organizations is a key differentiator for leadership expertise. The simple rate, volume, and pressure for change strongly influences the social fabric of organization—individuals in association with each other and the networks those relationship represent and occupy.

Benefits of Effective Relationships

- Provides a venue to create commitment to the organization, the work of healing and patient care, and to the team

- Supports the development of competence in team members to embrace and thrive in the rapidly changing health care environment

- Creates moral commitment among team members for quality service

- Provides a vehicle for discussion of complex situations and challenges

- Encourages the achievement and celebration of excellent outcomes

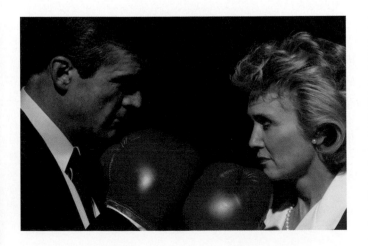

Note:

Poor relationships are costly to organizations and individuals—physically, mentally, and fiscally. The lack of social support impacts both work performance, adversely affects the immune system and ultimately one's health. Stressful social relationships rival smoking, high blood pressure, high blood cholesterol, obesity, and physical inactivity as risk factors for illness and early death. High levels of stress are related to the occurrence of herpes viruses, allergies, and cancer.

Five Stages of Relationship Development

In this section, an overview of the five stages of skill acquisition in relationship development are presented to assist leaders in recognizing the developmental stages of this interpersonal skill. Leaders continually work with others to develop their capacity and ability to meet the challenges of the workplace. In addition to acquiring the content or theory of a leadership skill, individuals need time and experience to progress to a high level of performance. The following stages, based on the work of Dreyfus and Dreyfus (2004), are typically evident as one learns a new process and acquires skills to expertly apply the theory.

Consider the experience of a new manager learning to develop effective relationships

1. Novice:
Individual + Theory Content

The novice is a student of the relationship's development. The theory and information are context free—and the student or learning leader strictly relies on rules to form relationships or to manage relationship difficulty.

2. Advanced Beginner:
Individual + Theory Content + Other Person

The advanced beginner has completed the workshop on relationships, and is beginning to apply content to real life situations following the maxims and rules learned in the workshop. A first-time manager can be considered an advanced beginner and will attempt some relationships and seek guidance in most employee situations.

3. Competent:
Individual + Content + Other Person + Issue

With increasing experience, the number of features and maxims is now overwhelming and the leader learns to adopt a hierarchical view of decision making, and skills of prioritization emerge. With additional experience and practice, the individual is able to form relationships with new employees and assist others in forming relationships based on maxims and rules with relative ease. The competent individual focuses on forming relationships as the means to achieve goals. An experienced manager can be considered a competent professional

4. Proficient:
Individual + Content + Other Person + Issue + Organization

The individual proficient in relationship skills is one who can initiate, modify, and sustain basic relationships with minimal assistance. The relationships are effective, predictable, and successful in most cases. Forming relationships is moving from reactive to proactive. The proficient leader knows the importance of relationships with employees and seeks out opportunities to strengthen the relationships. The focus of the competent individual is on integrating the work of individuals into the larger picture and with others in the organization. An experienced director or leader can be considered a proficient professional.

5. Expert:
Individual + Content + Other Person + Issue + Organization + Community

The expert relationalist forms effective relationships in all areas affecting the work, the community, professional organizations, and internal teams and departments. The expert is able to address adversarial situations effectively, facilitate consensus building, and avoid rumination about past events. The expert has fully integrated maxims and rules and uses them as references rather than roadmaps. The expert sees what needs to be done, then decides how to do it. The expert knows how to perform with calculating and comparing alternatives. The expert is able to form complex and competitive relationships in the most complex and challenging situations with successful outcomes. The expert routinely serves as a coach and mentor for those with less developed relationship skills.

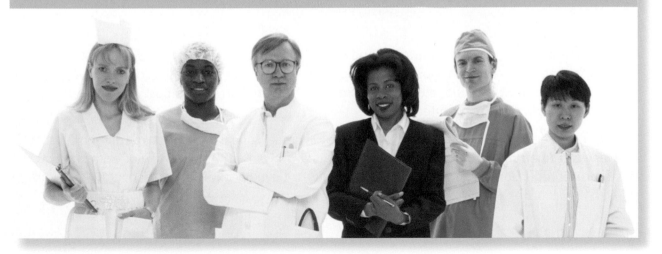

FOUR CHARACTERISTICS OF HEALTHY RELATIONSHIPS: OVERLAPPING AND INTERWOVEN

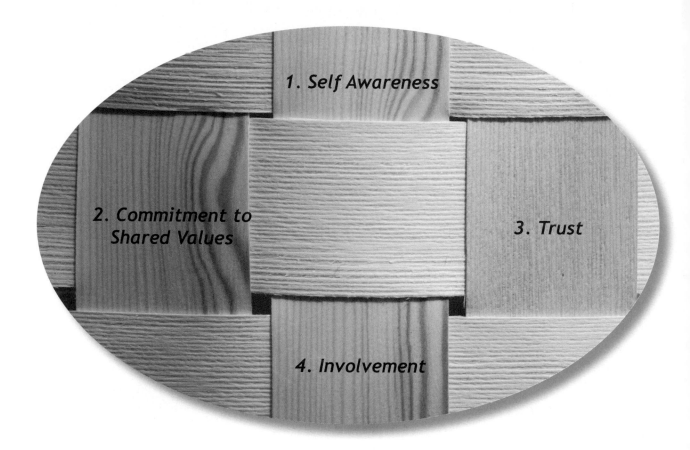

1. Self Awareness

2. Commitment to Shared Values

3. Trust

4. Involvement

Leaders are continually challenged to expand their thinking about relationships and determine how to ensure that these relationships are appropriate, timely, and productive. Relationships in the information age must be fluid, flexible, and more efficient than in the past given the increased complexity and availability of information.

Four common principles are identified as essential in creating healthy, effective relationships: self-awareness, commitment to shared values, trust, and involvement. An overview of each characteristic is presented, along with issues and strategies to develop excellence in overall relationship skills.

CHARACTERISTIC 1: SELF-AWARENESS

Self-awareness is about knowing what one knows and what one does NOT know, one's strengths and areas of opportunity for growth. No leader can be a banker, computer programmer, nurse, physician, researcher, and a nutritionist at the same time—and know all there is to know about each discipline! Leaders must also know their blind spots—the situations that are difficult to handle in spite of the best preparation.

Reflecting and examining one's shadow and assessment tools can provide differing levels of insight into personal relationship skills.

Leadership Reflection for Greater Self-Awareness

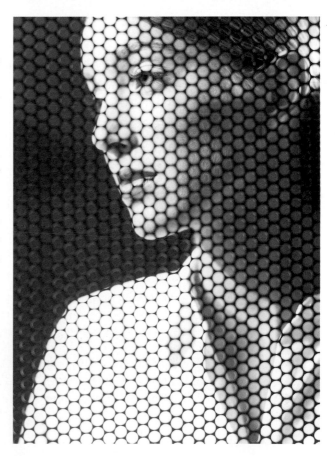

The skills of reflection for leaders can be invaluable. Leaders are wise to reflect on their technical performance and knowledge of leadership specific to building teams, coaching, mentoring, budgeting, and planning, but they also need to reflect on the reality that in spite of a high level of knowledge and skill, there is a need for comfort with the underdetermined nature of leadership; that is, the work is open to variations not accounted for by science or principles.

To maximize productivity, leaders need to reflect on current work and avoid the temptation to determine a collection of discrete performance proficiencies and a policy for every potential variation in practice. The emphasis should be on defining a constellation of factors that constitute the work of leadership. For example, certain principles and goals specific to the work of coaching can be learned; however, each coaching experience is different and requires customization in the application of skills. Working to create multiple coaching scripts is not the best use of leadership time.

KNOW YOUR SHADOW

Another avenue for self-awareness is one's personal shadow. Carl Jung (Taylor, 1999) described the shadow as a composite of personal characteristics and potentials that have been denied expression in life and of which a person is unaware; the ego denies the characteristics because they are in conflict and incompatible with a person's chosen conscious attitude. Leaders can gain insight into personal behaviors and expressions of values through shadow work. The shadow is an important source of hunches and helps to understand unexplainable actions and coping with problematic aspects.

Shadows can be identified by looking at what you project onto others. Often, when you deny a trait in yourself, you tend to be very aware of that trait in other people. You may react irrationally to one of these traits in someone else, becoming annoyed and irritated. However, one can also notice the traits that are admired in others. When you repeat a pattern of behavior involuntarily, it is a sign that your shadow is running the show.

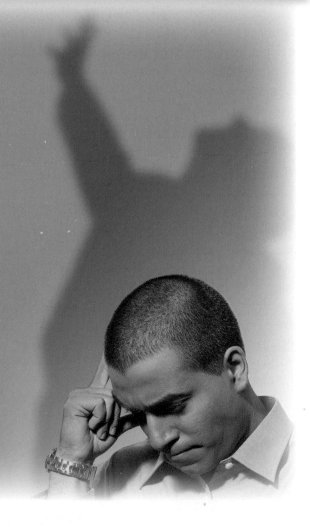

Leaders should consider exploring one's shadow to:

- Understand why one behaves in a certain way.

- Get help or support the unfolding of skills and abilities.

- Address feelings of fear, grief, anger, or shame.

- Change old patterns of behavior.

INDIVIDUALS WITH HIGH SELF-AWARENESS EXHIBIT MANY OF THE FOLLOWING BEHAVIORS:

- Are aware of personal values related to culture, religion, race, gender, etc.
- Articulate personal and professional boundaries specific to physical space, thoughts, sense of identity, and relationship with a higher power
- Communicate in an open style and questions frequently to gain greater understanding; communicates likes and dislikes
- Separate data from opinion in making decisions
- Value multiple perspectives and diversity of ideas
- Recognize the effect of verbal and nonverbal communication
- Do not talk down to others; uses language that is easily understood
- Strive to be concise in communication and avoids rambling on; does not filibuster or tolerate filibustering
- Know the purpose for the relationship and what is expected of each person

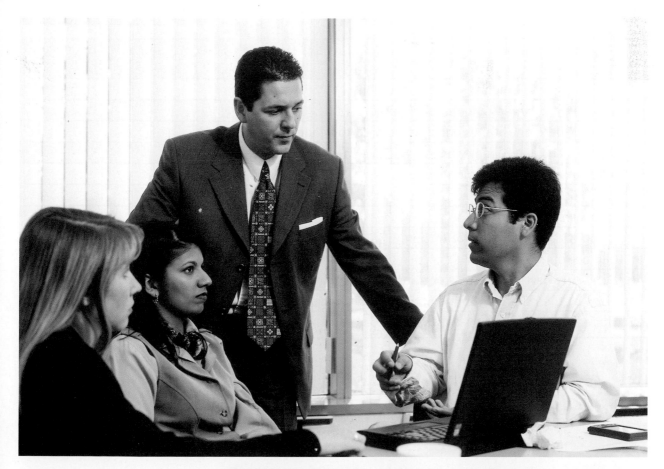

Building Relationships in the New Age of Work   609

VALIDATING YOUR PERSONAL LEVEL OF SELF-AWARENESS

How Am I Perceived by Others?

Reflect on the following 12 statements and rate your own performance for each item using the 1 to 5 rating scale. Request a colleague with whom you work closely to rate your performance in these 12 categories. Compare the ratings.

1. What are the areas of agreement?
2. What are the areas of differing perceptions?
3. What strategies can I use to change these perceptions?

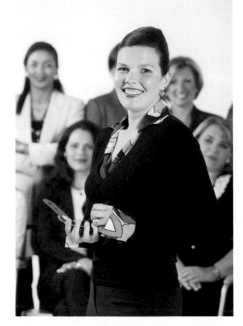

5 = Always; 4 = Most of the time; 3 = Some of the time; 2 = Seldom; 1 = Never; 0 = Not sure	Self	Colleague
1. Uses consensus building to make decisions		
2. Sensitive to feelings and beliefs of others		
3. Knows where one stands on issues related to gender and racial bias		
4. Opinionated and judgmental		
5. Able to see the bigger picture		
6. Tends to be unpredictable		
7. Emphasizes competition		
8. Is cynical and distrusting of others		
9. Can be relied on		
10. Genuinely participates in all duties/responsibilities		
11. Lives by the rules only and emphasizes following policies		
12. Shares personal opinions and willingness to learn others' opinions		

CHARACTERISTIC 2: A COMMITMENT TO SHARED VALUES

The work of health care is about effective, empathic services that require a community of clinicians who commit themselves to working together to meet myriad individuals' needs in health and illness. Healthy relationships among clinicians include those within or across disciplines and are grounded in common values.

These relationships begin with commitment to healing work. Teamwork, learning from and making use of the expertise of others, helping others learn and develop, integrating services at individual and systems levels, and setting aside issues of specialism, hierarchy, and privilege are necessary to support the work of health care.

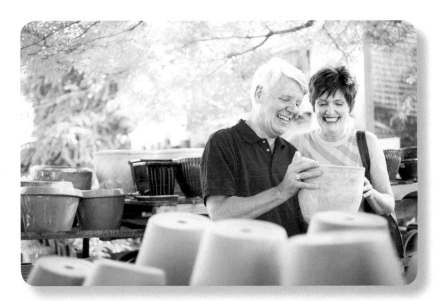

Healing Relationships: The Foundation for Health Care Work

- Reflect the nature, depth, degree of interaction and connection between self, others, nature, God/universe.

- Include the quality and characteristics of interactions that facilitate healing.

- Involve empathy, caring, love, warmth, trust, confidence, credibility, honesty, expectation, courtesy, respect, and communication.

(Dossey, 2005)

HEALING ENCOUNTER

A moment in time when two or more people come together and in that moment a change, insight, or connectedness is experienced. This change is recognized because of a transpersonal dimension that is an intersubjective human-to-human relationship in which one person affects and is affected by another.

Behaviors That Reflect a Commitment to Shared Values

- Able to identify common ground among members of the team, especially when common ground is not readily apparent

- Able to see the bigger picture

- Learns new skills as needed to meet the challenges of not only technology but also of changes in the social contract between employer and employees

- Works to facilitate the work of others to support shared goals

- Tends to be inclusive rather than exclusionary

- Walks the walk—is believable

- Pushes the edges and challenges the status quo to ensure that values are continually relevant

INFLUENCING SHARED VALUES

Multiple areas exist in which the leader's effective relationship skills can serve to influence the expression of shared values. These include the following:

- **Shared Values for Timeliness**

  Collaboration with information technology: ensuring that health information technology provides patient information at the right time to the right person and is a means to better quality, safety, and effectiveness, not an end in itself or a barrier to quality care.

- **Shared Values for Progress**

  The emerging work of the biomedical/genomic science innovations is considered and integrated when appropriate.

- **Shared Values for Quality**

  Quality patient care is continually assessed for the degree of personalization, safety, and effectiveness. The right care at the right time by the right provider is the ever-present, underlying value.

- **Shared Values for Evidence**

  A commitment to evidence-based principles is sustained through emphasis on delivering patient care that is based on the best available evidence for clinical interventions and use of technology that is based on helpfulness and usability for the patient.

When values are not congruent and team members are not in sync, the leader must be alert for the early signs of value misalignment. Some behaviors include the individual who is continually questioning his or her ability, unrealistic expressions of fear of failure, overemphasis on perfectionism, procrastination, and workaholism. Although each of these behaviors is not uncommon, it is when they are excessive that the leader must revisit core values and work to reestablish congruence with core values.

Expressions of "Individual Values"

- Every deadline is missed, but excuses seem legitimate.
- Individual is chronically late to work and early to leave, often leaving others with incomplete work.
- Needs constant attention, reassurance, and feedback; requires more time to manage than any other employee and work products are only mediocre.

ASSESSMENT OF VALUE DISCONNECTION

Often, when conflict emerges, there are subtle but significant value disconnections. Neither values nor goals are shared, resulting in unsatisfactory outcomes. Consider the experience between a leader and another person such as an external regulator (DHS, JCAHO) that did not go well. The leader expected to learn from the facility survey, to validate the organization's current status, and follow the guidelines of the surveying agency. But the surveyor has preconceived notions about the facility, has only limited time for the survey, is about to go on vacation, and is known for following the rules to the letter of the law.

Reflect on the encounter from the perspective of values and the degree to which values were common to both parties using the following self-awareness statements. Rate your perceptions and what you perceived as the actions of the other person using the 1 to 5 rating scale.

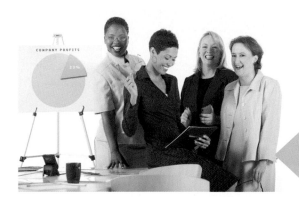

Unilateral, opinionated, and unpredictable

or

collaborative, open to dialog, predictable, and reliable?

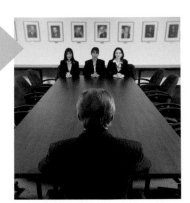

5 = Always   4 = Most of the time   3 = Some of the time
2 = Seldom   1 = Never   0 = Not sure

Self-Awareness Statements	Self	Power Person
1. Uses consensus building to make decisions		
2. Sensitive to feelings and beliefs of others		
3. Knows where one stands on issues related to gender and racial bias		
4. Opinionated and judgmental		
5. Able to see the bigger picture		
6. Tends to be unpredictable		
7. Emphasizes competition		
8. Is cynical and distrusting of others		
9. Can be relied on		
10. Genuinely participates in all duties/responsibilities		
11. Lives by the rules only and emphasizes following policies		
12. Shares personal opinions and willingness to learn others' opinions		

CHARACTERISTIC 3: TRUST

Trust has been called the ugly duckling of science—utterly condemned to be subjective, imprecise, and unreliable.

Why is it so difficult to develop good long-lasting relationships? Fear of disclosure, fear of failure, or a lack a accountability for performance? Is it lack of TRUST or something else? Certainly, trust is a large component of healthy relationships. Healthy relationships in an environment of continual and complex change require not only a high level of self-awareness and shared values but also that each leader is comfortable not knowing everything and is able to trust that colleagues have the same shared values and will perform to their best ability.

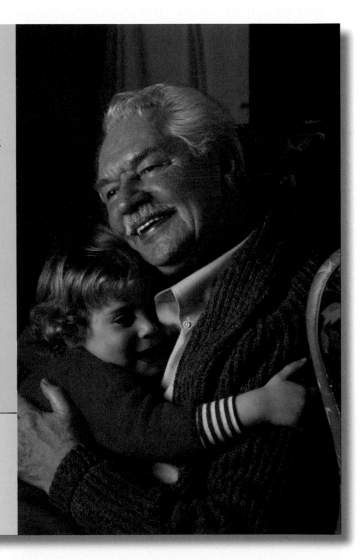

- Trust is that which an observer knows about an entity and can rely on to some extent (consider your spouse/partner or coworker).

- Trust is that which can be relied on without surveillance by the observer (to what degree can you trust your 16-year-old not to take the car when you are not at home?).

- Trust is received information that has a degree of belief that is acceptable to an observer.

- Trust depends on the observer; there is never absolute trust. Trust exists only as self-trust; trust on others will always have surprises; unexpected behaviors.

- Mutual trust is a two-way street in which you trust me and I trust you.

Note:

Trusting relationships cannot be bought or recruited from the outside; they must develop over time and through experience.

CAN I TRUST YOU? CAN YOU TRUST ME?

How do I know if I can trust someone? Certain behaviors reflect trust more than others. Consider the following trust-enhancing and trust-busting behaviors as you develop your relationships.

Trust-Enhancing Behaviors

- Sharing relevant information; be sure that work expectations are spoken, not unspoken. Unspoken work expectation leaves room for ambiguity and misinterpretation.

- Revealing concerns

- Working to understand others and their perspectives

- Reducing controls

- Allowing for mutual influence

- Clarifying mutual expectation

- Meeting expectations

- Letting employees know their work is valued

- Recognizing contributions not only by financial reward but also by presence, concern, and support of effective relationships

- Being realistically optimistic, recognizing that it is easy to be discouraged. Realizing that leaders cannot afford to wallow in pessimism because a negative attitude will inevitably have a negative effect on others.

- Sharing information regarding the rationale for changes and requesting input whenever possible. Sharing information even when it is not pleasant.

- Making eye contact

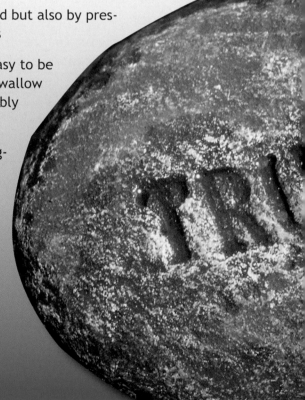

Trust Busters: Unhealthy Behaviors

- Making erroneous assumptions

- Keeping thoughts to oneself; avoiding discussion about sensitive issues

- Being insensitive to the beliefs and values of others

- Tending to be opinionated and judgmental; close-minded

- Expressing an opinion before a person has an opportunity to share an idea or opinion

- Interrupting another while speaking

- Avoiding discussion of sensitive issues in the group. Discussing or criticizing others when they are not present.

- Being too busy for dialog about controversial topics

- Being uninterested in the ideas and opinions of others

  - Encouraging competition—winners and losers

    - Being unpredictable

      - Retaliating when displeased with the actions of others.

        - Being frequently negative and cynical; the cup is half empty rather than half full

      - Working in isolation and then presenting ideas to others as complete

      - Living by the rules without exception

      - Being insensitive to interactions within a group

      - Sharing information only when forced

      - Preferring to do things him- or herself; seldom delegates

    - Having hidden agendas

CHARACTERISTIC 4: PURPOSEFUL INVOLVEMENT

Involvement is about being present and engaged in the moment, regardless of one's comfort level in the situation. Involvement in the information age also requires a new level of discretion in forming and sustaining relationships. Leaders must continually ask, which activities should I be involved in and to what degree should I be involved?. The management of vast amounts of information and increasing expectations requires new approaches for work efficiency and time management. When time is limited, purposeful encounters become critical to enhancing and extending relationships and to get the work accomplished. Haphazard and unplanned encounters decrease productivity and delay goal achievement.

Building Strategic Alliances for the Future

The work of health care in the information age requires new partnerships with disciplines that were once not believed essential to the success of health care operations. Alliances with competitors, vendors, and the numerous specialties within the technology world are now essential for success.

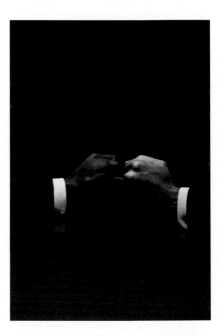

Expert leaders proactively develop relationships with colleagues in each discipline affecting the health care experience so that when the need is there the relationship facilitates efficient solution finding. Relationships are built one encounter at a time over time. When issues arise that need to be addressed by individuals from different perspectives, it is often too late to build the necessary relationships. Such relationships must be in place before they are needed to be effective in the accelerated technology world. To create strategic alliances, listening, presence, and compassion are essential.

Listening
Being present and focused with intention to understand what another person is expressing or not expressing

Presence
Relating to an individual in a way that reflects a quality of being with and in collaboration with rather than doing to

Compassion
The ability to be present for all levels of suffering; feeling the suffering of others

Building relationships with other disciplines, generations of workers, and within the policy arena are essential for success. Considerations for each alliance are discussed in this section.

Building Strategic Alliances with Discipline

The work of health care includes nearly every professional discipline! Examples are listed in the box below. Alliances with human factors researchers and ergonomic engineers are now essential to ensure effective work processes in the environment that is replete with personal computers, laptops, wireless, and mobile devices. Alliances with technology experts for hazardous waste management, and others support good work in the increasingly complex health care workplace.

Building Strategic Alliances with Generations

Building relationships with members of all generations is necessary for optimal teamwork and appropriate services. One area of opportunity is participation in professional associations. The involvement of all generations in professional associations has become both a challenge and an opporunity for better work processes. According to Reese (1999), the emerging workforce members are not joiners and do not become involved in professional organizations as members or leaders. Yet the work of standards setting and expectations for outcomes for each discipline must still be accomplished.

The work is to create new models of engagement for professional oversight that integrate the values of the profession and the values of the members of all generations. Continuing to entreat members of Generation X to join organizations that they view as bureaucratic and inconsequential is futile. Engaging Generation X to continue the work of the profession in a new way is the appropriate strategy. The sophisticated electronic, audio, and video technology has diminished the value of many of face-to-face meetings and large annual gatherings. This technology offers promise for the rethinking of professional organizations and the way in which the work is accomplished. Using discussion groups, chat rooms, and numerous other online tools involves all generations. This transformation will be especially important to sustain the core values of each profession and at the same time link professions in a virtual world.

Partnership Opportunities

- Clinical medicine
- Cognitive psychology
- Human factors
- Ergonomics/biomechanics
- Safety experts
- Industrial engineers
- Mathematicians/statisticians
- Computer science/ engineering
- Industrial design engineers

- Architects
- Fire science experts
- Interior designers
- Sociology experts
- Business experts
- Finance experts
- Communications
- Education
- Political science

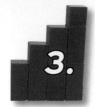

Building Strategic Alliances for Political Influence

Many relationships focus on influencing local, state, and national public policy as well as organizational policy. The focus of political relationships, whether internal to the organization or in the public arena, is on facilitating and ensuring that health care work occurs safely and is affordable. In the information age, more data are accessible to support positions, and communication with decision makers has changed. Access to videocam broadcasting of hearings and legislative sessions has allowed constituents to participate in ways that were once not possible. What continues to be a challenge for each health care leader is how to determine the most effective means of communication for each policymaker and legislator.

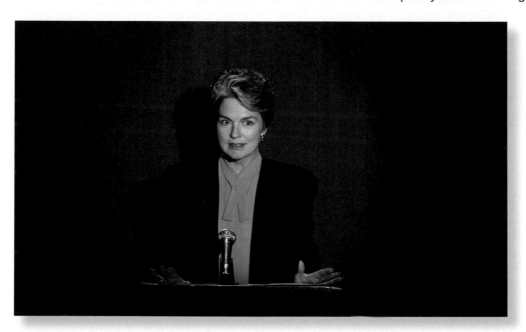

Specific Topics for Political Influence Include:

- Funding for safety initiatives.

- Technology implementation and standardization of applications and language.

- Mandates for value-based health care and outcome evaluation.

- National health care funding philosophy for patient care and education of providers.

- Provider role clarity.

- Health care research priorities.

COMMON BARRIERS TO EFFECTIVE RELATIONSHIPS

When one of these behaviors is identified, confront the issue and begin discussion to overcome and eliminate the barrier.

Bringing up unrelated issues

Holding a grudge—never forgive, never forget

Insisting that the problem is entirely the other person's fault

Being sarcastic

Being defensive

Being self-righteous and convinced you are right

Using the silent treatment

Disregarding the other person's feelings

Pretending nothing is wrong

Saying or doing things that are hurtful and cruel

References

Dossey, B. (2005). *Holistic nursing: A handbook for practice* (4th ed.). Sudbury, MA Jones and Bartlett.

Dreyfus, H. L., & Dreyfus, S. E. (2004). The ethical implications of the five-stage skill-acquisition model. *Bulletin of Science, Technology & Society*, 24(3), 251-264.

Reese, S. (1999). The new wave of GenX workers. *Business & Health*, 17, 19-24.

Taylor, E. (1999). *Shadow culture: Psychology and spirituality in America*. Washington, DC: Counterpoint.

Wheatley, M. J. (1999). *Leadership and the new science: Discovering order in a chaotic world*. San Francisco: Berrett-Koehler.

Suggested Readings

Benner, P. (2004). Using the Dreyfus model of skill acquisition to describe and interpret skill acquisition and clinical judgment in nursing practice and education. *Bulletin of Science, Technology & Society*, 24(3), 188-199.

Clancy, C. (2005). *Health information technology, quality of care and evidence-based medicine: An interlinked triad*. Annual symposium, American Medical Informatics Association, Washington, DC, October 25, 2005. Retrieved February 8, 2006, from www.ahrq.govinews/sp102505.htm

Leach, L. S. (2005). Nurse executive transformational leadership and organizational commitment. *JONA*, 35(5), 228-237.

Meyerson, D. E. (2001). Radical change, the quiet way. In: *The best of HBR on leadership: Stealth leadership*. Boston, MA: Harvard Business School Publishing Corporation.